Occupational Therapy in East Asia

This is the first major textbook on occupational therapy (OT) aimed at students and practitioners based in Asia.

Written by a team of authors mainly based in Hong Kong, the book is divided into four sections. Section I presents the history of OT in the region as well as those key theories which underpin it. Section II introduces the essentials of OT practice. From assessment through to evaluation and intervention, these chapters cover five key therapeutic areas in which occupational therapists work: providing support for sensory and motor functions, providing support for cognitive and perceptual issues, providing support for psychosocial issues, providing support for returning to home and the community (including the use of assistive technology), and providing support for returning to the workplace. Section III then details a range of case studies to show occupational therapists in action, while Section IV looks at how the field is developing, including the increasing use of AI and other technologies. Throughout the book, cultural factors specific to the region are highlighted.

An ideal resource for any student in Hong Kong, mainland China, Taiwan, or Singapore, this outstanding text is also a key reference work for practitioners in the region.

Hector Wing Hong Tsang, trained as an occupational therapist, amassed over ten years of clinical experience in psychiatric and geriatric rehabilitation before moving to The Hong Kong Polytechnic University in 1997. He was Head of the Department of Rehabilitation Sciences of the University from 2017 to January 2024 and is currently Chair Professor of Rehabilitation Sciences. He has focused on integrative medicine and psychiatric rehabilitation for people with severe mental illness for over 30 years.

Stella Wai Chee Cheng has been a Professor of Practice in Occupational Therapy at the Department of Rehabilitation Sciences, The Hong Kong Polytechnic University since 2018. She was the Chairperson of the Hong Kong Occupational Therapy Association from 2018 to 2024 and has been the Hong Kong Delegate to the World Federation of Occupational Therapists since 2016.

David Wai Kwong Man currently serves as the Vice President (Academic) at Tung Wah College, Hong Kong, bringing over 40 years of experience in occupational therapy and rehabilitation sciences. He formerly worked at the Department of Rehabilitation Sciences, The Hong Kong Polytechnic University. His specialization lies in cognitive rehabilitation, and he conducts research in basic neurosciences related to prospective memory, including leading clinical trials for individuals with cognitive decline. An internationally recognized scholar, David has held various leadership roles and made significant contributions to curriculum development, thereby enhancing academia.

Authored by many of the world's occupational therapy experts, the *Occupational Therapy in East Asia* textbook offers a comprehensive summary of foundational occupational therapy practice based on the latest empirical knowledge, combined with clear descriptions of state-of-the-art guidelines for how occupational therapy can be effectively provided in Asia. This is the ideal occupational therapy textbook.

Mark P. Jensen, *University of Washington, United States*

Tsang, Cheng, and Man's book, *Occupational Therapy in East Asia: Concepts, Principles and Practice* breaks new ground as a comprehensive go-to text for students studying occupational therapy. The topics and case studies are relevant, culturally grounded, and informed by cutting-edge East-meets-West scientific research. This text belongs on the shelf (or e-reader) of every student planning a career in occupational therapy, regardless of national origin.

Renée R. Taylor, *University of Illinois Chicago, United States*

As the first occupational therapy textbook published in Hong Kong, the book's East-meets-West cultural background and approach to rehabilitation make it highly recommended for use in occupational therapy education in mainland China.

Lijuan Ao, *Kunming Medical University, China*

Occupational Therapy in East Asia is an essential resource for students, uniquely addressing the intersection of cultural nuances and clinical practice. Its insightful case studies and East-meets-West rehabilitation approaches make it an invaluable guide for aspiring rehabilitation professionals across Asia and beyond.

Marco Pang, *The Hong Kong Polytechnic University, Hong Kong*

Occupational Therapy in East Asia

Concepts, Principles and Practice

Edited by Hector Wing Hong Tsang

With Stella Wai Chee Cheng and David Wai Kwong Man

Routledge
Taylor & Francis Group

LONDON AND NEW YORK

THE HONG KONG
POLYTECHNIC UNIVERSITY
香港理工大學

Designed cover image: Getty Images

First published 2026
by Routledge
4 Park Square, Milton Park, Abingdon, Oxon OX14 4RN

and by Routledge
605 Third Avenue, New York, NY 10158

Routledge is an imprint of the Taylor & Francis Group, an informa business

British Library Cataloguing-in-Publication Data
A catalogue record for this book is available from the British Library

ISBN: 978-1-032-72119-4 (hbk)
ISBN: 978-1-032-72120-0 (pbk)
ISBN: 978-1-032-72117-0 (ebk)

DOI: 10.4324/9781032721170

Typeset in Sabon
by KnowledgeWorks Global Ltd.

Contents

Figures and tables

Figures

Tables

Contributors

Sam Chi Chung Chan, Associate Professor at the Department of Rehabilitation Sciences, The Hong Kong Polytechnic University, is an occupational therapist specializing in rehabilitation for clients with spinal cord injuries, orthopedic conditions, and various medical conditions, such as stroke and dementia. His interests include cognitive rehabilitation for people with cognitive impairments and community-based rehabilitation programs for those with chronic conditions. He has published academic articles in various international journals, including *Frontiers in Human Neuroscience* and *PLoS ONE*.

Andy Shu Kei Cheng is a Professor of Occupational Therapy at Western Sydney University. He is a registered occupational therapist, chartered safety and health practitioner, and certified work capacity evaluator. He was the first Asian recipient of the Canadian Institutes of Health Research Scholarship for postgraduate training on the Work Disability Prevention CIHR Strategic Training Program at Université de Sherbrooke and the University of Toronto.

Stella Wai Chee Cheng has been a Professor of Practice in Occupational Therapy at the Department of Rehabilitation Sciences, The Hong Kong Polytechnic University since 2018. She was the Chairperson of the Hong Kong Occupational Therapy Association from 2018 to 2024 and has been the Hong Kong Delegate to the World Federation of Occupational Therapists since 2016.

Chi-Wen Chien is an Associate Professor at the Department of Rehabilitation Sciences, The Hong Kong Polytechnic University. His research expertise includes parent coaching, children's participation, and hand-skill assessment. He is also the developer of two online databases: the Children's Hand Skills Assessment Hub (https://childrenhandskills.com) and the Hub of Occupational Therapy Theory (https://ottheory.com).

Kenneth Nai-Kuen Fong is a Professor and Associate Head (Research, Innovation, and Knowledge Transfer) at the Department of Rehabilitation Sciences and Director of the Research Centre for Assistive Technology, The Hong Kong Polytechnic University. He is also a registered occupational therapist in Hong Kong, the UK, and the US and is currently the Editor-in-Chief of the *Hong Kong Journal of Occupational Therapy*.

Eddie Yip Kuen Hai is a Lecturer in the occupational therapy program at the University of Sunderland, UK. He formerly served as a Clinical Associate at The Hong Kong Polytechnic University. With over 25 years of work experience, he specializes in neurorehabilitation and the use of assistive technology. Eddie combines academic and clinical expertise to advance occupational therapy education and practice.

Soo Fung Ho is a Principal Occupational Therapist and Art Therapist at the Institute of Mental Health (IMH), Singapore. She oversees the provision of occupational therapy to forensic clients at IMH and the Changi Prison Complex. She has held management as well as teaching roles and currently provides art therapy to adults, children, and adolescents.

Kamaldin Bin Ibrahim is a Principal Occupational Therapist at the Department of Forensic Psychiatry, Institute of Mental Health, Singapore.

Cynthia Yuen Yi Lai is an Associate Professor at the Department of Rehabilitation Sciences, The Hong Kong Polytechnic University. She is the author of the *Sensory Processing and Self-regulation Checklist* (Heep Hong Society, 2013, 2018) and *Occupational Therapy – Keyboard Playing: Mix & Match* (Hong Kong Occupational Therapy Association, 2024).

Frank Ho-Yin Lai, Assistant Professor at Northumbria University in the UK, is a seasoned occupational therapy expert with extensive experience in education, clinical practice, and research. He excels at integrating evidence-based techniques, healthcare technology, and innovative caregiving approaches. He has led initiatives in capacity building and program design, advancing occupational therapy to tackle complex challenges and achieve lasting improvements in health outcomes and quality of life.

Johnny Wai Hon Lam is an Assistant Professor of Practice at The Hong Kong Polytechnic University. Being an occupational therapist specializing in developmental disabilities, he has extensive experience in pediatric rehabilitation. He is passionate about fostering the next generation of healthcare professionals through teaching occupational therapy courses at the university and running training workshops across Hong Kong, mainland China, Taiwan, and Macau. He has also been supervising clinical placements for various institutes since 2013.

Kino Chiu Kim Lam is an Assistant Professor of Practice at The Hong Kong Polytechnic University. Being the first Chinese practitioner certified in metacognitive therapy (MCT), he is a pioneer in the field. With over 17 years of clinical experience, he specializes in treating mental health disorders and actively promotes innovative therapeutic approaches to enhancing public mental health and well-being.

Vera Wai Man Lam is an Assistant Professor of Practice at the Department of Rehabilitation Sciences, The Hong Kong Polytechnic University. She holds a bachelor's degree in occupational therapy and a master's in applied psychology. With over 15 years of experience in psychiatry, she has provided recovery-oriented mental health services and led a research project funded by the Beat Drugs Fund Association. Currently, she is the Subject Leader for "OT in Psychosocial Practice" and was conferred the "Outstanding Young Teacher Award" in 2023/24.

Winnie Wing Tung Lam is a registered occupational therapist in Hong Kong. She did her MPhil at The Hong Kong University of Science and Technology, where she learned the application of AI and computer science. With her background in AI technology development, she pursued a PhD at The Hong Kong Polytechnic University, collaborating with clients and healthcare professionals to enhance the integration of technology in rehabilitation.

Benson Wui Man Lau is an Associate Professor at the Department of Rehabilitation Sciences, The Hong Kong Polytechnic University. His research interest is to elucidate the importance of neuroplasticity in emotions and behaviors. Using animal models that simulate human emotional and behavioral symptoms, including depression, anxiety, phobia, and sexual dysfunction, his studies explore the neurological basis of these symptoms and the mechanisms underlying the respective treatment methods, particularly rehabilitation treatment modalities.

Zoey Yutong Li is a PhD student at The Hong Kong Polytechnic University. She studies how traditional Chinese medicine (TCM) impacts symptoms, autonomic function, and brain activity in clients with depression, aiming to validate its effectiveness in promoting mental health and explore the potential mechanisms. She is also interested in exploring the relationship between autonomic nervous function and depression to identify new treatment approaches.

Phyllis Liang is an experienced occupational therapist who has worked in various healthcare and community contexts across Singapore and Australia. In the community setting, she has led high-impact strategic innovation, research, and digitalization. Previously, she was a Research Assistant Professor at Nanyang Technological University and led the clinical aspects of healthcare rehabilitation research. She has been awarded over $10 million in competitive grants and funds.

May Sok Mui Lim is an Associate Professor and the Assistant Provost (Applied Learning) at the Singapore Institute of Technology (SIT). She is the first occupational therapist in Singapore to be awarded a PhD qualification. She started the Bachelor of Science (Honors) in Occupational Therapy program at SIT in 2016 and now serves on various advisory boards and continues her clinical practice with young children with developmental delays.

Chung-Ying Lin is a Professor at the Institute of Allied Health Sciences, College of Medicine, National Cheng Kung University, Taiwan. His research expertise and interests are broad, including psychosocial, quality of life, health psychology and behaviors, and psychometrics with applied statistics. He has extensive experience and has been part of numerous international research collaborations, having published over 500 academic papers with an h-index of over 55.

Jessie Jingxia Lin is an Assistant Professor at the Department of Rehabilitation Sciences and an Internal Member of the Mental Health Research Centre, The Hong Kong Polytechnic University. She was trained as a psychiatrist and focuses on the early detection and intervention for psychiatric disorders.

Erin Yiqing Lu is a Research Assistant Professor at the Department of Rehabilitation Sciences, The Hong Kong Polytechnic University. She is a researcher with expertise in mind-body interventions for psychosocial rehabilitation. She has a track record of studying health *qigong* as a non-pharmacological approach for promoting psychological well-being and a healthy lifestyle. She is also interested in understanding the psychological and physiological mechanisms of mind-body interventions.

David Wai Kwong Man currently serves as the Vice President (Academic) at Tung Wah College, Hong Kong, bringing over 40 years of experience in occupational therapy and rehabilitation sciences. He formerly worked at the Department of Rehabilitation Sciences, The Hong Kong Polytechnic University. His specialization lies in cognitive rehabilitation, and he conducts research in basic neurosciences related to prospective memory, including leading clinical trials for individuals with cognitive decline. An internationally recognized scholar, David has held various leadership roles and made significant contributions to curriculum development, thereby enhancing academia.

Yogeswary Maniam is a Principal Occupational Therapist in the Early Psychosis Intervention Programme (EPIP), Institute of Mental Health, Singapore, and the author of the chapter on "Community Psychosocial Intervention in Early Psychosis" in the book *Early Psychosis Intervention: A Culturally Adaptive Clinical Guide*, edited by Eric Yu-hai Chen, Helen Lee, Gloria Hoi-kei Chan, and Gloria Hoi-yan Wong (Hong Kong University Press, 2013).

Bacon Fung Leung Ng is a Professor of Practice (Occupational Therapy) at the Department of Rehabilitation Sciences, The Hong Kong Polytechnic University. He is an experienced occupational therapist with his Doctor of Health Science degree conferred by The Hong Kong Polytechnic University and his Doctorate of Occupational Therapy by Chatham University in the US. He has published over 70 articles and over 70 conference papers. Details can be found on his personal website: http://www.baconng.org.

Bobby Hin Po Ng has over 30 years of clinical experience in Hong Kong's public hospital system. He was the Department Manager (Occupational Therapy) at Kowloon Hospital, managing a department with over 100 staff and an annual workload of more than 4,000 patients, before he started teaching at The Hong Kong Polytechnic University in 2021. He is also one of the very few local clinicians who is active in publication, with 17 academic publications.

Seiji Nishimura is affiliated with the Department of Rehabilitation Science, Faculty of Health Sciences, Institute of Medical, Pharmaceutical and Health Sciences, Kanazawa University, Japan. His specialty is rehabilitation in the field of upper limb and hand surgery.

Wendy Wing Yan So is a Senior Research Manager at The University of Hong Kong with a decade-long focus on mental health promotion across diverse contexts. Her work covers a broad array of initiatives, ranging from school to community-based settings. Wendy's expertise lies in implementing evidence-based practices and evaluating program effectiveness, with a strong focus on transforming research into practical applications.

Abby Jin Song is a Lead Occupational Therapist at the Second Affiliated Hospital of Kunming Medical University, China. She graduated from Boston University with an OTD and acquired OTR/L and CBIS in the US.

Sharon Fong Mei Toh, a Principal Occupational Therapist at Yishun Community Hospital, Singapore, specializes in neurorehabilitation and integration of technology into rehabilitation. She earned her MSc and PhD from The Hong Kong Polytechnic University, focusing on wearable technology in stroke rehabilitation. She has published extensively in renowned journals and led initiatives such as chairing The National Occupational Therapy Conference in Singapore in 2018. Her dedication lies in advancing rehabilitation through research, innovation, and leadership.

Hector Wing Hong Tsang, trained as an occupational therapist, amassed over ten years of clinical experience in psychiatric and geriatric rehabilitation before moving to The Hong Kong Polytechnic University in 1997. He was Head of the Department of Rehabilitation Sciences, The Hong Kong Polytechnic University from 2017 to January 2024, appointed Cally Kwong Mei Wan Professor in Psychosocial Health in 2018 and promoted to Chair Professor of Rehabilitation Sciences in July 2019. For the past three decades, he has focused on integrative medicine and psychiatric rehabilitation for people with severe mental illness (SMI). His research on vocational rehabilitation strategies for people with SMI and health *qigong* has attracted worldwide interest. He has secured more than HK$258 million research grants and produced more than 200 academic publications. His h-index is 57, with over 12,000 citations. He was a Visiting Professor at both Yale University and the University of Pennsylvania and is currently an Honorary Professor of The University of Hong Kong, as well as a Visiting Professor of Peking University and Shanghai Jiao Tong University. He was awarded the honor of Distinguished Professor of Nanshan Scholar by Guangzhou Medical University and is the lead consultant for the Rehabilitation Programme Plan of the HKSAR Government.

Chi Man Tsui is an occupational therapist by training. He obtained his bachelor's degree in occupational therapy from The Hong Kong Polytechnic University and returned to the university to complete his PhD in rehabilitation after obtaining a master's in medical sciences at The University of Hong Kong. Specializing in psychiatry, pediatrics, and geriatrics, his expertise in these areas supports his clinical practice, tertiary teaching, and research.

Shu-Mei Wang received awards for visiting research in the US. She had worked at the Department of Rehabilitation Sciences, The Hong Kong Polytechnic University. She currently serves as an Associate Professor at the Department of Long-term Care, the National Taipei University of Nursing and Health Sciences, Taiwan. As an occupational therapist, she specializes in psychiatric disorders, motor control, and AI applications. She was also the hospital supervisor for psychiatric occupational therapists.

Josephine Man-Wah Wong, Associate Professor of Practice at the Department of Rehabilitation Sciences, The Hong Kong Polytechnic University, specializes in orthopedic rehabilitation, particularly hand and upper limb rehabilitation. As an experienced occupational therapist, she has been a guest speaker at a number of international seminars, conferences, and practical workshops in various cities worldwide to talk about hand splinting skills, sharing her clinical experiences with undergraduates and postgraduates since 1997.

Ching-Yi Wu is the Associate Dean of the College of Medicine and a Professor at the Department of Occupational Therapy, Chang Gung University, Taiwan. She has been the Associate Editor of *OTJR: Occupation, Participation and Health* since 2017 and of *Biomedical Journal* since 2023. She has published more than 200 research papers in internationally renowned journals. She also edited *Contemporary Occupational Therapy: Overview and Ethics* (Chinese; He-Feng Book Store Co., Ltd., 2024) and *Evidence-based Occupational Therapy* (Chinese; He-Feng Book Store, 2020).

Yanwen Xu is the Director of the Rehabilitation Therapy Center, Wuxi Ninth People's Hospital Affiliated to Soochow University, China. He is also the Head of the Department of Occupational Therapy and the Head of the Bachelor of Science in Rehabilitation Therapy (Occupational Therapy) program at Nanjing Medical University. He is a chief therapist in China and the Chairman of the Occupational Therapy Committee of Jiangsu Association of Rehabilitation Medicine.

Melva Yin Mei Yip is an Assistant Professor of Practice at the Department of Rehabilitation Sciences, The Hong Kong Polytechnic University. She obtained her bachelor's degree in occupational therapy from The Hong Kong Polytechnic University and her master's in musculoskeletal medicine and rehabilitation from The Chinese University of Hong Kong. She has a wide range of clinical experiences, particularly in musculoskeletal, medical, and geriatric services.

Jack Jiaqi Zhang is a Research Assistant Professor at the Department of Rehabilitation Sciences, The Hong Kong Polytechnic University. With a background in occupational therapy, his research interests are in using transcranial magnetic stimulation along with multimodal neurophysiological and neuroimaging techniques to better understand the recovery process following various neurological and psychiatric conditions and to optimize rehabilitation outcomes.

Ya Zhou is a full-time teacher at the Department of Rehabilitation Occupational Therapy, School of Rehabilitation, Kunming Medical University, China. She has been teaching the core courses of "Occupational Therapy Theory", "Occupational Therapy Foundation", and "Pediatric Occupational Therapy" since 2019. She is also responsible for teaching the clinical internship program of "Pediatric Occupational Therapy". She is passionate about pediatric rehabilitation education and committed to promoting the development of pediatric rehabilitation in Yunnan.

Foreword

As a former Chairperson of the Departmental Advisory Committee who served for eight years at the Department of Rehabilitation Sciences, The Hong Kong Polytechnic University, it gives me great pleasure to write a foreword for this unique textbook – the first of its kind to be published in Hong Kong that targets a regional readership in East Asia. This comprehensive text covers occupational therapy (OT) topics both in breadth and depth across 13 chapters, ranging from the history of OT to its principles, concepts, and clinical applications. The content includes physical and cognitive assessments and the management of specific common disorders combined with illustrative case examples. The practical aspects of the book include communication, ethics, and legal documentation, which are essential parts of any clinical profession. A unique feature is the inclusion of cultural aspects and the use of Chinese techniques such as *qigong, tai chi,* and acupressure in the management of conditions. The list of authors is impressive, with a wide range of local and international expertise in OT and rehabilitation sciences. They all possess a solid background in teaching as well as considerable academic and clinical experiences. An extensive review of the content by a panel of local and international scholars prior to its final draft gives further credence to this textbook. The editors, led by Professor Hector Tsang, have structured the chapters with uniformity and continuity to make the book eminently readable, particularly to undergraduates and entry-level Master's program students of OT.

Professor Shu-Leong Ho
Honorary Professor
The University of Hong Kong and The Hong Kong Polytechnic University,
Hong Kong

Foreword

I am delighted to have been asked to write a foreword for this novel occupational therapy (OT) textbook, written particularly for the Asian and Chinese markets. The book is the first of its kind to specifically target the educational needs of undergraduate and post-graduate students in Hong Kong and throughout Asia. As such, it will provide a crucial foundation for introducing key concepts in OT and rehabilitation, professional principles, and essential components of practice. However, while this textbook is essentially aimed at supporting the student population, it will likely serve as an important refresher book for others to "dip in and out" of, allowing them to keep their knowledge base up to date.

The authors are distinguished colleagues at the Department of Rehabilitation Sciences, The Hong Kong Polytechnic University, and experts in OT and rehabilitation. They all have worked and have relevant experience in three key areas: clinical practice, research, and teaching. These aspects have thus informed both the presentation style and content of the book. Moreover, the authors have invited renowned experts from Asia and beyond to contribute their expertise to the various chapters.

In addition to covering key OT topics, the book includes relevant Asian cultural factors. It also includes the so-called "East-Meets-West" approach to rehabilitation; for example, outlining this principle in interventions such as *tai chi*, acupressure, and mindfulness. A real strength of the text is the inclusion of useful and clear figures to highlight key points, as well as case studies sited in Asian contexts. These concrete and practical examples bring the clinical situations to life, particularly for Hong Kong and Asian students.

This is a significant new OT textbook that has real potential to be a key source for many occupational therapists throughout Asia now and in the future. As an occupational therapist myself, I know the importance of investing in a solid and reliable textbook that can be used during study and after qualification. This book fulfills both these requirements.

Professor Avril Drummond
Professor of Healthcare Research
University of Nottingham, United Kingdom

Preface

Hector Wing Hong Tsang

The idea of preparing and publishing a textbook on occupational therapy (OT) first came to me when I assumed the role of the Head of the Department of Rehabilitation Sciences, The Hong Kong Polytechnic University (RS, PolyU) in 2017, and was thinking in terms of setting the strategic directions for the department, particularly the impact we planned to create over the coming years. This was an important task that held special meaning since my term of headship (from 2017 to January 2024) coincided with the 40th and 45th birthdays of RS, which was established in 1978.

In my strategic planning, I took into consideration RS's achievements in education: our OT and physiotherapy programs are highly ranked internationally and among the top in Asia. For example, according to EduRank's 2022 rankings, PolyU ranked No. 1 for the first time in China and Asia in medical-related specialties, including OT and physical therapy. In fact, RS's faculty members have established several strong and mature teaching teams and compiled numerous teaching materials in various OT fields over the past 45 years, such as in physical rehabilitation, neurorehabilitation, mental health, geriatrics, pediatrics, and the use of assistive technology. For OT education in Hong Kong, mainland China, and other parts of Asia, it has been a meaningful endeavor collecting these teaching materials and sharing them with OT teachers, students, and other stakeholders around the world, particularly in Asia.

More importantly, in terms of an essential principle in tertiary education, which emphasizes that teaching should be informed and supported by relevant research conducted in the local context, our faculty members have done a splendid job. First, we have continued to carry out culturally relevant OT research in Hong Kong, mainland China, and other Asian regions for the past three decades. This is reflected in our track record of securing both local and overseas research grants, as well as our number of publications and citation indices. For example, four of our OT scholars (Professor David Wai Kwong MAN, Professor Chetwyn Che Hin CHAN, Professor Benjamin Kay Yan YEE, and I) have been ranked as the World's Top 2% most-cited scientists by Stanford University, meaning that our OT colleagues have published numerous research papers that have had a significant impact in the scientific community. Second, RS has been organizing the Pan-Pacific Conference on Rehabilitation (PPCR) for more than two decades, which is now well known as an iconic biannual event since its inauguration in Guangzhou in 1998. The conference aims to foster multidisciplinary collaborations among rehabilitation professionals, academics, students, and healthcare administrators throughout Asia-Pacific, reflecting how RS has assumed a lead role in OT research and teaching in the region.

Despite all the above, as well as the establishment of numerous OT programs in universities across Asia, there was no textbook demonstrating RS's strengths in OT teaching and research. I therefore decided to publish an OT textbook targeting university students in Hong Kong, mainland China, and other parts of Asia, with a special focus on cultural factors in clinical practice and the East-Meets-West approach to rehabilitation.

I would like to take this opportunity to express our deepest appreciation to the following PolyU leaders who have provided strong and continuous support throughout the publication process: Professor Jin-Guang TENG (President), Professor Philip C. H. CHAN (former Interim President), Professor Timothy W. TONG (former President), Professor Wing-tak WONG (Deputy President and Provost), Professor Miranda LOU (Executive Vice President), Professor Kwok-yin WONG (Vice President [Education]), and Professor David SHUM (Dean of the Faculty of Health and Social Sciences). I am also grateful to the 19 external reviewers (whose names I cannot disclose because of the anonymous nature of the review process), who gave invaluable comments and suggestions for revising and enhancing the content.

Thanks to the contributions and efforts of the 38 authors and co-authors, we are delighted to present this OT textbook – the first of its kind in Asia. We hope it will contribute to OT education in Hong Kong, mainland China, and Asia at large, providing up-to-date knowledge, skills, and insights to OT students, teachers, and occupational therapists everywhere.

Introduction

Hector Wing Hong Tsang

Occupational Therapy in East Asia: Concepts, Principles and Practice is the first occupational therapy (OT) textbook published in Hong Kong designed to meet the learning needs of undergraduate and entry-level master's students in OT or rehabilitation sciences, both in Hong Kong and across Asia. The book is broadly divided into four sections, each covering a distinct OT theme, and further subdivided into 13 chapters, each focusing on a specific and essential OT topic. To provide readers with an overview before they explore each chapter in more depth, this introduction will briefly outline the content covered in all 13 chapters.

Due to space limitations, it would be difficult, if not impossible, for our writing team to cover all topics, issues, and trends relevant to clinical OT practice for entry-level therapists. Nevertheless, we have carefully selected the most essential OT theories, principles, and practices required for training aspiring occupational therapists, along with the cultural values and considerations underlying them. Additionally, each chapter includes a detailed reference list to guide readers seeking further information or research on the topic.

* * *

Section I – Introduction consists of two chapters: Chapter 1 – History, Principles, and Theories, and Chapter 2 – Documentation. **Chapter 1 – History, Principles, and Theories** introduces the history and illustrates the principles and theories of OT, particularly from an Asian perspective. It begins with the history of this profession in Hong Kong, mainland China, and Taiwan, respectively. Occupation, as the core concept of OT, is then introduced and discussed in an oriental context, with a focus on the productivity of persons with both physical and psychiatric disabilities. A review of the use of related models and frames of reference in OT for analyzing various clinical or disability conditions (such as physical and psychiatric conditions) commonly seen in clinical practices then follows. The Model of Human Occupation is used as an

DOI: 10.4324/9781032721170-1

example to explain how it can guide the application of traditional Chinese medicine in OT interventions. Then comes a discussion on the ways in which concepts of Chinese psychology affect Chinese people's views on disabilities, leading to stigmatization of those with intellectual disabilities and mental illnesses, respectively, which, in turn, undermines their behavioral health. Finally, a case example on traumatic brain injury is used to demonstrate how the East-Meets-West approach, which looks to apply Western OT theories and principles in the Chinese context, can be of practical help in guiding the assessment and provision of interventions in the rehabilitation process.

In **Chapter 2 – Documentation**, we will introduce the definition, importance, and types of documentation, as well as the characteristics of good professional documentation and ethical considerations for documentation related to OT practice. Documentation is important to OT in that occupational therapists are legally required to adhere to regulatory standards governing healthcare practice. Proper documentation ensures that occupational therapists meet these requirements by providing a clear record of the care provided to clients. Documentation plays a crucial role in treatment planning and evaluation, allowing occupational therapists to record initial assessments, set measurable goals, document interventions, and track progress over time. This information informs the ongoing planning and adjustment of treatment strategies to optimize client outcomes. It also allows occupational therapists to convey essential information about a client's condition, treatment plan, progress, and outcomes to other members of the healthcare team, thereby facilitating coordinated care. Occupational therapists' documentation supports quality assurance efforts and risk management within the professional practice. It provides evidence of adherence to best practices, helps identify areas for improvement, and mitigates legal risks by documenting the rationale behind clinical decisions and interventions. Strategically, documentation can contribute to research endeavors aimed at advancing professional development. Last but not least, documentation serves as a valuable educational resource for students and junior therapists.

Section II – Assessment, Evaluation, and Intervention expounds on the core principles and practices of OT in five chapters: Chapter 3 – Sensorimotor Functions, Chapter 4 – Cognitive Perceptual Functioning, Chapter 5 – Psychosocial Practice for Chinese Population, Chapter 6 – Return to the Home and Community, and Chapter 7 – Return to Work. **Chapter 3 – Sensorimotor Functions** reviews the principles and skills related to sensory and motor assessments, as well as the treatments used by occupational therapists for clients with sensorimotor dysfunctions. It starts with a guideline for sensory and motor assessments and identifies the various stages of occupational assessments: medical history, interview, and physical and functional assessments. After providing practical guidelines for assessing sensory functions and pain conditions, specific motor-related assessments for musculoskeletal and neurological conditions are outlined. This is followed by a description of various functional tests, including hand function tests, activity of daily living (ADL) assessments, and functional mobility assessments. The results of sensorimotor and functional assessments provide the basis for planning and implementing OT interventions using the biomechanical frame of reference. The principles of sensory interventions, such as sensory re-education, and motor interventions by means of remedial activities are then discussed. When sensory and motor functions are optimized, clients with musculoskeletal conditions will be given functional training, such as personal ADL training or mobility training. The chapter concludes with a case study of a client with a sensorimotor injury, demonstrating how assessment and intervention strategies are applied and justified.

Chapter 4 – Cognitive Perceptual Functioning provides occupational therapists and students with principles and methods for evaluating and treating individuals who have cognitive and perceptual deficits due to acquired brain injury such as stroke and traumatic brain injury. Cognitive-perceptual skills include information processing, integration, and action selection. These skills are vital for achieving functional independence after an acquired brain injury.

To ensure accurate identification and effective intervention, occupational therapists need a solid understanding of the assessment tools. This chapter presents examples of standardized assessment tools commonly used in Hong Kong and other countries, emphasizing their robust psychometric properties for evaluating acquired brain injury. It highlights the importance of cultural and linguistic factors during the administration of these tools. Additionally, non-standardized evaluation methods are discussed, drawing on relevant literature, clinical protocols, and experiences from both local and overseas sources. This chapter also explores treatment strategies, protocols, procedures, and specialized methods for addressing cognitive-perceptual issues, incorporating insights from literature, clinical studies, and practical experience. Treatment strategies are categorized based on individual needs and stages of recovery, utilizing restorative and functional adaptive/compensatory approaches. The chapter provides numerous examples illustrating the management of diverse cognitive-perceptual problems associated with acquired brain injury. By offering a comprehensive guide, this chapter helps occupational therapists effectively evaluate and treat individuals experiencing cognitive and perceptual deficits due to acquired brain injury.

Chapter 5 – Psychosocial Practice for Chinese Population covers psychosocial practice in the Chinese context. The psychosocial practice of OT is culturally relevant. For OT in Chinese communities, it is important to recognize indigenous health promotion techniques that can be complementary to conventional rehabilitation approaches. Interventions to address social and psychological issues that hinder Chinese people's rehabilitation should also be specific to the sociocultural values and environment. This chapter introduces the development of psychosocial practice in stress management, mental illness stigma, and social skills and employment over the past two decades. It then looks at how cultural roots shape perceptions of stress, contribute to the formation of stigma, and define desirable workplace social skills. Finally, the chapter presents and discusses efforts to reduce stress, combat stigma, and improve social skills for Chinese populations.

Chapter 6 – Return to the Home and Community reviews the role of OT in clients' return to their home and community. The return to the home or community is the ultimate goal of OT, and occupational therapists play a crucial role in planning and preparing for the discharge of clients admitted to hospitals. This chapter discusses common assessments used by occupational therapists for pre-discharge evaluations in hospitals, focusing on basic and instrumental activities of daily living, as well as home safety assessments. A step-by-step guide for discharge planning and preparation is also included to help inexperienced therapists in this important and complex intervention. Home assessment and environmental modification are other common interventions to help clients return to home. A case scenario is used to demonstrate the clinical reasoning process, and readers are expected to adopt similar approaches in other scenarios.

Chapter 7 – Return to Work presents an overview of the key concepts and components of rehabilitation programs for injured workers to allow them to have a safe and timely return to work. Returning to work after a work injury is a complex and multifactorial process, influenced by the nature of the injury, the medical treatment required, sociodemographic, psychological, and economic factors, ergonomic and psychosocial worksite variables, and employer policies. It is overly simplistic to view work status as being solely dependent upon the nature and severity of the clinical condition, or to assume that the ability to return to work is directly related to the trajectory of recovery from an injury. The focus of the traditional medical model may be too narrow to inform the various factors that can affect the return to work of injured workers, particularly those with chronic symptoms or work disabilities. There should be a move away from the purely medically determined approach toward a proactive and holistic one.

Section III – Case Illustration includes four chapters that provide illustrative case studies of four common clinical conditions or disorders: Chapter 8 – Musculoskeletal Injuries Related to Work Rehabilitation, Chapter 9 – Stroke, Chapter 10 – Developmental Disorders, and Chapter 11 – Schizophrenia. In **Chapter 8 – Musculoskeletal Injuries Related to Work Rehabilitation**, a case study of an individual with a scaphoid fracture in the right wrist that had undergone percutaneous screw fixation is used to illustrate how an occupational therapist carried out work rehabilitation, from analyzing critical work demands and conducting a functional capacity evaluation to designing a training program based on the work intention of the individual. We use our hands for almost everything. From cooking and cleaning to dealing with various work activities, our hands are some of our greatest tools and it is often not until they become injured or otherwise incapacitated that we really notice how much we use them. Occupational therapists play a pivotal role in the rehabilitation of musculoskeletal injuries, particularly those in the upper extremities. They also provide work rehabilitation for various musculoskeletal injury types affecting different parts of the body, helping injured individuals return to work.

Chapter 9 – Stroke first describes the etiology, symptoms, and complications of stroke, followed by the role of occupational therapists in stroke rehabilitation, the challenges faced by stroke survivors regarding community integration, and the challenges for caregivers who attend to family members who have had a stroke. The case studies at the end of this chapter describe the journeys of two clients suffering from a stroke. Firstly, during the acute phase of management after onset, and then from the subacute to chronic phases longitudinally to highlight the role of occupational therapists in the rehabilitation process.

Stroke, or cerebral vascular accident, is a sudden disease with complex causes, etiology, comorbidities, and a high mortality rate. Most importantly, stroke is the third leading cause for temporary to permanent disabilities, both physical and cognitive, which can affect an individual's quality of life in the long term. Approximately 80% of stroke survivors suffer from motor disabilities over one side of the body, but only 10–20% of these motor disabilities can be fully recovered from. Occupational therapists play a pivotal role in rehabilitating and supporting stroke survivors in their recovery journey, particularly in terms of overcoming obstacles in their ADL.

Chapter 10 – Developmental Disorders uses a case example of developmental disorders to illustrate the assessment and intervention processes related to pediatric rehabilitation. Developmental disorders are prevalent in pediatric OT, and children with these disorders often exhibit delayed or impaired motor, cognitive, self-care, or social skills compared to their same-age peers. This chapter focuses on a case study involving a four-year-old child with autism spectrum disorder, showcasing assessments and interventions from three Oriental regions: Taiwan, Hong Kong, and Singapore. The purpose is to highlight the regional variations in OT practices.

Despite these differences, there are common considerations that guide the provision of services. These considerations include adopting a family-centered approach, understanding child development, recognizing the role of caregivers/parents, and utilizing play as a means and end in therapy. By exploring these considerations, this chapter provides valuable insights for students in the early stage of their studies, helping them to gain a deeper understanding of pediatric OT and better prepare them for future clinical placement.

In **Chapter 11 – Schizophrenia**, the clinical practice of OT in Hong Kong and Singapore is described through a case study of a young man called Jeff, who had schizophrenia and received OT during the acute stage and the day hospital/outpatient stage. Jeff and occupational therapists collaborated and discussed intervention plans. In the acute stage, the therapists conducted interviews related to the stress-vulnerability model and assessments using the Montreal Cognitive Assessment and Allen's Cognitive Level Screen. Based on the results of these processes, the therapists collected information on Jeff's stressors, protective factors, and cognition. Interventions in the acute stage focused on illness and stress management. During the day hospital or outpatient stage, the therapists adopted both the Model of Human Occupation and the stress-vulnerability model to conduct interviews and assessments using the Interest Checklist, Role Checklist, VALPAR Component Work Samples, MATRICS Consensus Cognitive Battery, and Brief Assessment of Cognition in Schizophrenia. Interventions in the day hospital/outpatient stage aimed to support Jeff's engagement in his student, work, social, and leisure activities, as well as his illness and stress management. These interventions included individual sessions, involvement of peer support specialists, vocational training, Social Cognition and Interaction Training, cognitive training, leisure groups, caregiver groups, the Illness Management and Recovery program, health *qigong*, and discussion-based groups. This case illustration shows the Oriental cultural aspects of OT.

Section IV – Future Trends comprises two chapters: Chapter 12 – Evidence-Based Practice in Occupational Therapy and Chapter 13 – Use of Advanced Technologies in Occupational Therapy. **Chapter 12 – Evidence-Based Practice in Occupational Therapy** begins with a review of the definition and development of evidence-based practice, then outlines the evidence-based interventions in OT, and finally makes recommendations for enhancing and strengthening research in OT. There is often confusion as to how existing research data and findings should be interpreted and applied in clinical practice. This chapter also attempts to help readers consume and interpret research data and literature with a view to them evaluating the effectiveness of treatments and interventions in order to select the most appropriate evidence-based practice for their clinical application. The chapter concludes with a summary of how to use the knowledge as a practical guide to evidence-based practice.

Chapter 13 – Use of Advanced Technologies in Occupational Therapy introduces the adoption of assistive technology in OT assessments and interventions. Assistive technology, in a broad sense, is technology that supports people with disabilities, and is an important branch in OT. With recent advances in technology, its scope has become even greater, ranging from cutting-edge technologies such as mobile technology and telerehabilitation, healthcare and social robots, virtual reality, augmented and mixed realities, artificial intelligence, and ambient assistive technology with the use of the Internet of Things, to traditional assistive devices and orthotics used to help clients in their daily functioning, enhance their participation in self-care, work, and leisure activities, and facilitate or enhance their ability to carry out functional activities independently through mastery of the environment. This chapter describes various assistive technology models, with examples of both low and high technologies, as well as the clinical reasoning for using assistive technology in the context of OT. To help occupational therapists incorporate advanced technology into their future professional practice, this chapter introduces several cutting-edge technologies, including mobile technology and telerehabilitation, artificial intelligence, virtual reality, and emerging neuromodulation, neurophysiological, and neuroimaging techniques, with examples from published research in the local context.

Introduction

CHAPTER 1

History, principles, and theories

Hector Wing Hong Tsang, Cynthia Yuen Yi Lai,
Bacon Fung Leung Ng, Chi Man Tsui,
Kino Chiu Kim Lam, and Chung-Ying Lin

History of occupational therapy

History of occupational therapy in Hong Kong

The history of occupational therapy (OT) in Hong Kong dates back to 1949 when, according to Jenks (1988), the first handicraft instructor (a rattan worker) started working in the Mental Hospital on High Street on Hong Kong Island. This is commonly regarded as the start of OT service provision in Hong Kong. Since then, a series of key events track its professional development in the city. For example, in 1950, Dr. Uttley, the Acting Director of the Medical and Health Services, Mr. Brickford, the Medical Secretary, and Ms. Wallace Turner, a physiotherapist, formed a committee for the development of OT in Hong Kong. Three years later, in 1953, the committee employed a part-time occupational therapist. Starting in 1955, several OT departments were established in various hospital settings. However, it was 1960 to the late 1970s which saw a rapid development of OT service provision. There were 4 occupational therapists and 18 OT assistants in 1960, with the majority of the occupational therapists coming from England. During the 1960s, OT began to develop in the non-government sector, such as the John F. Kennedy Centre (for cerebral palsy), United Christian Hospital, Kwong Wah Hospital, and Caritas Hospital. By that time, the need for local occupational therapists was obvious and urgent. Under the provision of government scholarship, the first three local male Chinese students were sent to Australia to receive training as occupational therapists in 1967. In 1975, only 14 out of 19 OT positions were filled. Similarly, two female Chinese students were sent to Australia for training in 1971, and another two to England in 1972 under the same government scholarship scheme.

According to Wong and Fong (2013), there were several important milestones in the formation of the OT profession in Hong Kong in the late 1970s. First, there was an expansion of social welfare services after the release of the Government White Paper on Integrating the Disabled into the Community. This resulted in a remarkable increase

DOI: 10.4324/9781032721170-3

in rehabilitation facilities, OT, physiotherapy, and support services for people with mental and physical disabilities. Second, the implementation of a Government policy providing education for children with intellectual disabilities led to the offering of more subsidies in special schools. OT was thus extended to this demographic. Third, the first Higher Diploma program in OT was offered by The Hong Kong Polytechnic (now The Hong Kong Polytechnic University) in 1978 and recognized by the World Federation of Occupational Therapists (WFOT). Its first program leader was Mr. Philip Chan, and the first batch of 43 OT students graduated in 1981. Fourth, there was a fundamental change in the professional structure in Hong Kong. The Hong Kong Association of Occupational Therapists (HKAOT) was established in 1978 with 40 members. At that time, the first Chairman, Ms. Elsie White, was the OT Superintendent in the Medical and Health Department of the Hong Kong Government. The 1980s saw the OT profession gain increasingly more recognition from both public and international communities. In 1981, the Occupational Therapists Board (OTB) was established under the Supplementary Medical Professions Ordinance, Chapter 359, Laws of Hong Kong (Occupational Therapists Board, n.d.). In 1984, HKAOT was officially accepted as a full member of WFOT. In 1985, the first issue of the *Journal of the Hong Kong Association of Occupational Therapists* (former name of the *Hong Kong Journal of Occupational Therapy*) was published.

In the 1990s, OT further demonstrated its professional status and autonomy in Hong Kong. For example, the first private OT clinic was established in 1990.

According to documents available in the Department of Rehabilitation Sciences of The Hong Kong Polytechnic University (PolyU), the Professional Diploma in OT program at The Hong Kong Polytechnic was upgraded to the Bachelor of Science (BSc) degree program in 1991. In 1992, the first local postgraduate OT program, the Postgraduate Diploma in Health Care with specialization in OT, was launched. This was followed, in 1995, by the first OT postgraduate master's degree, the Master of Science in Health Care (OT). In 1998, the BSc in OT degree at PolyU was validated into an honors program, the BSc (Hons) in OT. In the same year, PolyU hosted the first Pan-Pacific Conference on Rehabilitation (PPCR). By the turn of the millennium, the OT profession in Hong Kong had become even more professional and impactful. For instance, the first Doctor of Philosophy in OT graduated in 2002. According to a survey conducted in 2004, the fields of practice among occupational therapists were physical rehabilitation (26.8%), psychiatric/psychosocial rehabilitation (25.5%), geriatric rehabilitation (21%), pediatric rehabilitation (16.4%), community rehabilitation (5.6%), and vocational/work rehabilitation (4.1%). Most were employed by the Hospital Authority (68.5%) or non-governmental organizations (NGOs) (24.5%); only a fraction (1.8%) worked in the private sector (Tse et al., 2005). In 2005, Dr. Kit Sinclair, a pioneer of OT education in Hong Kong, was elected President of WFOT (Wong & Fong, 2013). Two years later, in 2007, PolyU successfully launched a full-time Master of Science in OT program.

In the early 2010s, the expansion of OT services and education became more prominent. In fact, while the number of registered occupational therapists reached 1,400 in 2010, demand was outweighing supply. The first entry-level Master in OT (MOT) program in Hong Kong was launched in 2011 under sponsorship from the Social Welfare Department to support NGO services. In 2012, in line with the four-year undergraduate curriculum, PolyU admitted its first cohort of four-year BSc (Hons) in OT students to replace the three-year program, and the intake number was increased to 90. In 2013, Tung Wah College launched its first self-financed BSc (Hons) in OT.

In Hong Kong, PolyU continues to play a leading role in OT education and research. To cultivate the integration of East and West approaches in rehabilitation sciences, as well as to nurture future leaders, the Department of Rehabilitation Sciences of PolyU launched its Summer Overseas Exchange Scholarship Scheme (SOESS) in 2013 (Tsang, 2015). With a strong background in rehabilitation and research, academic staff in OT contributed to government-commissioned projects (e.g., the Persons with Disabilities and Rehabilitation Programme Plan) to benefit the community (Faculty of Health and Social Sciences, 2018). In 2020, the first-ever university-based OT clinic in Hong Kong, the Tam Wing Fan Rehabilitation Service Centre (Occupational Therapy), was officially opened, boasting cutting-edge equipment (Department of Rehabilitation Sciences, 2020). In 2021, the Chair Professor and the then Head of the Department of Rehabilitation Sciences, Prof. Hector Tsang, was ranked among the world's top 2% most-cited scientists (Subject Field: Psychiatry), according to Stanford University (Department of Rehabilitation Sciences, 2021).

As of December 2021, there were 2,778 registered occupational therapists, including 2,164 Part I and 614 Part II (those who shall not practice except under supervision from a Part I registered occupational therapist) in Hong Kong (Occupational Therapists Board, n.d.). The major milestones in the local training of occupational therapists are summarized in Table 1.1.

History of occupational therapy in mainland China

The development of the OT profession in mainland China stemmed from rehabilitation medicine. Co-organized by the Ministry of Health and the World Health Organization Collaborating Centre, the first training course on rehabilitation medicine was launched in 1983 (Chen, 2001). To allow the training to be sustainable and more intensive, Dr. Harry Fang, a renowned orthopedic surgeon in Hong Kong and the founder of the Hong Kong Society of Rehabilitation, successfully urged the World Health Organization in 1989 to financially support a ten-year project to establish formal training for rehabilitation doctors on the mainland (Wong & Li-Tsang, 2010). The focus was primarily on physical rehabilitation for neurological and orthopedic conditions (Zhuo, 1999). Such development in rehabilitation training enhanced awareness of the need to create a professional rehabilitation workforce on the mainland. A breakthrough came around 2000 when rehabilitation personnel there started receiving formal OT education (Zhuo, 2006). Figure 1.1 shows this shift (Moy, 2018; Wong & Li-Tsang, 2010).

Table 1.1 The major milestones in the local training of occupational therapists

Year	Milestones
1978	Launched Higher Diploma in OT at The Hong Kong Polytechnic.
1991	Upgraded to Bachelor of Science in OT at The Hong Kong Polytechnic.
1998	Validated into Bachelor of Science (Honors) in OT at PolyU.
2011	Launched Master in OT at PolyU.
2013	Launched Bachelor of Science (Honors) in OT at Tung Wah College.

First group of rehabilitation therapists went to places such as Hong Kong, Japan, Australia, and Canada to study accredited OT programs and then obtain OT registration status.

Some university graduates in rehabilitation therapy selected OT as their specialism and then learned OT knowledge and skills through continuous education.

Some three-year diploma in rehabilitation therapy programs covering various therapeutic modalities including OT skills were offered in junior colleges, colleges, and universities in Guangzhou, Shanghai, Hubei, and Anhui.

Some prestigious tertiary institutes offered advanced rehabilitation training. For example, Sun Yat-Sen University developed a three-year diploma program and a five-year degree program in rehabilitation therapy.

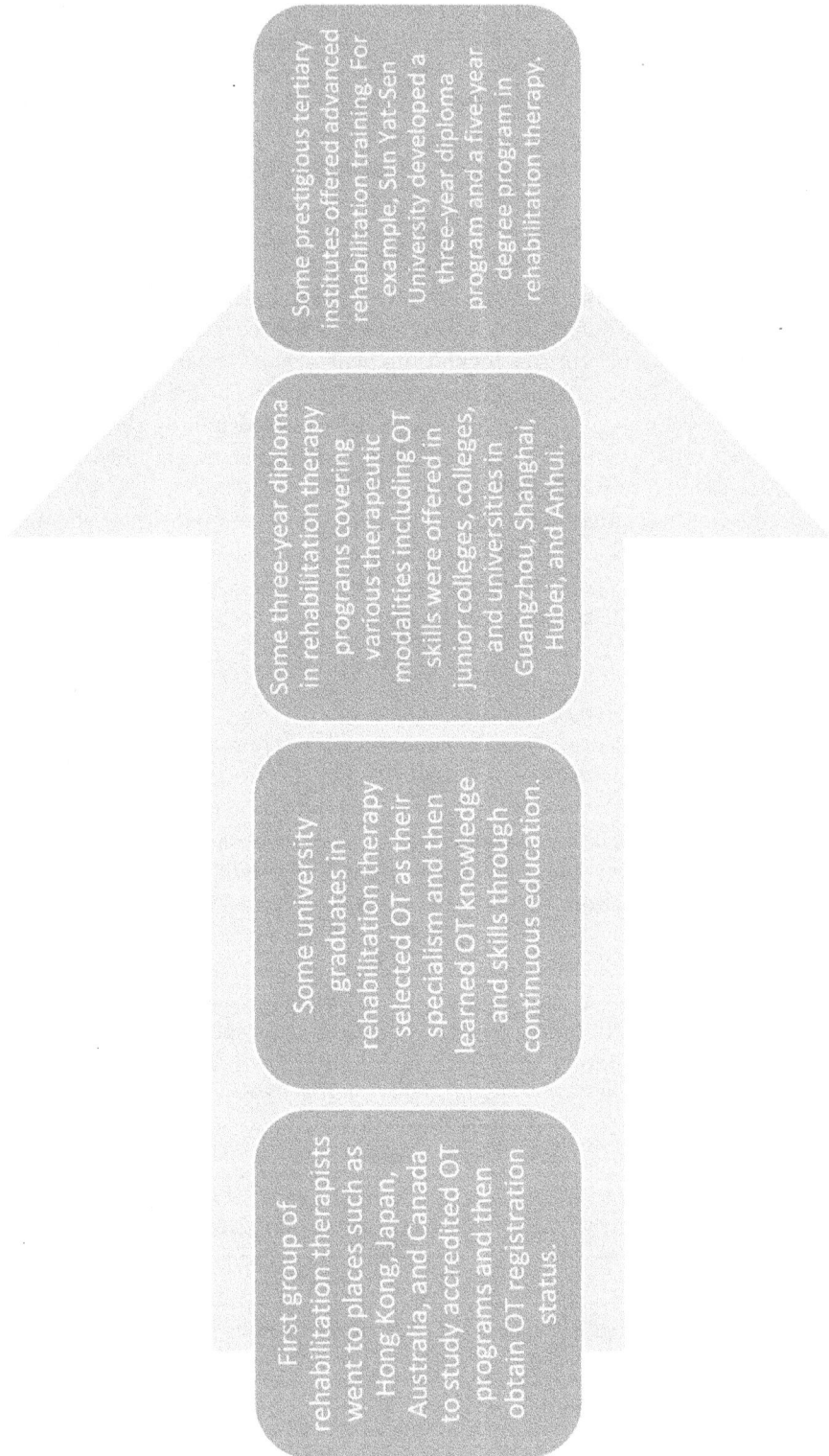

Figure 1.1 Formal OT education received by rehabilitation personnel in mainland China around 2000

While such rehabilitation medicine programs helped relieve the severe shortage of rehabilitation therapists on the mainland, the training did not clearly distinguish between OT and physiotherapy. As such, no specialization of these professional disciplines was made (Erlandsson, 2011) until the launch of the first local four-year undergraduate degree program in OT at the Capital Medical University in 2002 (World Federation of Occupational Therapists, n.d.).

The critical moment for local formally trained occupational therapists came in 2008 after an earthquake in Sichuan. There was a huge and urgent need for OT rehabilitation services due to the sudden emergence of a large number of victims with both physical conditions (such as traumatic brain injuries, fractures, and amputations) and psychological conditions (such as post-traumatic stress) (Lee, 2014). Jointly establishing the Institute for Disaster Management and Reconstruction (the first of its kind on the mainland), PolyU and Sichuan University initiated in 2013 the first master's-entry OT program accredited by WFOT for practicing rehabilitation therapists with an undergraduate degree in rehabilitation therapy or with relevant working experience (Shi & Howe, 2016). This accredited program also shaped the scope of OT services by providing the knowledge and skills necessary for all specialties, including psychiatric and geriatric. With the increasing need for an OT workforce throughout the mainland, more OT programs have been launched. Indeed, the OT profession in China obtained full membership in WFOT in 2018. There are currently nine accredited local undergraduate OT programs across China, such as in Beijing, Sichuan, Kunming, and Guangzhou (World Federation of Occupational Therapists, n.d.).

The above indicates the steady growth of OT and its services in mainland China. Nevertheless, strategic planning in healthcare policies is necessary for tackling the challenges that come with further increasing the number of OT professionals and expanding the scope of OT services. In doing so, access to rehabilitation for people with various disabilities across China can be maximized (Lavine & Greiner, 2020).

History of occupational therapy in Taiwan

OT in Taiwan developed after Japan conceded Taiwan to the Nationalist Government after 1945. At that time, several psychiatric centers (e.g., Xikou Psychiatric Center [former name of Taoyuan Psychiatric Center] and Jen Chi Hospital) provided a limited range of treatments and interventions involving the concept of OT (Huang et al., 2009). Moreover, several hospitals (e.g., National Taiwan University Hospital and Cheng Hsin Hospital) operated a Department of Occupational Therapy to provide OT services. However, an official title for OT practitioners in hospitals was not used until 1989. Various titles had been used up until that point, including nursing assistant, occupational instructor, occupational assistant, and technician. In 1989, the title of "occupational therapist" began being used in Taipei City Psychiatric Center. To ensure the quality of OT practitioners, certification of OT was legislated in May 1997 and the first central examination for OT certification was implemented in July 1998 (Chen-Sea, 2000; Tsai et al., 2017). In addition, the Taiwan Occupational Therapy Association was established in 1982 and the Occupational Therapists Union was established in 2001 to oversee the career development and rights of occupational therapists in Taiwan.

Despite OT practitioners having provided services in hospitals since 1945, Taiwan's education system did not include OT teaching or training until 1970. The first

Table 1.2 Undergraduate programs in OT at various institutes in Taiwan since 1988

Year	Institute
1970	National Taiwan University (First undergraduate program in OT within the Department of Rehabilitation Medicine, which was later developed to be the School of OT in 1992)
1988	Chung Shan Medical University (formerly Chung Shan Medical College)
1989	Kaohsiung Medical University (formerly Kaohsiung Medical College)
1990	National Cheng Kung University
1994	Chang Gung University
2003	I-Shou University
2004	Fu Jen Catholic University
2016	Asia University
2022	Da-Yeh University

undergraduate program in OT in Taiwan was established within the Department of Rehabilitation Medicine of National Taiwan University. At that time, the Department offered two undergraduate programs: OT and physical therapy. Subsequently, more OT undergraduate programs were developed and launched by other institutions, as summarized in Table 1.2 (Chen-Sea, 2000; Huang et al., 2009).

Additionally, two junior college programs in OT were launched at Jenteh Junior College of Medicine and Shu-Zen Junior College of Medicine and Management. To improve the research excellence of OT professionals, several graduate OT programs have been established at National Taiwan University (master's and doctorate programs), National Cheng Kung University (master's and doctorate programs), Chang Gung University (master's program), Chung Shan Medical University (master's program), and Kaohsiung Medical University (master's and in-service master's programs).

Principles and theories of occupational therapy

Occupation in the Oriental context

Occupation refers to any activities that a person engages in during daily life, including activities of daily living (ADLs) such as eating and cooking, productivity activities such as education and work, leisure pursuits, and essential periods of rest and sleep (American Occupational Therapy Association, 2020). While productivity is obviously contextual and bound to corresponding environments with embedded cultural and socio-economic factors (Serrat, 2019), other occupations such as ADL and leisure pursuits are also culturally relevant. In other words, engagement in these occupations is likely to be determined by the diverse cultural and socio-economic backgrounds of the individuals.

To illustrate cultural influence, eating as an ADL in a Chinese family will be used here as an example. During mealtime, family members always sit around a table to share dishes instead of having their own sets of food and drink. While adherence to dining etiquette is expected in every culture, Chinese people have particular concerns regarding this. Sharing dishes often implies interaction among family members. Interestingly, especially in the past, unnecessary talking or chatting was generally not encouraged (although not strictly prohibited). In Chinese culture, talking while eating is considered impolite, which is reflected in the saying, "not to talk when eating". Additionally, the proper use of eating utensils, particularly chopsticks, is highly emphasized. Ineffective use of chopsticks not only looks awkward but also makes it difficult to pick up food, which may end up dropped onto the table or floor, leading to waste. Older adults often find the wastage of food unacceptable, which is likely due to the hardships they faced in the past. Even today, Chinese people in rural areas keep leftover food for use in the next meal.

In terms of play and leisure, Confucianism still heavily influences societies in Asia, such as China, Japan, and Korea. For example, even in Hong Kong where people have taken on more Western values, parents still believe that "hard work is rewarding while play is unbeneficial". It is therefore unsurprising to note that the time allocated to kids for play is insufficient (ChinaDaily Asia, 2016). The situation is even worse for those with disabilities (Beckett et al., 2020), while provision of physical environments to facilitate play is limited (Shen et al., 2018).

As for work, it has long been regarded in both the East and West as an essential component of human life, forming one's socio-economic status and his/her connection with society (Hutchison, 2003). In turn, this contributes to one's psychological wellness and quality of life (Dich et al., 2019; Weziak-Bialowolska et al., 2020). Influential for centuries, Confucianism and East Asian collectivism have continued to shape and guide cultural values, in particular, the perception and nurturing of people's social roles (e.g., the worker role) in Oriental regions, including mainland China, Hong Kong, Macau, Taiwan, Singapore, Malaysia, Japan, and Korea (Allen et al., 2015; Cho & Choi, 2018; Neville, 2000). In contrast to Western contexts, family members are expected to be interdependent in order to create a strong family unit, which serves as a fundamental building block of society. Each member, particularly males, is required to fulfill culturally expected responsibilities that are essential for developing and maintaining their social and economic roles, in which work is of utmost importance as it significantly contributes to the financial stability of both their immediate family and their primary family, including aging parents (Huang, 2011; Lai & Surood, 2009). This ideology can account for the importance of getting employed or re-employed regardless of one's situation, including health (Ross, 2007). In Hong Kong, for example, the Employees Retraining Board plays a role in re-employment. It aims to offer training courses to two major groups to help them rejoin the labor force: (1) those at the sub-degree educational level or below who are unemployed or underemployed, and (2) those with health-related conditions (Employees Retraining Board, n.d.). The Selective Placement Division in the Labour Department also contributes by offering practical support to the second group, such as employment counseling and guidance, as well as follow-up services for monitoring work progress (Labour Department, n.d.).

The following paragraphs aim to illustrate how occupational therapists with Oriental perspectives facilitate people with various needs to engage in their occupations. Examples will be used in the discussion that will focus primarily on productivity but will also briefly cover occupations of ADL and leisure.

OT around the globe is a well-recognized rehabilitation profession devoted to therapeutically facilitating service users with various conditions to enter, resume, and sustain work through interventions of work/vocational rehabilitation (Moll et al., 2003). Work rehabilitation and vocational rehabilitation usually refer to interventions for those with physical and mental conditions, respectively. The former covers conditions such as work injuries and traumatic brain injuries, and the latter targets those with mental illnesses, learning disabilities, autistic spectrum disorders, etc.

Regarding work rehabilitation, return-to-work programs for injured workers under work injury management have become increasingly popular in Asian countries nowadays after almost two decades of development in the Western world (Costa-Black et al., 2011). Active and organized engagement of stakeholders, including injured workers, employers, and healthcare professionals, is central to making return-to-work programs successful. Thus, it is necessary to understand and embed their beliefs, perceptions, expectations, and roles in return-to-work in the planning, implementation, and evaluation of the interventions (MacEachen et al., 2006). Singapore, like many other Asian countries, is eager to provide effective and culturally specific return-to-work programs based on the results of numerous research studies. For instance, a randomized controlled trial (Tan et al., 2016) in Singapore attempted to investigate if an emerging return-to-work coordination model could facilitate earlier return-to-work in comparison with usual hospital standard care. This model involved the establishment of a new professional role called a "return-to-work coordinator", which was taken on by occupational therapists with clinical experience in work rehabilitation and additional training in areas such as effective disability management, legislation and disability management, advanced clinical skills, and case management. The aim was to sharpen return-to-work coordination through structured contact between the injured workers (mainly with fractures to the upper or lower limbs) and employers, including earlier contact with the employers, frequent updates on the injured workers' progress, and detailed advice on work adaptation, such as alternative work duties and environmental modifications. The results showed that those participating in the return-to-work coordination program could return to work ten days earlier than those receiving standard hospital care, and that a greater number of the former were able to return to modified jobs.

As for vocational rehabilitation for people with severe mental illness (SMI), there have been various research studies in a number of regions across China. In the study by Tsang et al. (2013) on caregivers' perspectives on the perceived rehabilitation needs of individuals with schizophrenia in Hong Kong, work was considered by the female caregivers to be most important. A similar study (Li et al., 2013) conducted in Wuxi on the perceived rehabilitation needs of people with schizophrenia also showed that productivity was considered crucial. The need for gaining employment was closely correlated with another rehabilitation need about finance in these two studies. It is reasonable, particularly in Asian regions, that caregivers, especially mothers, are expected to be responsible for nurturing children so that they can ultimately earn a living not only for themselves but also for the family (Malhotra & Sachdeva, 2005). This is in line with the influence of Confucianism discussed earlier. If those with SMI can get a job with a stable income upon receiving effective vocational rehabilitation interventions, such as Integrated Supported Employment (Tsang et al., 2009), the financial burden on both the individuals and their families will likely be relieved to a certain extent. In turn, this can contribute to their psychological wellness. The findings about the perceptions of these two types of stakeholders in Chinese societies strengthen the belief that return-to-work interventions under vocational rehabilitation have become critical in psychiatric rehabilitation to enable recovery in Chinese cultural contexts (New Life Psychiatric Rehabilitation Association, n.d.; Tsang & Chen, 2007). Specializing in vocational rehabilitation, occupational therapists are well equipped to help individuals with psychiatric conditions tackle both internal and external challenges in seeking and maintaining jobs (King & Lloyd, 2007). Ongoing research into effective interventions to improve vocational outcomes, along with measures such as strengthening the OT workforce, should help consolidate strategies for successfully implementing vocational rehabilitation in Asian regions. This aims to re-engage individuals with SMI in meaningful productivity roles, thereby enhancing their recovery (Li et al., 2015).

In terms of ADL, those with difficulties in doing any of these activities should receive interventions. As with many other tasks involving multiple skills, dining requires one to have at least fundamental fine motor competency to use eating utensils as well as basic social manners. However, children with learning disabilities, for example, may not be able to use chopsticks properly or understand table manners clearly. Occupational therapists in special schools would provide ADL and social skills training to improve, as much as possible, children's manipulation of chopsticks and table manners, respectively.

Occupational therapists are well-positioned to advocate play as an important occupation for children. In fact, play has been proven globally to be both pleasurable and productive in the general development of children, including those with special needs (Humphry, 2002). This may help to counter the traditional Chinese belief that play is unhelpful. Occupational therapists are experienced in investigating the impacts of the human environment (e.g., parents' perceptions about play) and physical environment (e.g., the availability of a play infrastructure) on children's accessibility to play (Ray-Kaeser & Lynch, 2017). This highlights that, in addition to clinical duties, occupational therapists in Oriental regions need to execute another important role – the advocate for play as an indispensable occupation of children.

To sum up, occupations have unique Oriental contexts. Occupational therapists contribute by helping individuals with various health-related conditions to engage in their meaningful occupations. The sharing of valuable clinical experiences throughout Asia and other regions via scholarly activities such as conferences and clinical visits, together with further research on effective intervention models and protocols, should facilitate the development and advancement of OT, thereby widening the coverage of services geographically as well as strengthening their effectiveness and cultural relevancy.

Chinese psychology and stigmatization of disabilities and behavioral health

This section attempts to describe and discuss the views of Chinese people regarding disabilities from a psychological perspective, as well as the impacts of stigmatization on behavioral health. These will have an influence on the understanding and practice of OT assessments and interventions developed in Western countries. In addition, this section looks to explain the unique features of practice guidelines or techniques developed in Hong Kong and other places that share common views on disabilities and chronic illnesses.

The biographical experiences of individuals determine the way they perceive and portray reality and the world around them (Berger & Luckmann, 1966). As the term "biographical" means something related to one's life, it implies that the experience is both individualized and culturally dependent. Every society is likely to possess its own unique socio-economic features, hence, people growing up in a particular environment have been significantly immersed and influenced accordingly. Such lived experiences help shape a person's basic understanding of how the world works and what is expected of themselves and others, establishing a set of values for typification that guide their actions. Typification, similar to stereotyping, refers to the process of relying on general knowledge rather than direct personal knowledge to build a set of oversimplified and often unfair beliefs or ideas about a group. This process assumes that all individuals within the group, especially those who are underprivileged, share identical characteristics. The resulting ideology influences how society interacts with and perceives these individuals as a whole (Crossman, 2017).

Such constructs and actions are so securely internalized that they resist change. This may be particularly obvious in Chinese culture where people still quite firmly believe in fate and destiny, and usually have numerous taboos. In Chinese societies, the general public tends to hold a stereotype associated with the term "mental handicap" (or, the older term, "mental retardation"). In addition to several adjectives commonly used to encompass all types of handicap, regardless of the level (mild, moderate, severe, profound), such as "foolish", "incapable", and "dependent", it is common for some people to attribute an individual's intelligence abnormality to the evils incurred by his/her ancestors. Stereotyping of this group of people is even extended to sexuality, which is highly individualized in nature. Two extreme myths exist (Levy & Packman, 2004). One is that sexual desire is hindered in every individual with a mental handicap due to abnormal sexual development, and so all of them are asexual. The other myth is that their uncontrollable nature, caused by brain malformation, leads to an unexpectedly high sexual desire. As proper satisfaction of sexual desire is a significant component in sexuality, which contributes to behavioral health and, in turn, mental wellness (Flynn et al., 2016), these types of misconceptions could make their parents, guardians, or other stakeholders neglect the importance of promoting their sexual health, thus undermining their quality of life. This situation may still be particularly true in contemporary China and among the more conservative older generation in Hong Kong, forming a prolonged prohibitive cultural pattern that prevents Chinese people from dealing with any sexual topics or issues (Lieber et al., 2009).

A correlation exists between collectivism in Chinese culture and typification or stereotyping. In Chinese societies, family members are expected to be interdependent and must fulfill cultural responsibilities to establish and maintain their socio-economic roles. This is essential for forming a strong family, which serves as a fundamental unit that integrates into the community (Huang, 2011). Under collectivism, it is reasonable to infer that any of the family members with even a slight variation to the norm is likely to affect not only himself/herself but also the whole family. Such variations, specifically those pertaining to health and which are overt in nature (e.g., an abnormal appearance resulting from Down Syndrome or bizarre behaviors caused by autistic spectrum disorder) or which threaten social identity (e.g., those with SMI), are subject to the stereotype that they are "no good". In turn, this commonly results in stigma and discrimination.

Take SMI as an example. Stigma is usually due to poor understanding or fear (Corrigan & Watson, 2002). Negative perceptions of mental disorders, especially SMI, still exist in Chinese societies despite an increase in their awareness and acceptance of the medical nature of such types of illness (The Lancet, 2016). This seems contradictory. When the etiology of mental illness is shown to have a physiological basis, it suggests that those with mental illness likely have their biological mechanisms altered. This indicates that the illness is somewhat objective in nature, similar to how a disturbance in the endocrine system can lead to diabetes. Given this objectivity, there is little justification in blaming or fearing anyone with mental illness.

The stigma attached to SMI, such as schizophrenia, is clear in mainland China. Tsui and Tsang (2017) found that in both urban and rural regions of Wuxi (a city in China), discrimination against people with schizophrenia was regarded by those with this condition and their caregivers as a significant obstacle in community reintegration and in return-to-work to the open market. Both groups were frustrated by the common phenomenon of being looked down on by others in the community simply because of the mental illness. They also commented that the only reason why employers hesitated to recruit those with mental illness was their fear of being held responsible for any actions stemming from the employees' mental health issues, although they lacked understanding of the actual problems. It is not surprising that stigma arises when people learn that someone has a mental illness, and discrimination continues even in the absence of any symptoms (Byrne, 2000).

Family psychoeducation has been found to be effective in improving the caring attitudes and skills of family caregivers in mainland China (Ran et al., 2003). One of the key goals of this type of psychoeducation is to encourage and empower caregivers to give family members with mental illness vital coping skills (e.g., assertive and problem-solving skills) for managing challenging situations in daily life and the workplace (Lucksted et al., 2012). Sadly, it is likely that the caregivers' fear of being stigmatized deters them from joining family psychoeducation programs (Li et al., 2017). Occupational therapists no doubt play an important role in family psychoeducation. They should thus assess the caregivers' fear of stigma in advance to see if it might affect their willingness or eagerness to receive psychoeducation. Tackling this fear prior to commencing the education program is crucial for ensuring their subsequent level of participation and maximizing the outcomes.

The above arbitrary generalizations show the existence of serious stigma in Chinese culture concerning individuals with SMI and their significant others, including family members. The impacts of this deserve attention. For instance, it is common to find that accessibility to mental health services is severely limited, which, in turn, undermines the recovery process and outcomes (American Psychiatric Association, n.d.). Under the influence of collectivism in Chinese culture, the intention and attempt to avoid shame to oneself and the whole family may deter individuals with mental health problems from freely expressing their perceived needs and concerns about recovery. Worst still, when those with mental illness have been influenced by these public attitudes and suffer the negative consequences for themselves and their families, they may eventually come to believe that others' negative perceptions are true and that they deserve the public's adverse reactions. They might then internalize such stigma and become self-stigmatized, which can hinder their recovery by decreasing hope and self-esteem. This decline in self-worth may alarmingly lead to lower adherence to medical and rehabilitation interventions (Yanos et al., 2020). A study in Hong Kong (Fung et al., 2007) found a close correlation between self-stigma and psychosocial intervention compliance. Specifically, those with more serious self-stigma had poorer adherence to psychosocial intervention. They tended to believe the stereotypes that they were troublemakers and useless, and thus no treatment would work, further reducing their self-esteem.

A range of strategies should be utilized to address these issues. In terms of the general public, measures such as organizing campaigns and making use of mass media to tackle the stigma of mental illness by minimizing the stereotypes should be incorporated into mental health policy (Jenkins, 2003). Regarding individual-based interventions focusing on self-stigmatization, the first self-stigma reduction program was recently developed in Hong Kong. This program employs various techniques such as psychoeducation, cognitive behavioral therapy, social skills training, and motivational interviews (Fung, 2010). It has been found to be effective (Fung et al., 2011) and can be culturally adapted for use in other Chinese societies, taking into account their socio-economic contexts.

In summary, individuals with disabilities, including the mentally handicapped and those with mental illness, have been suffering from stigmatization or have had their behavioral health undermined due to the influence of Chinese culture. Although culture is likely resistant to change, occupational therapists together with other stakeholders should collaborate to devise potentially effective strategies to tackle the associated challenges. (Note: Chapter 5 of this book comprises two sections that further discuss mental illness and public stigma, as well as self-stigma of mental illness.)

Models and frames of reference in the Oriental context

Concepts of models, theories, and frames of reference in practical use

A website "HOTheory" (https://ottheory.com/index.php/) created by Dr. Chi-Wen Chien's team, with support from the Teaching Development Grant from PolyU (project code: LTG16-19/SS/RS3), has gathered useful information on models, theories, and frames of reference (FORs) associated with OT. Given that detailed information can be reviewed and obtained from the website, this section will simply illustrate some commonly used theories and FORs in the Oriental context.

Theories, models, and FORs all belong to the concept of theoretical knowledge, which is defined as "a set of ideas or concepts that occupational therapists use to guide their actions during the assessment and intervention process" (Chien, n.d.). More specifically, a theory is defined as "a plausible or scientifically acceptable general principle or body of principles offered to explain phenomena" (Merriam-Webster, n.d.b); a model is defined as "a symbolic representation of concepts or variables, and interrelationships among them" (Polit & Beck, 2010, p. 560); and a FOR is defined as "a set of ideas, conditions, or assumptions that determine how something will be approached, perceived, or understood" (Merriam-Webster, n.d.a). Under these definitions, we can consider that theories and models are broader concepts than FORs and are better for identifying the needs and problems of a client. A FOR incorporates elements of both theories and models, but its primary purpose is to provide practical guidelines for OT practitioners in designing appropriate interventions supported by theory. In absence of model answers, occupational therapists should rely on their clinical reasoning and experience to evaluate and justify which model(s) or FOR(s) to adopt based on their understanding and analysis of the core principles and details. A number of commonly adopted models will be introduced below, followed by some descriptions of various FORs.

Model of Human Occupation

The Model of Human Occupation (MOHO) developed by Prof. Gary Kielhofner and his colleague (1980) describes how individuals interact with their living environment to generate and modify their occupations, with such interaction presenting a dynamic open cycle system. There are basically three subsystems in an individual: volition, habituation, and performance. Volition includes personal causation, interests, and values which initiate an individual's actions. Habituation refers to internalized roles and habits which maintain an individual's daily routines and action patterns. Performance concerns an individual's skilled actions on daily tasks. MOHO is often used as a conceptual model to analyze an individual's overall conditions and help OT practitioners identify potential problems and set treatment goals. It can also be applied to any populations, including children, adolescents, adults, and older people; however, OT practitioners use MOHO more in a psychiatric setting than in a physical setting.

Person-Environment-Occupation and Person-Environment-Occupation-Performance models

The Person-Environment-Occupation (PEO) model developed by Prof. Mary Law and her colleagues (1996) emphasizes how an individual engages in occupations and displays occupational performance with the interactions between the person, environment, and occupation. Therefore, the PEO model emphasizes the domains of the person (i.e., demographics of the person, the person's cultural background, self-concept, role, personality, sensory capabilities, cognition, physical capacity, and health), environment (i.e., various environments including cultural, physical, social, institutional, and socioeconomic environments in which the person lives), and occupation (i.e., daily tasks or activities that the person engages in to achieve or meet with self-maintenance, expression, and well-being). A Person-Environment-Occupation-Performance (PEOP) model was later proposed to strengthen the PEO model with the addition of "performance" (Baum et al., 2015). Similar to the PEO, PEOP emphasizes the person, environment, and occupation, while adding the importance of occupational performance resulting from the interaction among the person, environment, and occupation. PEO and PEOP are often used as a conceptual model to analyze an individual's overall conditions and help OT practitioners identify potential problems and set treatment goals. Both can be applied to any populations, including children, adolescents, adults, and older people; however, OT practitioners use PEO and PEOP more in a physical setting than in a psychiatric setting.

Canadian Model of Occupational Performance and Canadian Model of Occupational Performance and Engagement

The Canadian Model of Occupational Performance (CMOP) and the Canadian Model of Occupational Performance and Engagement (CMOP-E) developed by Prof. Elizabeth Townsend and her colleague (2007) emphasize three main components: the person (located in the center with spirituality surrounded by the affective, physical, and cognitive abilities of the person), occupation (located in the intermediate circle, which links the person and environment and includes self-care, producibility, and leisure), and environment (located in the outermost circle and including various environments for the person: physical, social, cultural, and institutional environments). Additionally, the CMOP and CMOP-E are often used with the Canadian Occupational Performance Measure (COPM) (Law et al., 1990) because COPM can help identify the difficulties in a client's occupational performance. CMOP and CMOP-E can be applied to any populations, including children, adolescents, adults, and older people; however, OT practitioners use CMOP and CMOP-E more in a physical setting than in a psychiatric setting.

Kawa model

The Kawa model developed by Dr. Michael Iwama and his colleagues (2009) uses the metaphor of a river (i.e., "kawa" in Japanese) to indicate an individual's human life. The Kawa model emphasizes the person's subjective reports using a metaphor commonly used by Eastern people – "a river is like a human life". There are various elements in this model, including water (i.e., the life energy of the person), the river banks and bottom (i.e., the physical environment and social context of the person), rocks (i.e., issues such as the problems and difficulties encountered by the person), driftwood (i.e., the personal attributes, resources, and good features of the person), and space (i.e., how OT practitioners can work on the person's rocks, river banks and bottom, and driftwood to create space for water flow).

In addition to the aforementioned models, there are various FORs for OT practice.

Biomechanical frame of reference

This is a remedial approach applied to pediatric, adolescent, adult, and older populations. It targets physical disabilities or neurological disorders (McMillan, 2011).

Rehabilitative and compensatory frame of reference

This is a compensatory approach which assumes that the individual's functional abilities cannot be improved but their occupational performance can be enhanced (Addy, 2006; Gillen, 2014). It can be applied to pediatric, adolescent, adult, and older populations under the condition that they should have sufficient cognitive abilities to learn the compensatory techniques.

Behavioral frame of reference

This is a remedial approach focusing on techniques such as behavior modification (i.e., providing rewards or punishment to shape human behaviors), reinforcement (i.e., providing a set of situations/conditions to increase or decrease the behavior engagements), extinction (i.e., removing the reinforcement), forward chaining (i.e., separating the behaviors into several steps and modifying the behaviors from the first step), backward chaining (i.e., separating the behaviors into several steps and modifying the behaviors from the last step), systematic desensitization (i.e., teaching relaxation techniques for the individuals to control anxiety-eliciting stimuli), and the token economy (i.e., using mediums of exchange to shape behaviors) (Stein, 1983). It can be applied to pediatric, adolescent, adult, and older populations, with a focus on appropriate behaviors that can lead to better occupational performance instead of functional abilities.

Cognitive behavioral frame of reference

This is a remedial approach that focuses on four aspects of life experience: thoughts (i.e., whether the individual has negative distorted thoughts), emotions (i.e., the negative distorted thoughts lead to negative feelings), physiological responses (i.e., the negative emotions trigger the individual's somatic problems such as sweating and heart-beating), and behaviors (i.e., the negative distorted thoughts, negative emotions, and somatic problems induce the individual's inappropriate behaviors to cope with these uncomfortable feelings) (Duncan, 2011). One common intervention approach adopted by occupational therapists based on this FOR is the ABCDE model, which has been developed as a guide to help individuals break their negative distorted thoughts and subsequently modify their inappropriate behaviors. The ABCDE model has five stages: the activating event, beliefs, consequences, disputation of the beliefs, and effective new approach (Ellis, 1991). It can be applied to pediatric, adolescent, adult, and older populations and is often used in people with mental illness.

Psychodynamic frame of reference

It is a remedial approach which originates from Dr. Sigmund Freud's idea that emotions and psychic energy are needed to help individuals achieve basic needs and maintain social relationships. Under this concept, explorative and supportive approaches can be utilized. In the explorative approach, OT practitioners may bring the individual's conflicts from an unconscious to a conscious level, that is, to let the individual review his/her past and identify what life events caused his/her disabilities. In the supportive approach, OT practitioners may keep the conflicts hidden and undisclosed. Instead, they will attempt to strengthen the ego defense mechanism in the individual to resolve his/her problems without dealing with conflicts on the conscious level (Creek, 2014). It can be applied to pediatric, adolescent, adult, and older populations and is often used in helping people with mental illness.

Sensory integration frame of reference

This is a remedial approach with a focus on how a child's learning and adaptive behaviors interact with their sensory systems, including the visual, tactile, proprioceptive, vestibular, and auditory systems. Sequencing, bilateral integration, praxis, postural-ocular control, sensory discrimination, and sensory modulation all help children achieve satisfactory performance given that they can improve the outcomes of self-regulation, postural control maintenance, organized behaviors, and self-esteem/self-efficacy development. It is often applied to pediatric and adolescent populations who have sensory processing disorder (Schaaf et al., 2010).

Acquisitional frame of reference

This is a remedial approach that emphasizes the process of teaching and learning through the medium of activities. It also stresses the importance of the environment, where the individual processes his/her teaching and learning, the functional behaviors that he/she is required to perform, and the learned skills that the individual has acquired. The concept of the acquisitional FOR is that people can learn new skills through repeated interactions with the environment given that behaviors are responses to the environment. Subsequently, the learned skills can equip the individual to achieve satisfactory participation (Luebben & Royeen, 2010). It is often applied to pediatric and adolescent populations who need to shape their skills and behaviors.

Table 1.3 highlights the core principles of the aforementioned FORs.

Table 1.3 The core principles of various FORs

FOR	Core principle
Biomechanical	Training range of motion, strength, and endurance to deal with impairments that limit occupational performance.
Rehabilitative and compensatory	Using compensatory techniques or adaptations to maximize occupational performance.
Behavioral	Shaping an individual's behaviors into desired behaviors.
Cognitive behavioral	Modifying inappropriate behaviors by breaking negative distorted thoughts.
Psychodynamic	Achieving basic needs and maintaining social relationships by relieving tension within a person's psyche.
Sensory integration	Interacting with sensory systems to achieve learning and adaptive behaviors.
Acquisitional	Facilitating the process of teaching and learning through the medium of activities and the environment.

Model of Human Occupation and traditional Chinese medicine

Traditional Chinese medicine

Traditional Chinese medicine (TCM) is an ancient form of medicine developed from Chinese philosophy. One of the most famous books in TCM is *Huangdi Neijing*, which was published over 2,000 years ago. It offers systematic descriptions of TCM's diagnostic, treatment, and health preservation strategies. TCM emphasizes disease prevention and the slowing down of disease progression. The health preservation strategies of TCM can be classified into nine categories: psychological, *qi*, food, health *qigong*, prenatal care, temporal variation, aging, herbal medicine, and sex counseling (Tan, 2009). Body constitution is an important factor in understanding a person's sub-health situation before providing treatment. Body equilibrium and balance among the Three Treasures (i.e., essence, *qi*, and mind) can be restored through various treatment strategies, such as *tuina*, herbal medicine, acupuncture, scrapping, cupping, diet, tea, and health *qigong* (Zhong & Ng, 2018). Over a hundred systematic reviews have been published to prove the effectiveness of health *qigong* in improving physical and psychological functions in the health groups and disease groups of cardiovascular, metabolic, pulmonary, depression, and cancer clients (Ng, 2022; Ng et al., 2013; Ng et al., 2014).

Figure 1.2 shows the commonalities and differences between MOHO and TCM and was developed based on a previous conference presentation (Ng, 2012). At the center is a human being living between the sky and the earth. MOHO and TCM share commonalities in their core philosophies and intended outcomes, while their differences lie in the assessment structures and treatment processes.

Commonalities

The holism and system approach

TCM emphasizes the importance of considering the age-related pre-morbid body constitution of an individual before treatment planning. This echoes MOHO, which focuses on the human as an individual and his/her daily occupational activities and

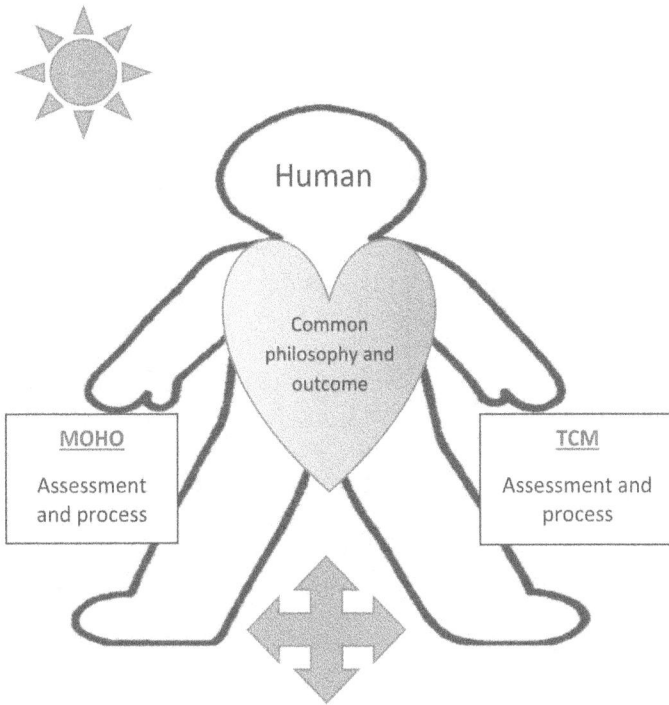

Figure 1.2 Conceptual commonalities and differences between MOHO and TCM

interactions with the environment. In TCM treatment, the focus is on considering the dynamic interactions among the Three Treasures to restore balance. The Occupational Questionnaire in MOHO highlights the importance of gathering information about an individual's daily patterns and lifestyle related to occupational activities. This focus on the habituation subsystem aims to achieve a meaningful balance among work, self-care, and leisure (Ng & Tsang, 2019). Both MOHO and TCM consider an individual's choices and needs. They focus on the time, place, and person, and emphasize the dynamic interaction as a whole instead of being separate from the environment. The harmony between the internal system and external environment in TCM is similar to the system theory of MOHO. Both adopt system and dynamic approaches.

TCM and MOHO share the philosophy that harmony with the environment is crucial. In TCM, nature is classified into *yin* or *yang*, while food nature is classified into heating or cooling. Consuming excessive amounts of heating foods will affect body constitution and create an imbalance, potentially leading to disease. In MOHO, the balance between an individual's performance and his/her life role expectations can be assessed using the Role Checklist. This tool helps identify areas of deficit, value distortions, and gaps to prioritize for treatment based on individual needs. Balance and harmony with the environment are common outcomes of both TCM and MOHO.

The humanist and client-centered approach

MOHO emphasizes the volition, habituation, and performance subsystems of an individual, as well as their interaction with the human and non-human environment. TCM offers an individualized approach that considers multiple occupational performances when offering treatment. TCM uses syndrome differentiation as a comprehensive approach, providing personalized recommendations based on age, body constitution, disease progression, and health preferences. Both TCM and MOHO emphasize the individual in the treatment philosophy instead of focusing on the disease.

Wellness habit and meaningful life

MOHO promotes the importance of occupational roles and habits in the habituation subsystem, which, in turn, promotes wellness. Furthermore, MOHO emphasizes personal causation, valued goals, and interest in the volition subsystem, which highlights the importance of a meaningful life. The use of the Occupational Self Assessment (OSA) reflects the uniqueness of the client's values and their priorities for change. The Volitional Questionnaire and the Interest Checklist used in MOHO are good examples that focus on habits and a meaningful life. In TCM, it is emphasized that individuals should perform appropriate activities according to their age, sex, body constitution, and temporal variation during the midnight-to-noon ebb and flow to preserve health (Ng, 2017; Tan, 2009). Both TCM and MOHO support the formation of a healthy lifestyle and lifestyle reconstruction. A preliminary study evaluating the effectiveness of a lifestyle modification program that incorporates circadian patterns based on an East-Meets-West approach for reducing the risk of pre-clinical metabolic syndrome in adults showed positive outcomes (Ng, 2017; Ng & Tsang, 2015; Ng & Tsang, 2024). MOHO and TCM share a core concept of prevention and health preservation, which aids in preventing relapses and diseases.

Pragmatic, problem, and asset focus

There are numerous publications related to the application of MOHO in clinical practice, and practical examples were published in the book *Conceptual Foundations of Occupational Therapy Practice* (Kielhofner, 2009). In the local Chinese context, MOHO is a well-known practice model that guides OT practice in Hong Kong (Liu & Ng, 2008). In Hong Kong, the Role Checklist is used to identify problems and assets, and to explore indications for treatment. The use of the Model of Human Occupation Screening Tool (MOHOST) and the Occupational Circumstances Assessment Interview and Rating Scale (OCAIRS) provides comprehensive problem and asset identification. MOHO is firmly grounded in the psychiatric field in Hong Kong, having been used for years in child and adolescent populations with intellectual disabilities, as well as in adult psychiatry. Similarly, in TCM, a pragmatic approach which considers the availability of treatment options is used flexibly when selecting meridian points and herbal formulas. Daily food ingredients such as ginger and spring onion roots are sometimes selected for TCM treatment. The strategies for balancing the Five Elements (wood, fire, earth, metal, and water) involve analyzing their strengths (assets) and weaknesses (problems) and promoting harmony through inter-growth and inhibition.

In Hong Kong, occupational therapists use the system approach and activities during treatment. Culturally relevant activities, such as health *qigong* and Chinese tea therapy, have been integrated into rehabilitation in Hong Kong for many years. With a deeper understanding of the philosophy of TCM and MOHO, the selection of activities could be expanded to suit clients' needs and maximize treatment benefits.

Similar to biology, psychology, and sociology, occupation is also regarded as a science. Occupational science, rooted in system theory and the holistic approach, emerged in 1989 and has been providing empirical knowledge to the OT profession ever since. Occupational therapists are encouraged to promote the uniqueness of their profession using a consistent communication model, with MOHO being an excellent choice. Health *qigong* coaches in Hong Kong are trained for both physical and psychiatric rehabilitation, as well as health promotion. In pain management, common OT strategies include positioning to maximize function, activity analysis and synthesis, ergonomics, edema control, splintage, and fascia massage. These strategies align with the TCM philosophy of nurturing genuine *qi* and facilitating its flow along meridians to improve health and function. TCM employs various massage techniques on the body's energy meridians to relieve blockages and pain.

Differences

Assessment structure and tools

The assessment and treatment packages of MOHO have been developed for years, as shown on the MOHO website, which is a useful resource platform for occupational therapists (MOHO-IRM Web, 2024). There are around 20 assessment tools with over 20 translated versions, as well as useful training packages such as the Remotivation Process. These assessment tools provide psychometric properties with validation and research support, such as the Occupational Questionnaire (OQ), Role Checklist, OSA, OCAIRS, and Assessment of Communication and Interaction Skills (ACIS).

TCM practitioners adopt a different structure and gather clients' information through four diagnostic methods (inspection, listening and smelling, inquiring, and palpation) and the Eight Principles (*yin*, *yang*, external, internal, hot, cold, weak, and strong) in response to the internal body constitution, external environment (wind, cold, heat, dampness, dryness, and fire), and seasonal temporal changes (Curran, 2008). Various treatment models can be adopted, such as the Syndrome Differentiation of Six-channels Theory, Syndrome Differentiation of *Zang-fu*, Syndrome Differentiation of *Qi*-blood-body fluid, and Syndrome Differentiation of *Sanjiao* Theory (Lu et al., 2004). The assessment structure of TCM is developed from induction, phenomenology, survival analysis, and syndrome comparison, which is completely different from MOHO.

Treatment process

MOHO uses activities as the primary intervention and adopts a system approach, as discussed in *Conceptual Foundations of Occupational Therapy Practice* (Kielhofner, 2009). It focuses on occupation and the use of therapeutic activities. The mind and body are considered to be connected in MOHO. The development of a new occupation can regenerate the lost function of a person (Kielhofner, 2009). In the treatment process, all three subsystems (volition, habituation, and performance) and environmental factors (physical, social, cultural, economic, and political) are considered when evaluating occupational competence, occupational engagement, and changes in occupational identity.

On the other hand, TCM has both active and passive modes of treatment modalities. For example, acupuncture and *tuina* are passive modes of treatment, while health *qigong* is an active treatment modality. TCM treatment involves managing the energy of the Three Treasures. Compared to MOHO, TCM offers more detailed insights into the significance of temporal variations and provides extensive descriptions of health preservation and preventive medicine. This is particularly evident in its approach to chronic conditions such as pre-metabolic symptoms.

Case example illustrating the use of the East-Meets-West approach in the treatment of a clinical condition

Case details

John is a 40-year-old man who suffered a traumatic brain injury (TBI) after a road traffic accident about a year ago. Prior to the accident, John was a certified accountant. He is currently receiving outpatient OT and has not returned to work.

John's parents, who live with him, reported that his personality has changed dramatically. Before the accident, John was an active, friendly person with a good sense of humor. Now he spends most of the day watching television. He does not participate in family activities unless pushed to do so. He appears passive and depressed. He rarely initiates conversations and appears to have lost his sense of humor. Moreover, he is disorganized and unable to get things done when cued to start tasks. John said to his parents, "I feel blue! I am not able to cope with anything difficult and complex!" John shows typical depressive symptoms, such as feeling tired, sick, heavy, hopeless, and sad most of the time. He spends a lot of time engaging in ruminative thinking. For example, he mentioned trying hard to think about "why he suffered from the traffic accident" and "why he can't function as well as in the past". Sometimes John shows irritability and anger. He finds that everything seems harder to do, and feels that life is not worth the effort. The prolonged emotional state of sadness has significantly interrupted John's leisure life. He does not spend time playing football or going on short trips around Hong Kong.

John was diagnosed with major depressive disorder (MDD). He is aware that being on extended sick leave is unsustainable and that he has to deal with the family's financial burden due to a mortgage on the house in which he is living with his parents. As a result, John feels extremely stressed as he used to be the family breadwinner. His psychosocial needs for rehabilitation can be understood by adopting MOHO (Table 1.4).

Depressive disorder is frequently found in primary care and general hospital practice but it often goes undetected. Unrecognized depressive disorder may lead to slow recovery and could worsen the prognosis. The low rate of help-seeking behavior, particularly among males, might contribute, in part, to the undertreatment. In 2010, there were 1,008 registered deaths attributable to suicide, with 62.4% of these cases committed by males. This may indicate that males suffering from problems in their daily lives tend not to seek help even when conditions worsen, reflecting a difference in the characteristics of help-seeking behavior between men and women.

Socialization takes place when society transforms female and male human beings into social women and men from childhood. Significant others, such as our parents, teachers, classmates, and siblings, influence our concept of the role of men, which echoes the cultural value that men are "strong". Society is not ready for men to become

Table 1.4 MOHO showing John's primary problems and psychosocial rehabilitation needs

	Client's major problems	Client's psychosocial rehabilitation needs
Volition		
Personal causation Example: "I am not able to cope with anything difficult and complex!"	■ Feeling vulnerable, lacking control, and tending to give up. ■ Failing to assume responsibility, or doing so in a passive manner. ■ The prolonged emotional state of sadness has significantly interrupted John's leisure life.	■ Self-efficacy. ■ Mood regulation.
Values Example: John finds that everything seems harder to do, and feels that life is not worth the effort.	■ Loss of sense of control with limited life goals. ■ Loss of meaning or value in most activities.	■ New meaningful life goals.
Interests Example: John does not spend time playing football or going on short trips around Hong Kong.	■ Decreased participation in activities and interests. ■ Failing to find enjoyment in activities, and only participating in activities to pass the time.	
Habituation		
Roles Unsatisfactory role performance.	■ Total disruption. ■ Lack of roles to play.	■ Role re-building (resuming the roles of worker and breadwinner in the family).
Habits Example: John only engages in a sedentary lifestyle, such as watching TV at home.		■ Active exercising. ■ Healthy lifestyle re-design.
Performance		
Psychomotor skills	■ Significant slowing down of psychomotor speed and low energy level.	
Process skills	■ Unable to handle various tasks at the same time. ■ Finding it difficult to concentrate, think clearly, or solve problems.	
Communication skills	■ Negative interaction styles, such as lack of assertiveness, demanding, and passivity.	

sick or seek medical assistance. On the other hand, it is acceptable for women to have diseases and request medical assistance and interventions. The cultural value that men need to be "strong" could make them less motivated to seek help or think of their problems as just a "moody period" rather than a mood disorder. John, who used to be the breadwinner in his family, is under a huge amount of stress since suffering from depression. Nevertheless, he still expresses the wish of resuming his worker role.

East-Meets-West approach

OT is a type of allied health service in Western medicine. Traditional OT treatments consist of physical, sensory, mental, and communication activities. Occupational therapists also use Chinese health exercises as treatment interventions to develop or recover certain abilities of clients. These health exercises are East-Meets-West approaches in rehabilitation (The Hong Kong Polytechnic University, 2018).

Based on the MOHO framework, John's personal causation and performance subsystems were explored in an initial interview. John expressed that he wanted to improve his sleep problem and ease his tension so that he could have better energy restoration to prepare for his return-to-work. For personal causation, he had adequate insight that depression had caused a continuous worsening of his mental condition. He wanted to be capable of doing his job as he was the breadwinner in his family and valued the role highly. He needed a relaxation and self-management approach so that he could relieve his stress on his own as he still did not want to disclose the details of his illness (he held the cultural value that men are "strong"). In addition, it was difficult for him to seek help psychosocially (low help-seeking behavior) and he expected a more advanced and speedy rehabilitation. Besides the initial interview, the MOHOST (MOHO-IRM Web, 2024) was used as a key reference in John's initial assessment. MOHOST is an assessment which addresses the majority of MOHO concepts (volition, habituation, skills, and environment), allowing a therapist to obtain an overview of the client's occupational functioning. MOHOST measures the occupational participation of the client, and occupational participation is defined as self-care, productivity, and leisure.

In this case, the occupational therapist made the following recommendations to John: using an East-Meets-West approach, John will be treated holistically, that is, both mind and body. Relaxation techniques and self-management programs will be conducted, including the Health *Qigong* Eight-section Brocades (*Baduanjin* 八段錦), an advanced psychological intervention using metacognitive therapy (MCT), and an occupational lifestyle redesign (OLSR) program.

Relaxation techniques using the Health Qigong Eight-section Brocades (Baduanjin 八段錦)

Qigong has long been regarded as a mind–body intervention in TCM, with *qi* literally meaning vital energy within the body, and *gong* meaning training and practice (Tsang et al., 2002). The free flowing of *qi* within the meridian system is essential for good health, whereas its blockage can result in illness. The aim is to enhance one's self-healing ability when recovering from diseases or one's self-defense ability to guard against diseases.

John was invited to participate in a group training class on *Baduanjin* exercise every Tuesday morning during his residual sick leave. The *Baduanjin qigong* training program requires John to attend 12 practice sessions, each 45 minutes in length, under the instruction of a certified health *qigong* master. It is conducted in the OT unit of a day hospital. Each 45-minute session comprises a 10-minute warm-up, a 25-minute *qigong* (*Baduanjin*) exercise, and a 10-minute cool-down exercise. Using the eight criteria for judging the "safe practice" of the health *qigong* protocol, which are adapted from the American College of Sports Medicine (2005) and Niemeyer (1980), John was confirmed to be fit enough to perform the exercise.

Advanced psychological intervention using metacognitive therapy

MCT is a third-wave psychotherapy for the treatment of emotional disorders. There is a large body of evidence showing that self-regulatory strategies, specifically those linked to cognitive attentional syndrome (CAS; e.g., worry), are associated with vulnerability to emotional disorders and are predictors of traumatic stress. The effects of individual MCT treatment techniques and of full treatment packages have been evaluated in several studies. The methodologies used include single-case replication series, experimental reversal designs, open trials, and randomized controlled evaluations (Clark & Wells, 1995; Clark et al., 2003; Fisher & Wells, 2008; Simons et al., 2006; Wells & King, 2006; Wells & Papageorgiou, 2001; Wells & Sembi, 2004; Wells et al., 2008).

In addition to attending health *qigong* training classes, John also receives psychological intervention on a weekly basis. Each intervention session lasts for approximately one hour. John has noticed that he has a "CAS" style of thinking since suffering from TBI. He believes that his mental condition has worsened due to this toxic style of thinking, which has further developed into depressive thinking and poor mental wellness. After eight sessions of psychological intervention by MCT, John now spends less time ruminating and is more motivated to re-engage in former hobbies.

Occupational lifestyle redesign

According to Leung (2014), OLSR is a process which requires active and conscious effort to explore, experiment, and develop new habits. It also involves the internalization of old or new daily activities in terms of self-care, home maintenance, work, leisure, and social and spiritual activities. These can be prioritized and incorporated into a new lifestyle in which physical and mental health can be maintained, spirit nurtured, personal growth facilitated, and meaning and happiness fostered. OLSR includes weekly goal setting and activity implementation according to the improvement of targeted life domains.

The intervention program for John also includes OLSR treatment which targets life role reinforcement and functional enhancement across four life domains, such as re-engaging in work life or rebuilding a healthy social circle. John's life role is the breadwinner and son in his family. Since suffering from TBI and depression, his work capability has deteriorated. Furthermore, due to his mental health condition, he is unable to sustain a job as it demands a significant amount of concentration. John is encouraged to plan the steps necessary to enhance his rehabilitation process, reinforcing his life role and allowing him to restore his work capacity in alignment with his original job as quickly as possible.

Summary

This chapter introduces the history of OT in Hong Kong, China, and Taiwan. It also covers the principles and theories of OT, particularly regarding Chinese cultural influences. Occupations as the major area of focus in OT practice are illustrated through a review of the commonly adopted OT theoretical models and FORs. A comparison between MOHO and TCM is used to illustrate the influence of Chinese culture on OT practice in the Oriental context. The East-Meets-West approach is further elaborated through the case study of a TBI sufferer.

References

Addy, L. M. (2006). *Occupational therapy evidence in practice for physical rehabilitation.* Blackwell Publishing.

Allen, T. D., French, K. A., Dumani, S., & Shockley, K. M. (2015). Meta-analysis of work–family conflict mean differences: Does national context matter? *Journal of Vocational Behavior, 90*, 90–100. https://doi.org/10.1016/j.jvb.2015.07.006

American College of Sports Medicine. (2005). *ACSM's guidelines for exercise testing and prescription* (7th ed.). Lippincott Williams & Wilkins.

American Occupational Therapy Association. (2020). Occupational therapy practice framework: Domain and process (4th ed.). *American Journal of Occupational Therapy, 74*(Suppl. 2), 7412410010p1–7412410010p87.

American Psychiatric Association. (n.d.). *Stigma, prejudice and discrimination against people with mental illness.* Retrieved July 27, 2022, from https://www.psychiatry.org/patients-families/stigma-and-discrimination

Baum, C. M., Christiansen, C. H., & Bass, J. D. (2015). The Person-Environment-Occupation-Performance (PEOP) model. In C. H. Christiansen, C. M. Baum, & J. D. Bass (Eds.), *Occupational therapy: Performance, participation, and well-being* (4th ed., pp. 49–56). SLACK Incorporated.

Beckett, A. E., Encarnação, P., Chiu, C.-Y., & Ng, S. T. M. (2020). Play for disabled children in Taiwan and Hong Kong: Parent perspectives. *Journal of Disability Studies in Education, 1*(2021), 90–120. https://doi.org/10.1163/25888803-bja10005

Berger, P. L., & Luckmann, T. (1966). *The social construction of reality: A treatise in the sociology of knowledge.* Doubleday & Company.

Byrne, P. (2000). Stigma of mental illness and ways of diminishing it. *Advances in Psychiatric Treatment, 6*(1), 65–72. https://doi.org/10.1192/apt.6.1.65

Chen, Z. W. (2001). Rehabilitation over the past 20 years in China. *Chinese Journal of Convalescent Medicine, 10*(5), 1–4.

Chen-Sea, M. J. (2000). The development and prospect of occupational therapy in Taiwan. *Journal of Occupational Therapy Association R.O.C., 18*, 72–80. https://doi.org/10.6594/JTOTA.2000.18.07

Chien, C. W. (n.d.). *What is theoretical knowledge relevant to occupational therapy?* HOTheory. Retrieved December 16, 2021, from https://ottheory.com/about-theoretical-knowledge#:~:text=Theoretical%20knowledge%20is%20a%20set%20of%20ideas%20or,of%20learning%20process%20to%20become%20an%20occupational%20therapist

chinadailyasia.com. (2016, October 8). Survey shows kindergartens lack sufficient play time. *ChinaDaily Asia.* https://www.chinadailyasia.com/hknews/2016-10/08/content_15507542.html

Cho, E., & Choi, Y. (2018). A review of work-family research in Confucian Asia. In K. M. Shockley, W. Shen, & R. C. Johnson (Eds.), *The Cambridge handbook of the global work–family interface* (pp. 371–385). Cambridge University Press. https://doi.org/10.1017/9781108235556.020

Clark, D. M., Ehlers, A., McManus, F., Hackmann, A., Fennell, M., Campbell, H., Flower, T., Davenport, C., & Louis, B. (2003). Cognitive therapy versus fluoxetine in generalized social phobia: A randomized placebo-controlled trial. *Journal of Consulting and Clinical Psychology, 71*(6), 1058–1067. https://doi.org/10.1037/0022-006X.71.6.1058

Clark, D. M., & Wells, A. (1995). A cognitive model of social phobia. In R. G. Heimberg, M. R. Liebowitz, D. A. Hope, & F. R. Schneier (Eds.), *Social phobia: Diagnosis, assessment, and treatment* (pp. 69–93). Guilford Press.

Corrigan, P. W., & Watson, A. C. (2002). Understanding the impact of stigma on people with mental illness. *World Psychiatry, 1*(1), 16–20. https://www.ncbi.nlm.nih.gov/pmc/articles/PMC1489832/

Costa-Black, K. M., Cheng, A. S. K., Li, M., & Loisel, P. (2011). The practical application of theory and research for preventing work disability: A new paradigm for occupational rehabilitation services in China? *Journal of Occupational Rehabilitation, 21*(Suppl. 1), S15–S27. https://doi.org/10.1007/s10926-011-9296-2

Creek, J. (2014). Approaches to practice. In W. Bryant, J. Fieldhouse, & K. Bannigan (Eds.), *Creek's occupational therapy and mental health* (5th ed., pp. 50–71). Churchill Livingstone.

Crossman, A. (2017). *What is typification?* ThoughtCo. Retrieved July 27, 2022, from https://www.thoughtco.com/typification-3026721

Curran, J. (2008). The Yellow Emperor's classic of internal medicine. *BMJ, 336*(7647), 777. https://www.bmj.com/content/336/7647/777.2

Department of Rehabilitation Sciences, The Hong Kong Polytechnic University. (2020). Opening ceremony of OT Clinic. *Impact, Winter 2020 Newsletter*, 1. https://www.polyu.edu.hk/rs/-/media/department/rs/content/about-rs/rs-at-a-glance/newsletter/2020/winter-2020.pdf

Department of Rehabilitation Sciences, The Hong Kong Polytechnic University. (2021). Four RS scholars have been ranked among top 2% of scientists in the world. *Impact, Summer 2021 Newsletter*, 1. https://www.polyu.edu.hk/rs/-/media/department/rs/content/about-rs/rs-at-a-glance/newsletter/2021/polyu_impact-summer2021.pdf

Dich, N., Lund, R., Hansen, Å. M., & Rod, N. H. (2019). Mental and physical health effects of meaningful work and rewarding family responsibilities. *PLoS ONE, 14*(4), e0214916. https://doi.org/10.1371/journal.pone.0214916

Duncan, E. A. S. (2011). The cognitive behavioural frame of reference. In E. A. S. Duncan (Ed.), *Foundations for practice in occupational therapy* (5th ed., pp. 153–164). Churchill Livingstone.

Ellis, A. (1991). The revised ABC's of rational-emotive therapy (RET). *Journal of Rational-Emotive and Cognitive-Behavior Therapy, 9*, 139–172. https://doi.org/10.1007/BF01061227

Employees Retraining Board, Hong Kong SAR Government. (n.d.). *Training courses*. Retrieved July 11, 2022, from https://www.erb.org/training_courses/erb_courses/manpower_development_scheme/en/

Erlandsson, G. (2011). Article commentary: Cultural differences in hand rehabilitation. *Hong Kong Journal of Occupational Therapy, 21*(2), 88–91. https://doi.org/10.1016/j.hkjot.2011.12.001

Faculty of Health and Social Sciences, The Hong Kong Polytechnic University. (2018, March 16). *Government commissions PolyU to provide consultancy service in formulating new Rehabilitation Programme Plan.* https://www.polyu.edu.hk/fhss/news-and-events/news/2018/20180316/?sc_lang=en

Fisher, P. L., & Wells, A. (2008). Metacognitive therapy for obsessive–compulsive disorder: A case series. *Journal of Behavior Therapy and Experimental Psychiatry, 39*(2), 117–132. https://doi.org/10.1016/j.jbtep.2006.12.001

Flynn, K. E., Li, L., Bruner, D. W., Cyranowski, J. M., Hahn, E. A., Jeffery, D. D., Reese, J. B., Reeve, B. B., Shelby, R. A., & Weinfurt, K. P. (2016). Sexual satisfaction and the importance of sexual health to quality of life throughout the life course of U.S. adults. *Journal of Sexual Medicine, 13*(11), 1642–1650. https://doi.org/10.1016/j.jsxm.2016.08.011

Fung, M. T. (2010). *Stages of change, self-stigma, and treatment compliance among Chinese adults with severe mental illness* [Unpublished doctoral dissertation]. The Hong Kong Polytechnic University. http://theses.lib.polyu.edu.hk/handle/200/6022

Fung, K. M. T., Tsang, H. W. H., & Cheung, W. M. (2011). Randomized controlled trial of the self-stigma reduction program among individuals with schizophrenia. *Psychiatry Research, 189*(2), 208–214. https://doi.org/10.1016/j.psychres.2011.02.013

Fung, K. M. T., Tsang, H. W. H., Corrigan, P. W., Lam, C. S., & Cheng, W. M. (2007). Measuring self-stigma of mental illness in China and its implications for recovery. *International Journal of Social Psychiatry, 53*(5), 408–418. https://doi.org/10.1177/0020764007078342

Gillen, G. (2014). Occupational therapy interventions for individuals. In B. A. B. Schell, G. Gillen, M. E. Scaffa, & E. S. Cohn (Eds.), *Willard & Spackman's occupational therapy* (12th ed., pp. 322–341). Lippincott Williams & Wilkins.

Huang, P. C. C. (2011). The modern Chinese family: In light of economic and legal history. *Modern China, 37*(5), 459–497. https://doi.org/10.1177/0097700411411554

Huang, M. T., Chen, W. S., & Chen, C. P. (2009). *Theory and practice of occupational therapy in mental health.* Wu-Nan Book Inc.

Humphry, R. (2002). Young children's occupations: Explicating the dynamics of developmental processes. *American Journal of Occupational Therapy, 56*(2), 171–179.

Hutchison, E. D. (2003). *Dimensions of human behavior: The changing life course* (2nd ed.). Sage Publications, Inc.

Iwama, M. K., Thomson, N. A., & Macdonald, R. M. (2009). The Kawa model: The power of culturally responsive occupational therapy. *Disability and Rehabilitation, 31*(14), 1125–1135. https://doi.org/10.1080/09638280902773711

Jenkins, R. (2003). Supporting governments to adopt mental health policies. *World Psychiatry, 2*(1), 14–19. https://www.ncbi.nlm.nih.gov/pmc/articles/PMC1525068/

Jenks, P. H. L. (1988). *The history and development of HKOTA.* Hong Kong Occupational Therapy Association. https://hkota.org.hk/history

Kielhofner, G. (2009). *Conceptual foundations of occupational therapy practice* (4th ed.). F.A. Davis Company.

Kielhofner, G., & Burke, J. P. (1980). A model of human occupation, part 1. Conceptual framework and content. *American Journal of Occupational Therapy, 34*(9), 572–581.

King, R., & Lloyd, C. (2007). Vocational rehabilitation. In R. King, C. Lloyd, & T. Meehan (Eds.), *Handbook of psychosocial rehabilitation* (pp. 143–158). Blackwell Publishing Ltd.

Labour Department, Hong Kong SAR Government. (n.d.). *Selective placement division.* Retrieved July 14, 2022, from https://www.labour.gov.hk/eng/service/content3.htm

Lai, D. W. L., & Surood, S. (2009). Filial piety in Chinese Canadian family caregivers. *International Journal of Sociology of the Family, 35*(1), 89–104. http://www.jstor.org/stable/23028802

Lavine, D., & Greiner, B. (2020). Occupational therapy in mainland China: Status, challenges, and future directions. *Annals of International Occupational Therapy, 3*(1), 38–44. https://doi.org/10.3928/24761222-20190813-04

Law, M., Baptiste, S., McColl, M., Opzoomer, A., Polatajko, H., & Pollock, N. (1990). The Canadian Occupational Performance Measure: An outcome measure for occupational therapy. *Canadian Journal of Occupational Therapy, 57*(2), 82–87. https://doi.org/10.1177/000841749005700207

Law, M., Cooper, B., Strong, S., Stewart, D., Rigby, P., & Letts, L. (1996). The Person-Environment-Occupation model: A transactive approach to occupational performance. *Canadian Journal of Occupational Therapy, 63*(1), 9–23. https://doi.org/10.1177/000841749606300103

Lee, H. C. (2014). The role of occupational therapy in the recovery stage of disaster relief: A report from earthquake stricken areas in China. *Australian Occupational Therapy Journal, 61*(1), 28–31. https://doi.org/10.1111/1440-1630.12106

Leung, K. F. (2014). *Coaching and occupational lifestyle redesign.* Queen Elizabeth Hospital.

Levy, H., & Packman, W. (2004). Sexual abuse prevention for individuals with mental retardation: Considerations for genetic counselors. *Journal of Genetic Counseling, 13*(3), 189–205. https://doi.org/10.1023/B:JOGC.0000028158.79395.1e

Li, D., Li, S. M. Y., Tsang, H. W. H., Wong, A. H. H., Fung, K. M. T., Tsui, M. C. M., Chung, R. C. K., Yiu, M. G. C., Tam, K. L., & Lee, G. T. H. (2013). Development and validation of perceived rehabilitation require questionnaires for caregivers of people with schizophrenia. *International Journal of Psychiatry in Clinical Practice, 17*(4), 264–272.

Li, Q., Li, D., Tsui, M. C. M., & Zhang, G. (2015). Is mainland China ready to implement vocational rehabilitation to re-engage its people with schizophrenia in meaningful worker roles? *International Journal of Social Psychiatry, 61*(2), 205–206. https://doi.org/10.1177/0020764014561308

Li, W., Zhang, L., Luo, X., Liu, B., Liu, Z., Lin, F., Liu, Z., Xie, Y., Hudson, M., Rathod, S., Kingdon, D., Husain, N., Liu, X., Ayub, M., & Naeem, F. (2017). A qualitative study to explore views of patients', carers' and mental health professionals' to inform cultural adaptation of CBT for psychosis (CBTp) in China. *BMC Psychiatry, 17*(1), 131. https://doi.org/10.1186/s12888-017-1290-6

Lieber, E., Chin, D., Li, L., Rotheram-Borus, M. J., Detels, R., Wu, Z., & Guan, J., National Institute of Mental Health (NIMH) Collaborative HIV Prevention Trial Group. (2009). Sociocultural contexts and communication about sex in China: Informing HIV/STD prevention programs. *AIDS Education and Prevention, 21*(5), 415–429. https://pubmed.ncbi.nlm.nih.gov/19842826/

Liu, K. P. Y., & Ng, B. F. L. (2008). Usefulness of the Model of Human Occupation in the Hong Kong Chinese context. *Occupational Therapy in Health Care, 22*(2–3), 25–36. https://doi.org/10.1080/07380570801989333

Lu, A. P., Jia, H. W., Xiao, C., & Lu, Q. P. (2004). Theory of traditional Chinese medicine and therapeutic method of diseases. *World Journal of Gastroenterology, 10*(13), 1854–1856. https://dx.doi.org/10.3748/wjg.v10.i13.1854

Lucksted, A., McFarlane, W., Downing, D., & Dixon, L. (2012). Recent developments in family psychoeducation as an evidence-based practice. *Journal of Marital and Family Therapy, 38*(1), 101–121. https://doi.org/10.1111/j.1752-0606.2011.00256.x

Luebben, A. J., & Royeen, C. B. (2010). An acquisitional frame of reference. In P. Kramer & J. Hinojosa (Eds.), *Frames of reference for pediatric occupational therapy* (3rd ed., pp. 461–488). Lippincott Williams & Wilkins.

MacEachen, E., Clarke, J., Franche, R.-L., & Irvin, E., Workplace-based Return to Work Literature Review Group. (2006). Systematic review of the qualitative literature on return to work after injury. *Scandinavian Journal of Work, Environment & Health, 32*(4), 257–269. https://doi.org/10.5271/sjweh.1009

Malhotra, S., & Sachdeva, S. (2005). Social roles and role conflict: An interprofessional study among women. *Journal of the Indian Academy of Applied Psychology, 31*(1–2), 37–42.

McMillan, I. R. (2011). The biomechanical frame of reference in occupational therapy. In E. A. S. Duncan (Ed.), *Foundations for practice in occupational therapy* (5th ed., pp. 179–194). Churchill Livingstone.

Merriam-Webster. (n.d.a). Frame of reference. In *Merriam-Webster.com dictionary*. Retrieved December 16, 2021, from https://www.merriam-webster.com/dictionary/frame%20of%20reference

Merriam-Webster. (n.d.b). Theory. In *Merriam-Webster.com dictionary*. Retrieved December 16, 2021, from https://www.merriam-webster.com/dictionary/theory

MOHO-IRM Web. (2024). *Translated MOHO assessments*. Retrieved July 3, 2024, from https://moho-irm.uic.edu/resources/translations.aspx

Moll, S., Huff, J., & Detwiler, L. (2003). Supported employment: Evidence for a best practice model in psychosocial rehabilitation. *Canadian Journal of Occupational Therapy, 70*(5), 298–310. https://doi.org/10.1177/000841740307000506

Moy, M. (2018). Development of health rehabilitation in mainland China: From traditional Chinese medicine to modern Western rehabilitation methods. *Independent Study Project (ISP) Collection, 2759*. https://digitalcollections.sit.edu/isp_collection/2759

Neville, R. C. (2000). *Boston Confucianism: Portable tradition in the late-modern world*. State University of New York Press.

New Life Psychiatric Rehabilitation Association. (n.d.). *Recovery-oriented service*. Retrieved July 11, 2022, from https://www.nlpra.org.hk/en/theme_recovery

Ng, B. F. L. (2012, February 24–26). *East meets West – What it means to occupational therapy* [Invited symposia]. 2012 International Occupational Therapy Conference, The Hong Kong Polytechnic University, Hong Kong, China.

Ng, B. F. L. (2017). *Effect on lifestyle modification using complementary and alternative medicine approach to reduce the risk of those with pre-clinical metabolic syndrome* [Unpublished doctoral dissertation]. The Hong Kong Polytechnic University. Retrieved July 14, 2022, from https://theses.lib.polyu.edu.hk/handle/200/9283

Ng, B. F. L. (2022). *Baduanjin training 9_2_2022*. Dr Bacon Ng Personal Website. Retrieved Feb 11, 2022, from www.baconng.org

Ng, B. F. L., Ho, R. T. H., Chan, J. S. M., Ng, S. M., Lau, B. W. M., So, K. F., Wang, C. W., Wong, N. W. Y., Ho, J. W. M., Ng, B. H. P., Tsang, H. W. H., Ziea, E. T. C., & Chan, C. L.

W. (2013). Clinical implications of health qigong on patients with chronic diseases. *Research in Complementary Medicine*, 20(Suppl. 1), 34.

Ng, B. F. L., & Tsang, H. W. H. (2015, October 23–24). *Using the Model of Human Occupation to conceptualize & develop a lifestyle modification program in primary health care* [Short paper session]. The Fourth International Institute on the Model of Human Occupation, Indiana University-Purdue University, Indianapolis, Indiana, United States.

Ng, B. F. L., & Tsang, H. W. H. (2019, September 27–29). *The use of occupational questionnaire in lifestyle modification of primary health care* [Paper presentation]. The Sixth International Institute on Kielhofner's Model of Human Occupation, University of Illinois Chicago, Illinois, United States.

Ng, B. F. L., & Tsang, H. W. H. (2024). East and West lifestyle modification for health promotion during the ageing process. In K. N. K. Fong, & K. W. Tong (Eds.), *Ageing care in the community: Current practices and future directions* (pp. 37–64). City University of Hong Kong Press.

Ng, B. F. L., Tsang, H. W. H., Ng, B. H. P., & Ziea, E. T. C. (2014, October 29–November 1). *An overview of evidences related to systematic reviews of qigong* [Oral poster presentation session]. The 6th Global Conference of the Alliance for Healthy Cities, Hong Kong SAR, China.

Niemeyer, L. O. (1980). *Cardiac rehabilitation: Practice and treatment guidelines for occupational therapists and other health professionals*. Fred Sammons, Inc.

Occupational Therapists Board. (n.d.). *About us – Functions*. Retrieved February 28, 2022, from https://www.smp-council.org.hk/ot/en/content.php?page=abt_func

Polit, D. F., & Beck, C. T. (2010). *Essentials of nursing research: Appraising evidence for nursing practice*. Lippincott Williams & Wilkins.

Ran, M. S., Xiang, M. Z., Li, S. X., Shan, Y. H., Huang, M. S., Li, S. G., Liu, Z. R., Chen, E. Y. H., & Chan, C. L. W. (2003). Prevalence and course of schizophrenia in a Chinese rural area. *Australian & New Zealand Journal of Psychiatry*, 37(4), 452–457. https://doi.org/10.1046/j.1440-1614.2003.01203.x

Ray-Kaeser, S., & Lynch, H. (2017). Occupational therapy perspective on play for the sake of play. In S. Besio, D. Bulgarelli, & V. Stancheva-Popkostadinova (Eds.), *Play development in children with disabilities* (pp. 155–165). De Gruyter Open Ltd. https://doi.org/10.1515/9783110522143

Ross, J. (2007). *Occupational therapy and vocational rehabilitation*. John Wiley & Sons Ltd. https://onlinelibrary.wiley.com/doi/book/10.1002/9780470988213

Schaaf, R. C., Schoen, S. A., Roley, S. S., Lane, S. J., Koomar, J., & May-Benson, T. A. (2010). A frame of reference for sensory integration. In P. Kramer, & J. Hinojosa (Eds.), *Frames of reference for pediatric occupational therapy* (3rd ed., pp. 99–186). Lippincott Williams & Wilkins.

Serrat, O. (2019). *Contextual factors in working*. Retrieved July 11, 2022, from https://www.researchgate.net/publication/331959963_Contextual_Factors_in_Working

Shen, Y. J., Ramirez, S. Z., Kranz, P. L., Tao, X., & Ji, Y. (2018). The physical environment for play therapy with Chinese children. *American Journal of Play*, 10(3), 328–358. https://scholarworks.utrgv.edu/coun_fac/57/

Shi, Y., & Howe, T. H. (2016). A survey of occupational therapy practice in Beijing, China. *Occupational Therapy International*, 23(2), 186–195. https://doi.org/10.1002/oti.1423

Simons, M., Schneider, S., & Herpertz-Dahlmann, B. (2006). Metacognitive therapy versus exposure and response prevention for pediatric obsessive–compulsive disorder: A case series with randomized allocation. *Psychotherapy and Psychosomatics*, 75(4), 257–264. https://doi.org/10.1159/000092897

Stein, F. (1983). A current review of the behavioral frame of reference and its application to occupational therapy. *Occupational Therapy in Mental Health*, 2(4), 35–62. https://doi.org/10.1300/J004v02n04_03

Tan, X. (2009). *Chinese medicine health preservation research*. People's Medical Publishing House Co., Ltd.

Tan, H. S. K., Yeo, D. S. C., Giam, J. Y. T., Cheong, F. W. F., & Chan, K. F. (2016). A randomized controlled trial of a Return-to-Work Coordinator model of care in a general hospital to facilitate return to work of injured workers. *Work*, 54(1), 209–222.

The Hong Kong Polytechnic University. (2018, January). *An East meets West approach in rehabilitation*. excel@PolyU. https://www.polyu.edu.hk/cpa/excel/en/201801/viewpoint/v1/index.html

The Lancet. (2016). The health crisis of mental health stigma. *The Lancet*, *387*(10023), 1027. https://doi.org/10.1016/S0140-6736(16)00687-5

Townsend, E. A., & Polatajko, H. J. (2007). *Enabling occupation II: Advancing an occupational therapy vision for health, well-being, & justice through occupation*. CAOT Publications ACE.

Tsai, A. Y., Chang, L. H., Chou, Y. C., & Mao, H. F. (2017). The adversity and vision of occupational therapy in Taiwan – The focus groups of occupational therapy leaders. *Journal of Taiwan Occupational Therapy Association*, *35*(2), 146–168. https://doi.org/10.6594/JTOTA.2017.35(2).02

Tsang, H. (2015). Summer Overseas Exchange Scholarship Scheme (SOESS). *Impact, Autumn 2015 Newsletter*, 1. https://www.polyu.edu.hk/rs/-/media/department/rs/content/about-rs/rs-at-a-glance/newsletter/2015/2015-impact_autumn2015_v6_preview.pdf

Tsang, H. W. H., Chan, A., Wong, A., & Liberman, R. P. (2009). Vocational outcomes of an integrated supported employment program for individuals with persistent and severe mental illness. *Journal of Behavior Therapy and Experimental Psychiatry*, *40*(2), 292–305. https://doi.org/10.1016/j.jbtep.2008.12.007

Tsang, H. W. H., & Chen, E. Y. H. (2007). Perceptions on remission and recovery in schizophrenia. *Psychopathology*, *40*(6), 469. https://doi.org/10.1159/000108128

Tsang, H. W. H., Cheung, L., & Lak, D. C. C. (2002). Qigong as a psychosocial intervention for depressed elderly with chronic physical illnesses. *International Journal of Geriatric Psychiatry*, *17*(12), 1146–1154. https://doi.org/10.1002/gps.739

Tsang, H. W. H., Li, D., Tsui, M. C. M., Chung, R. C. K., Wong, A. H. H., Li, S. M. Y., Fung, K. M. T., & Yiu, M. G. C. (2013). The perceived rehabilitation needs of people with schizophrenia in Hong Kong: Perspectives from consumers and care-givers. *Administration and Policy in Mental Health and Mental Health Services Research*, *40*(3), 179–189. https://doi.org/10.1007/s10488-011-0394-4

Tse, A. Y. K., Cheng, S. W. C., Li-Tsang, C. W. P., Chan, S. Y. C., Tsang-Lau, A. K. P., So, G. S. P., Chiu, A. S. M., Tam, S. C. W., Yu, E. C. L., Chan, E. P. S., & Chui, D. Y. Y. (2005). Survey of occupational therapy practice in Hong Kong in 2004. *Hong Kong Journal of Occupational Therapy*, *15*(1), 16–26. https://doi.org/10.1016/S1569-1861(09)70030-0

Tsui, M. C. M., & Tsang, H. W. H. (2017). Views of people with schizophrenia and their care-givers towards the needs for psychiatric rehabilitation in urban and rural areas of mainland China. *Psychiatry Research*, *258*, 72–77. https://doi.org/10.1016/j.psychres.2017.09.052

Wells, A., & King, P. (2006). Metacognitive therapy for generalized anxiety disorder: An open trial. *Journal of Behavior Therapy and Experimental Psychiatry*, *37*(3), 206–212. https://doi.org/10.1016/j.jbtep.2005.07.002

Wells, A., & Papageorgiou, C. (2001). Brief cognitive therapy for social phobia: A case series. *Behaviour Research and Therapy*, *39*(6), 713–720. https://doi.org/10.1016/S0005-7967(00)00036-X

Wells, A., & Sembi, S. (2004). Metacognitive therapy for PTSD: A preliminary investigation of a new brief treatment. *Journal of Behavior Therapy and Experimental Psychiatry*, *35*(4), 307–318. https://doi.org/10.1016/j.jbtep.2004.07.001

Wells, A., Welford, M., Fraser, J., King, P., Mendel, E., Wisely, J., Knight, A., & Rees, D. (2008). Chronic PTSD treated with metacognitive therapy: An open trial. *Cognitive and Behavioral Practice*, *15*(1), 85–92. https://doi.org/10.1016/j.cbpra.2006.11.005

Weziak-Bialowolska, D., Bialowolski, P., Sacco, P. L., VanderWeele, T. J., & McNeely, E. (2020). Well-being in life and well-being at work: Which comes first? Evidence from a longitudinal study. *Frontiers in Public Health*, *8*, 103. http://doi.org/10.3389/fpubh.2020.00103

Wong, R. S. M., & Fong, K. (2013). Celebrating the 35th anniversary: A brief history of occupational therapy in Hong Kong. *Hong Kong Journal of Occupational Therapy*, *23*(1), 1–3. https://doi.org/10.1016/j.hkjot.2013.08.002

Wong, S. K. M., & Li-Tsang, C. W. P. (2010). Development of hand rehabilitation in mainland China. *Hong Kong Journal of Occupational Therapy*, *20*(1), 19–24. https://doi.org/10.1016/S1569-1861(10)70054-1

World Federation of Occupational Therapists. (n.d.). *WFOT approved education programmes*. Retrieved July 23, 2022, from https://wfot.org/programmes/education/wfot-approved-education-programmes

Yanos, P. T., DeLuca, J. S., Roe, D., & Lysaker, P. H. (2020). The impact of illness identity on recovery from severe mental illness: A review of the evidence. *Psychiatry Research, 288,* 112950. https://doi.org/10.1016/j.psychres.2020.112950

Zhong, L. L. D., & Ng, B. F. L. (2018). Healthcare preventive approaches in Chinese medicine. *The Hong Kong Medical Diary, 23*(10), 27. https://www.fmshk.org/database/hkmd/hkmd201810.pdf

Zhuo, D. H. (1999). Bone and joint decade 2000–2010 and the role of rehabilitation medicine. *Chinese Journal of Rehabilitation Medicine, 14*(6), 241–243.

Zhuo, D. H. (2006). Present situation and future development of occupational therapy in China. *Hong Kong Journal of Occupational Therapy, 16*(1), 23–25. https://doi.org/10.1016/S1569-1861(09)70036-1

Documentation

Cynthia Yuen Yi Lai, Frank Ho-Yin Lai, Stella Wai Chee Cheng, Chung-Ying Lin, Ya Zhou, and Abby Jin Song

Definition of documentation

Documentation in occupational therapy (OT) is required by practice settings, laws, regulatory and payer requirements, external accreditation programs, and professional associations when occupational therapists provide services within specified time frames, formats, and established standards (American Occupational Therapy Association, 2018, 2021). OT practitioners identify the types of documentation required and record all necessary components of the services provided within their scope of practice (American Occupational Therapy Association, 2015a). Documentation of OT services should be maintained in a reader-oriented, legally signed, accurate, clear, factual, specific, and timely fashion, which will be explained in detail in a later section. In Hong Kong, failure to maintain adequate client records is considered a violation of professional responsibilities toward clients (Occupational Therapists Board Hong Kong, 2023).

The American Occupational Therapy Association (AOTA) Standards of Practice for Occupational Therapy (2015b) states that an OT practitioner documents the OT services and "abides by the time frames, formats, and standards established by practice settings, federal and state laws, other regulatory and payer requirements, external accreditation programs, and AOTA documents" (p. 4). These requirements apply to both electronic and written forms of documentation, although they may vary considerably by practice setting and facility. The AOTA Occupational Therapy Code of Ethics (2015a) states that OT practitioners "shall promote fairness and objectivity in the provision of occupational therapy services" (p. 5) and "shall provide comprehensive, accurate, and objective information when representing the profession" (p. 6). In accordance with the AOTA Standards of Practice for Occupational Therapy, documents should record the therapy sessions provided within the scope of practice, including the synthesis of evaluation results, intervention plans within the time frames and formats, changes in the client's performance and capacities, and for transitioning the

DOI: 10.4324/9781032721170-4

client to another type or intensity of service or discontinuing services when the client has achieved identified goals, reached maximum benefit, or does not desire to continue services (American Occupational Therapy Association, 2021).

Importance of documentation

OT documentation not only describes the services being provided but also gathers the information to ensure the therapy is completed in a safe and effective manner (American Occupational Therapy Association, 2018). More importantly, it paves the way for OT practitioners to develop clinical reasoning and may also be used as an interdisciplinary communication tool to promote client-centered care. The documents should concisely and accurately describe the client's current status, evaluation results, intervention plans, justification for OT services, the client's response to OT services, outcomes, and recommendations. OT practitioners synthesize the information about clients' occupational profiles, as well as the rationale for the effectiveness of the services provided through documentation (American Occupational Therapy Association, 2018).

From the legal perspective, OT documentation is a tool for practitioners to defend themselves or their clients when they are put on the stand. From the reimbursement perspective, the documentation is required to demonstrate the value of OT services for which the insurance companies are paying. For example, Medicare and Medicaid require the enhancement of a client's Functional Independence Measure (FIM) score to reimburse a rehabilitation stay in the United States. City insurance and provincial insurance in some parts of mainland China require evidence showing improvements in the client's body functions and FIM scores for reimbursement. From the perspective of intra- and inter-team communication, documentation serves as a clear record of the client's status, occupational history, evaluation results, intervention plans, therapeutic response, etc., allowing team members to effectively provide client-centered care.

Types of documentation

Documentation types may be identified differently or combined and reorganized to meet the specific needs of the client and the setting. All facets of OT clinical practice, including individual and group therapies, must be documented. The clinical record is a legal document that records the events, choices, interventions, and plans made during the OT–client interaction. Documentation of OT practice is maintained in a professional and legal fashion (i.e., complete, concise, accurate, timely, legible, clear, grammatically correct, and objective) for each client served (American Occupational Therapy Association, 2018). Generally speaking, clinical records may include a screening report, evaluation report, re-evaluation report, intervention plan, contact report, progress report, transition plan, and discharge/discontinuation report according to the AOTA Guidelines for Documentation of Occupational Therapy (American Occupational Therapy Association, 2018). A specific type of documentation should be identified by practitioners to meet the specific needs of their clients or settings (American Occupational Therapy Association, 2018). We will now list the essential components of each type of documentation.

Screening report

Screening identifies people in an apparently healthy population who are at higher risk of a health problem or condition. It allows early treatment or intervention to be offered, thereby reducing the incidence or mortality of the health problem or condition within the population (WHO Regional Office for Europe, 2020). Screening occurs when an individual is referred for an assessment to determine their need for OT services. Therefore, a screening report should contain referral information (services requested and the reason for referral), client information (the client's occupational history, experiences, and performance; health status; and applicable medical, educational, and developmental diagnoses, precautions, and contraindications), a brief occupational profile (the reason for seeking OT services; areas of occupation in which the client is successful or challenged; contexts and environments that support or hinder occupational performance [e.g., patterns of living, interests, values]; medical, educational, and work history; the client's priorities; and targeted goals), assessment results, and recommendations (professional judgments regarding the need for a complete OT evaluation based on the results of the assessments) (American Occupational Therapy Association, 2018). In some clinical settings, the screening report may be referred to as a triage for prioritization before admission to the comprehensive service unit. For example, an early education and training center may have a meeting with the children and parents before admission to the center. In that meeting, a team of professionals (e.g., a social worker, occupational therapist, physiotherapist, speech therapist, and teacher) will interview the parents and conduct assessments of the children. The team would discuss and compile a screening report with brief reports from all parties after the meeting. The screening report of OT may contain the date of the intake assessment, referral information, client information, a brief occupational profile, assessment results (e.g., developmental assessment and functional assessment), recommendations (e.g., provision of OT or not, mode of service suggested, or requirement for more in-depth assessments of certain aspects, etc.), and signatures. Another example of when a screening report is needed is when a referral to OT is made with specific concerns. For instance, a 6-year-old child is referred for OT screening with the concern of poor visual motor skills, sensory processing abilities, and fine motor skills. After spending time with the child, additional information can be gathered through a parental interview, and the Beery-Buktenica Developmental Test of Visual-Motor Integration (Beery-VMI), Sensory Processing and Self-regulation Checklist (SPSRC; Figure 2.1), and Hong Kong Preschool Fine Motor Developmental Assessment (HK-PFMDA; Figure 2.2) can be used to collect the necessary data. A screening report should then be generated, incorporating all the information obtained along with professional judgments regarding the child's need for school OT services. If it is decided that OT is required, other types of documentation will follow.

Evaluation report and re-evaluation report

The evaluation report should include referral information, client information (a description of the client's occupational history, experiences, and performance; health status and previous services required and accessed; and applicable medical, educational, and developmental diagnoses, precautions, and contraindications), an occupational profile (the reason for OT services; areas of occupation in which the client is successful or challenged;

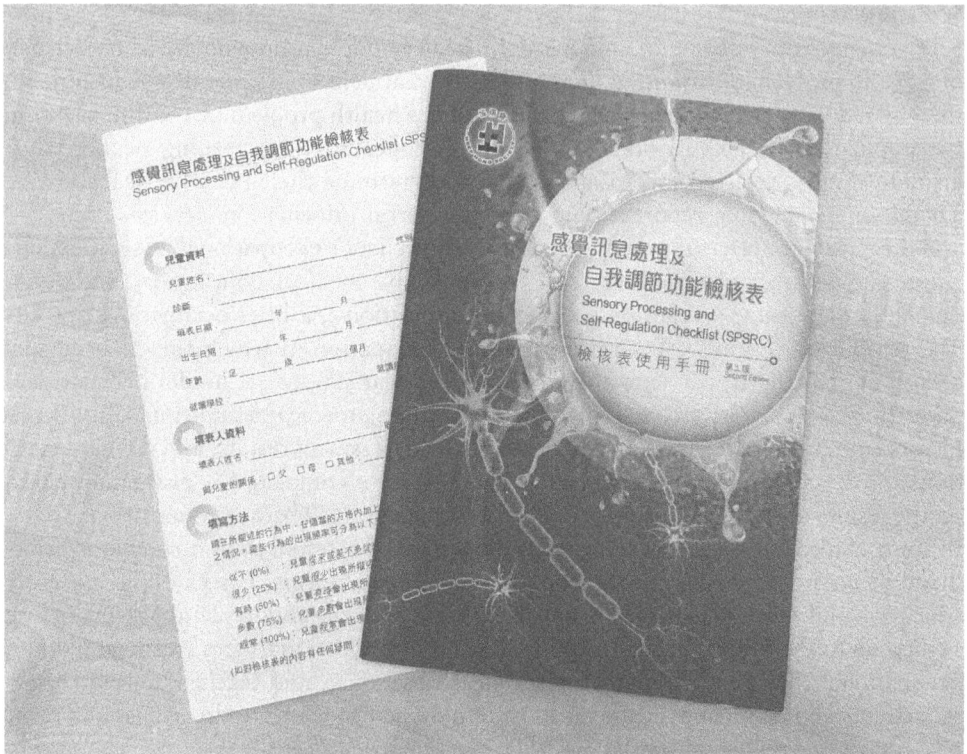

Figure 2.1 Sensory Processing and Self-regulation Checklist, a standardized assessment for quantifying sensory processing abilities of children

contexts and environments that support or hinder occupational performance; medical, educational, and work history; occupational and psychosocial history [e.g., patterns of living, interests, values]; the client's priorities; and targeted goals; see the example depicted in Appendix 2.1), assessment results, analysis of occupational performance (analysis of occupational performance and identification of factors that support or hinder performance and participation [objective and measurable identification of performance skills, performance patterns, contexts and environments, activity demands, outcomes from standardized or non-standardized assessments, and client factors]; an interpretation and summary of the occupational profile and occupational performance issues; identification of targeted areas of occupation and occupational performance to be addressed; and expected outcomes; see the example depicted in Appendix 2.2), and judgments regarding the necessity for specialized OT services or other services.

In some cases, re-evaluations are needed to revise the treatment plans or fulfill the reimbursement requirements. A re-evaluation report should include re-evaluation results and everything mentioned above in the evaluation report except the referral information.

From the evaluation results and relevant analyses, occupational therapists should then create the intervention plan, sometimes referred to as the "plan of care". This should contain the client's information, intervention goals, intervention approaches and types of intervention to be used, service delivery mechanisms, plans for discharge, and outcome measures (American Occupational Therapy Association, 2018) (Appendix 2.1).

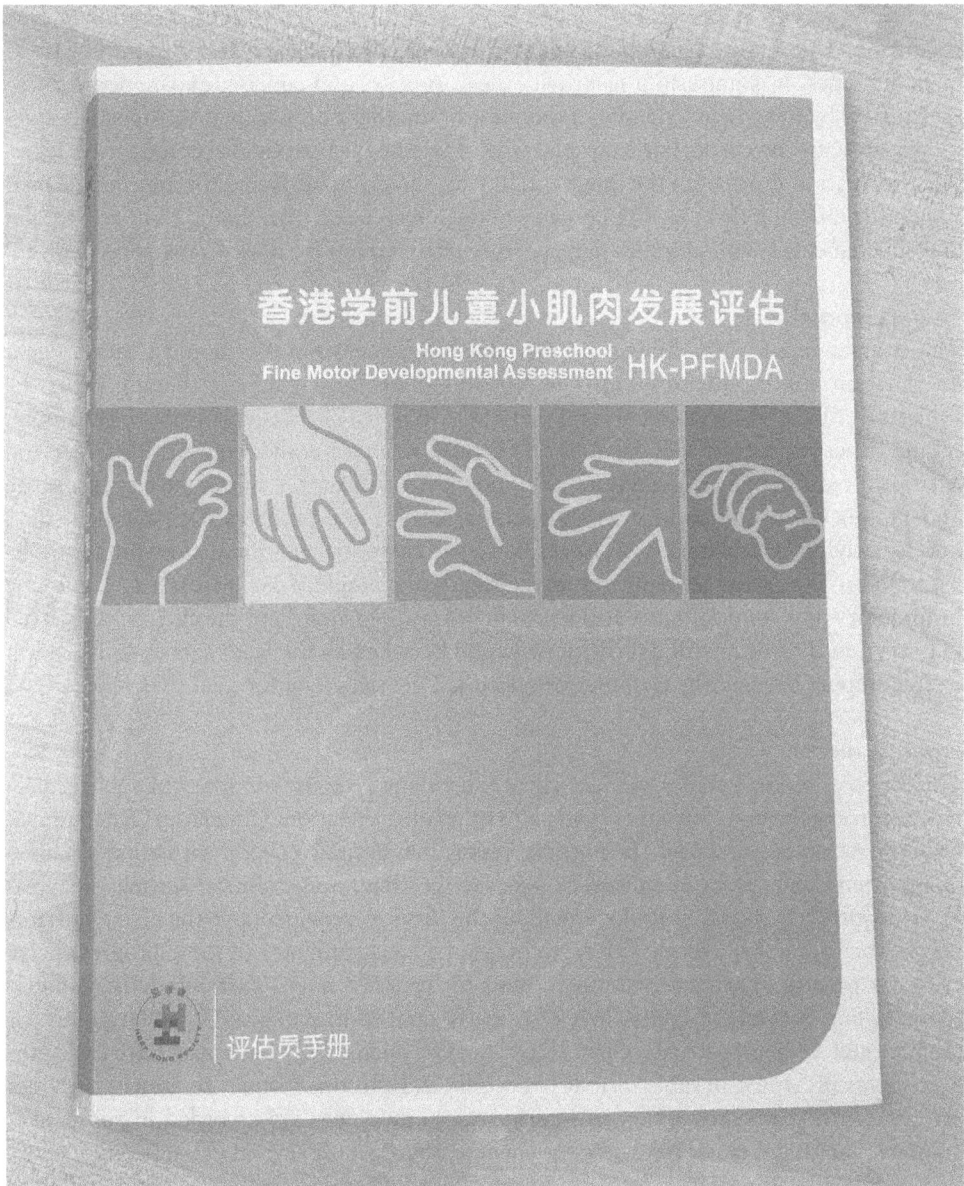

Figure 2.2 Hong Kong Preschool Fine Motor Developmental Assessment, a standardized assessment for evaluating fine motor skills of children

Intervention plan

The intervention plan should contain client information, treatment objectives, treatment period, mode of intervention, name of staff responsible for delivering the service, treatment activities (e.g., procedures and duration), equipment required, and safety precautions. Depending on the client's service needs, the mode of intervention could vary from direct service on a regular basis to consultation on demand. For direct service, a description of the service format is recommended (e.g., on an individual or group basis), along with the frequency of service (e.g., once a week or once every two weeks), duration of each treatment session (e.g., 60 minutes per session), and the sequence and duration of treatment activities. It is important to provide clear, precise, and concise information for further review by the case occupational therapist or another occupational therapist who will follow up with the client. For example, when the case occupational therapist is on leave, the information written on the intervention plan should be sufficient for another occupational therapist to follow up. The contents of the intervention plan should be in text format and supplemented with graphics (e.g., posture of the client) for illustration as needed.

Contact report

The contact report, also known as the "daily treatment notes", should contain client information and the therapy log. The most common format for the therapy log is the subjective, objective, assessment, and plan (SOAP) note. The frequency of progress note-taking varies by country and depends on the purpose of the contact report. Medicare and Medicaid require one progress note every ten days of therapy, while some city insurance and provincial insurance in mainland China require one progress note every 14 days upon receiving rehabilitation services. For legal cases, occupational therapists may be asked to provide a contact report upon request. For example, a client suffered a traumatic brain injury as a result of a car accident two years ago. Since then, the client has received OT services. The occupational therapist would be asked by the legal agency to provide a contact report because the client has received OT services over the past two years.

Progress report

The progress report usually includes client information, goals, summary of services provided, current client performance, and plans or recommendations (American Occupational Therapy Association, 2018). The progress report may contain client information obtained or reported during a case conference (or case meeting). Some clinical settings in Hong Kong require a progress note documenting the services provided and the client's performance each time they receive OT services, as well as a summary of these progress notes every six months. There are various formats for progress notes, particularly in pediatric services. For example, progress notes can be organized in paragraphs, bullet points, or table format. In some settings, clients receiving OT on a weekly basis may have their progress notes presented in table format (Appendix 2.3). In this format, treatment activities are listed in the first column, while performance outcomes are recorded in subsequent columns, making it easier to review the client's progress over several OT sessions.

Transition plan and discharge/discontinuation report

When a client is transitioning to the next stage of rehabilitation, a transition plan is needed. This should include client information, the client's current status, the transition plan, and any recommendations. After a client is discharged from the current rehabilitation facility or has decided to discontinue the ongoing OT services, practitioners are required to provide a discharge/discontinuation report, which includes client information, a summary of the intervention process, and any recommendations (American Occupational Therapy Association, 2018). For instance, when a child is discharged from a special childcare center and then admitted to a special school, the occupational therapists in the two settings must communicate to ensure the smooth transition of OT services.

In addition to the abovementioned clinical records, there are other documents for specific purposes, such as medical-legal reports and occupational therapist reports for candidates applying for special examination allowances. For example, the Hong Kong Examinations and Assessment Authority will consider special examination arrangements for students with special educational needs who are sitting for the Hong Kong Diploma of Secondary Education Examination (HKDSE, a public examination). Those students applying for special examination arrangements need to provide substantial evidence explaining how the deficits (e.g., fine motor deficits) affect their functional performance (e.g., copying speed; Figure 2.3) and how the recommended special examination arrangements (e.g., extra time allowance) could benefit them.

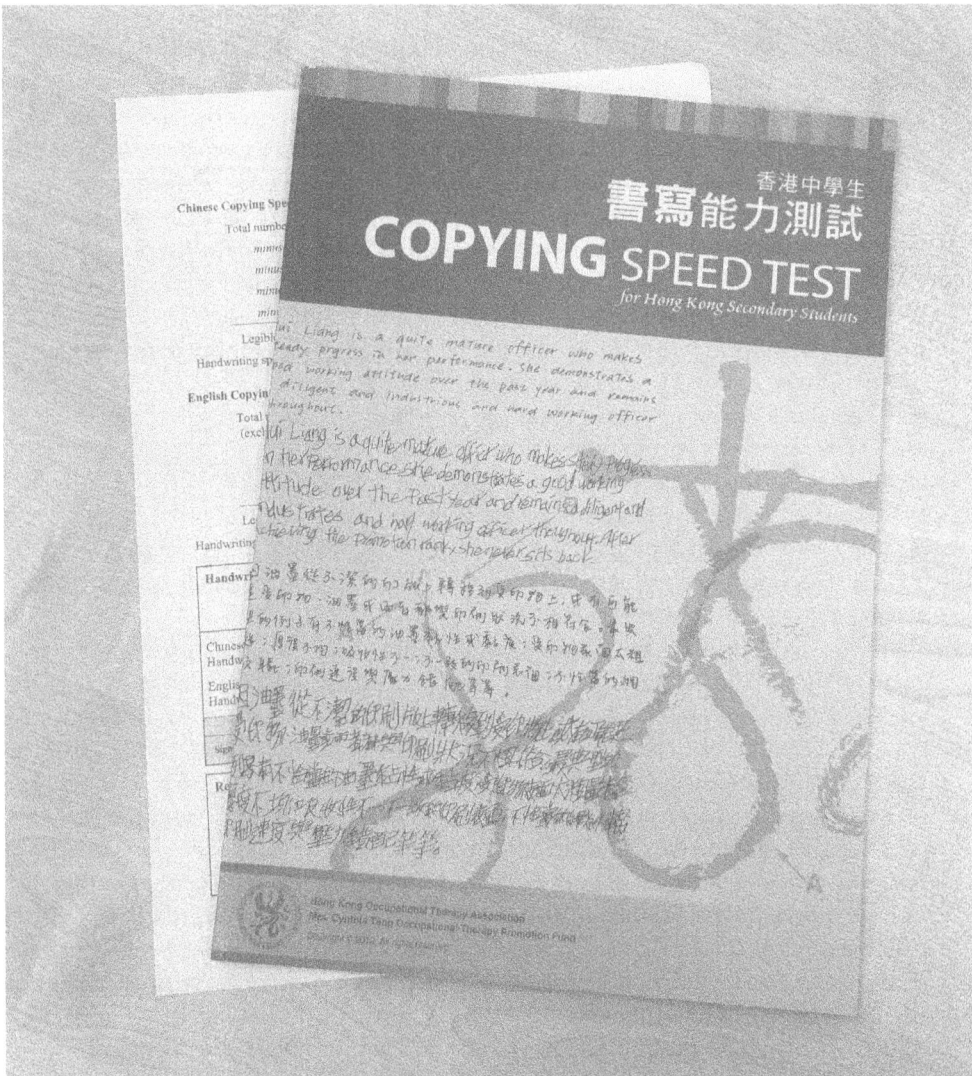

Figure 2.3 Copying Speed Test for Hong Kong Secondary Students, a standardized assessment for documenting clients' functional performance in copying speed

There are also documents needed for the administrative management of an OT department, including client payment records, service unit regulations, employee contracts and job descriptions, appraisal forms, etc. Since this chapter focuses on clinical records, readers are encouraged to observe the practices of specific clinical settings and consult literature on business management. The format, language, and choice of words will vary depending on the purpose and type of communication.

Characteristics of good professional documentation

While documentation is a valuable communication tool, it also plays a crucial role in constructing clients' occupational profiles and evaluating the effectiveness of services. Below are the key characteristics of effective professional documentation for these purposes.

(1) *Reader-oriented*: Occupational therapists should ensure that a document serves its purpose. The choice of words and format of a document depends on its readers. For example, a daily clinical document reporting a client's progress would be different from a discharge summary report. An expert report used in legal proceedings would be different from a home program document sent to clients or their caregivers. The information should also be organized in such a way as to help the reader better understand the content. For example, the clinical documentation of initial assessments may include the following information in a logical sequence:
- Reason(s) for referral or OT
- Background information on the client, such as demographic data, diagnosis, past medical history, social background, etc.
- The client's subjective complaints
- OT assessments and findings
- Interpretation of the assessments
- Treatment objectives and intervention plan
- Signature and credentials

(2) *Timely*: Documentation created as soon as possible after an event is generally more reliable than records based on memory.

(3) *Accurate*: Occupational therapists should ensure that the information written is accurate to the best of their knowledge. For instance, the subjective experience of the client should not be presented as objective observation by the therapist. In addition to content, the accuracy of the record's date is equally important. Documentation of the client's performance should be written in chronological order to give a clear account of the progress. If corrections need to be made to a clinical document, the therapist should strike through the incorrect information and sign next to the change.

(4) *Factual*: Documentation should be based on facts, not subjective feelings or interpretations. Any judgmental comments indicating bias or prejudice toward the client should be avoided. As a general rule, no comments should be made about other professionals. If the information is provided by a third party or the client, it should be specified and quoted.

(5) *Specific*: Treatment goals, objectives, and intervention plans should be specific in terms of the time, duration, frequency, context, and expected outcomes. This helps people, such as the referrer and the multidisciplinary team, understand the OT provided to the client.

(6) *Clear*: To avoid any misunderstanding or clinical errors, a clear presentation of information is essential. The method of documentation (e.g., handwriting) and the choice of language (e.g., abbreviations and professional OT terminology) can impact the clarity of the presentation. For example, handwriting in written records should be legible. The use of abbreviations can result in ambiguity, similar to poor handwriting. As a best practice, abbreviations should be avoided whenever possible. Only those abbreviations accepted by the facility should be used. Additionally, there are numerous languages spoken across various countries and even within the same country in Asia. The terminology used in OT can differ among Asian countries and even between cities within a single country. It is recommended to refer to the official websites of public bodies, regulatory boards, or OT organizations in the relevant Asian countries or cities for guidance (Appendix 2.4). Apart from these websites, the World Federation of Occupational Therapists (WFOT) website is a useful resource for searching WFOT's member organizations and related information (https://wfot.org/membership/organisational-membership/member-organisations-profiles).

(7) *Signatures and credentials*: All documentation should be signed by the occupational therapist. Documents written by OT students or assistants should also be countersigned by the supervising occupational therapist. This is not only a display of accountability but can also ensure a correct line of communication in case of doubt.

After constructing the client's profile, applying the standard framework and terminology that describes the OT process and domain is a key aspect of professional OT documentation. The standard terminology can be obtained from OT theories, models, and frames of reference (please refer to Chapter 1 of this book). These resources are extremely useful in guiding the documentation of OT processes systematically. For instance, if a clinical setting utilizes the Model of Human Occupation (MOHO; see Chapter 1) or the sensory integration frame of reference (see Chapter 1), it is advisable to organize the documentation (e.g., assessment results) according to these models or theories and to report the findings using the appropriate terminology. Additionally, OT practitioners will often collaborate with professionals in other disciplines. In such cases, applying the standard terminology adopted across disciplines is also important. For example, the International Classification of Functioning, Disability and Health (ICF; World Health Organization, n.d.) is commonly applied by various disciplines in clinical practice. ICF was officially endorsed by the World Health Organization in May 2001 as the international standard for measuring people's health and disabilities. Readers can access this website for more details: https://www.who.int/standards/classifications/international-classification-of-functioning-disability-and-health.

Good documentation is essential for establishing evidence-based practice in OT. Assessments form the foundation for intervention, and the data collected during assessments play a crucial role in supporting evidence-based practice. As previously mentioned, the information documented must be accurate, clear, and specific as it contributes to a data pool for further aggregation and analysis. It is important to obtain and document informed consent from the client for any data analysis. When standardized assessments are used, they enhance the accuracy and objectivity of data collection and interpretation. However, many standardized assessments used in clinical practice are developed in Western countries, and there is a lack of translated and validated versions for use in some Asian countries. To resolve this problem, local universities might consider conducting community-based participatory research to develop standardized assessments or validate the translated versions of standardized assessments. This could help establish the evidence-based practice of OT in Asian countries.

Occupational therapists are required to handle clients' documents correctly. For example, rehabilitation organizations in mainland China have internal guidelines on handling clients' records (e.g., rehabilitation training files comprising assessments, training plans, training records, re-evaluations and summaries, and evaluations of training outcomes). The guidelines for using clients' rehabilitation training files are summarized as follows:

(1) Managers at all levels should be familiar with the contents of the rehabilitation training files and how to use them. Additionally, rehabilitation offices for individuals with disabilities at all levels should apply these training files consistently.
(2) Users should receive training before using the rehabilitation training files to ensure the files are used correctly.
(3) The information in the rehabilitation training files should be completed in a timely, objective, and accurate manner, and the files should be maintained properly.

Certain organizations have rules governing the protection of confidentiality (e.g., documents are stored in a password-protected computer and storage device), the duration of record keeping (e.g., at least three years for retrieval of records), and the methods of disposing of old records (e.g., hard copies are shredded).

Each facility or clinical team might have their own rules on documentation. Occupational therapists should always observe and follow these guidelines. Furthermore, regulations governing the practice of occupational therapists in various countries often include guidelines on documentation.

Ethical considerations for documentation

OT documentation is a valuable tool that supports OT services and demonstrates how well occupational therapists adhere to the code of ethics. OT takes a holistic approach, addressing individuals' well-being and quality of life by considering sensory, psychosocial, cognitive, physical, and other aspects of performance in various contexts. By taking these factors into account, occupational therapists help their clients engage fully in everyday activities, thereby enhancing their overall well-being and quality of life (American Occupational Therapy Association, 2005).

Occupational therapists must adhere to a code of ethics that outlines their responsibilities toward clients, other professionals and employees (e.g., medical doctors, physiotherapists, nursing personnel), and both local and global communities (World Federation of Occupational Therapists, 2016). There are seven longstanding core values in the OT profession: altruism, equality, freedom, justice, dignity, truth, and prudence (American Occupational Therapy Association, 2020). Moreover, there are six principles in the OT profession that guide practitioners in making appropriate decisions in accordance with the highest ideals: beneficence, non-maleficence, autonomy, justice, veracity, and fidelity (American Occupational Therapy Association, 2020).

OT documentation should not be viewed merely as routine paperwork; it is a vital component of the healthcare system, akin to other medical reports. The preparation of OT reports must adhere to the code of ethics. According to the Code and Principles established by the American Occupational Therapy Association (2020), professional behavior encompasses various considerations, including honesty, communication, ensuring the common good, competence, confidential and protected information, conflict of interest, impaired practitioner, sexual relationships, payment for services and other financial arrangements, and resolving ethical issues.

(1) *Honesty* guides OT practitioners to be honest with themselves and those with whom they interact or contact. Moreover, OT practitioners should know their strengths and limitations to adhere to honesty. Under the professional behavior of honesty, the principles of veracity, autonomy, duty, beneficence, and procedural justice should be met (American Occupational Therapy Association, 2020).

(2) *Communication* guides OT practitioners to understand the importance of communication across all aspects, including electronic, verbal, and written communication. Under the professional behavior of communication, the principles of veracity, duty, beneficence, non-maleficence, fidelity, and procedural justice should be met (American Occupational Therapy Association, 2020).

(3) *Ensuring the common good* guides OT practitioners to increase their awareness of their social responsibilities in terms of occupational practice to promote the common good. Under the professional behavior of ensuring the common good, the principles of duty, fidelity, and procedural justice should be met (American Occupational Therapy Association, 2020).

(4) *Competence* guides OT practitioners to provide services within their areas of competence and to subsequently take advantage of any opportunities to expand or update their competence. Under the professional behavior of competence, the principles of duty, beneficence, non-maleficence, and autonomy should be met (American Occupational Therapy Association, 2020).

(5) *Confidential and protected information* guides OT practitioners to protect and keep safe any and all confidential information. In other words, information should not be shared in any way without appropriate consent. For example, information is shared on a need-to-know basis and only with individuals responsible for decision-making. Under the professional behavior of confidential and protected information, the principle of confidentiality should be met (American Occupational Therapy Association, 2020).

(6) *Conflict of interest* guides OT practitioners to avoid any potential conflict of interest, whether real or perceived, to maintain the integrity of interactions. Under the professional behavior of conflict of interest, the principles of non-maleficence, veracity, procedural justice, and fidelity should be met (American Occupational Therapy Association, 2020).

(7) *Impaired practitioner* guides OT practitioners to report any OT personnel who are unable to perform their duties properly or competently after their impairments are reasonably accommodated. The main reason for this behavior is to ensure that no harm is caused to any parties (e.g., clients, students, and colleagues) related to the OT personnel who are impaired. Under the professional behavior of an impaired practitioner, the principle of non-maleficence should be met (American Occupational Therapy Association, 2020).

(8) *Sexual relationships* guide OT practitioners to avoid any sexual relationships during professional interactions, as such behavior is considered a form of misconduct. Under the professional behavior of sexual relationships, the principle of non-maleficence should be met (American Occupational Therapy Association, 2020).

(9) *Payment for services and other financial arrangements* guides OT practitioners to avoid promising or guaranteeing any specific outcomes for OT services. Under the professional behavior of payment for services and other financial arrangements, the principles of procedural justice and beneficence should be met (American Occupational Therapy Association, 2020).

(10) *Resolving ethical issues* guides OT practitioners to use the resources available to identify any potential conflicts or ethical dilemmas and to subsequently resolve them. Under the professional behavior of resolving ethical issues, the principles of duty, fidelity, and procedural justice should be met (American Occupational Therapy Association, 2020).

Box 2.1 discusses the code of ethics for OT practitioners in Hong Kong and Taiwan.

Box 2.1 Code of ethics for OT professionals in practice in Hong Kong and Taiwan

In Hong Kong, the Code of Practice of the Occupational Therapists Board has provided guidance for registered occupational therapists since 1998 and was revised in 2023 (Occupational Therapists Board Hong Kong, 2023). The document outlines the conduct and ethical standards that OT practitioners in Hong Kong are expected to follow in their daily and professional practices.

In general, it adheres to the Code of Ethics proposed by the American Occupational Therapy Association (2020). Specifically, the document includes Part I (Basic Ethical Principles That Suggest What a Registered Occupational Therapist Should Do), Part II (Meaning of "Misconduct in a Professional Respect"), Part III (Convictions and Forms of Professional Misconduct Which May Lead to Disciplinary Proceedings), and Part IV (Sections Extracted from the Supplementary Medical Professions Ordinance, Cap. 359) (Occupational Therapists Board Hong Kong, 2023). For example, occupational therapists in Hong Kong are obliged to observe the Code of Practice of the Occupational Therapists Board Hong Kong in their daily practice. In the Code, a significant part is dedicated to "Professional Communication and Information Dissemination" (Occupational Therapists Board Hong Kong, 2023).

In Taiwan, the code of practice and professional ethics for OT have been established since 1983, with modifications made in 1990 and 2002 (Occupational Therapists Union of The Republic of China, n.d.). This document outlines the expected professional behaviors of OT practitioners and how they should adhere to ethical standards in their daily practices. Similar to the Code of Practice of the Occupational Therapists Board Hong Kong, this guidance aligns with the Code of Ethics proposed by the American Occupational Therapy Association (2020). Specifically, the document is organized into three chapters: Chapter I (The Relationships Between OT Practitioners and Their Service Recipients), Chapter II (The Social Responsibilities of OT Practitioners), and Chapter III (The Relationships Between OT

Practitioners and Their Colleagues/Other Professionals) (Occupational Therapists Union of The Republic of China, n.d.). Within these chapters, there are 13 items (six in Chapter I, two in Chapter II, and five in Chapter III) addressing the principles of justice, autonomy, veracity, fidelity, non-maleficence, confidentiality, duty, and beneficence.

Summary

In this chapter, we introduce the importance of documentation, the types of documentation, the characteristics of good professional documentation, and the ethical considerations for documentation related to OT practice. Documentation plays an essential role throughout the OT process and contributes to evidence-based practice, which, in turn, benefits client care and professional development in the long run.

Appendix 2.1 Example of an evaluation report in OT practice

Occupational Therapy Evaluation Report
Room/Bed no.:
Name: Gender/Age: Date of birth:
Diagnosis:
Medical history:
Insurance: Patient class:
Name of occupational therapist:

Occupational profile
Name of informant:
Reason for seeking service:
Current concerns:

Prior level of function

- ADL:
- IADL:
- Functional mobility:
- History of falls:
- Employment/Daily routine:
- Patterns of engagement in occupations:

Context or environment

- Self-care assistance available at home: {Lives with ...}
- Assistive device or medical equipment already at home:
- Things that support/inhibit desired occupations:

Appendix 2.1 Example of an evaluation report in OT practice (*continued*)

Client's interests and values:

Client's/Family's goal statements:

Priority of outcomes:

Comments:

Occupational performance			
(1) Occupations and contexts to be managed:			
(2) Assessment			
Assessment tool	Performance	Client factor	Context & environment
(3) Comments on client's performance on the desired occupations:			
(4) Hypothesis of occupational performance strengths and weaknesses:			

Appendix 2.1 Example of an evaluation report in OT practice (*continued*)

Goal	
Intervention goal: (Client's desired outcome)	Outcome measure method:

Appendix 2.2 Quick tips on writing an evaluation report in OT practice

Work Capacity Evaluation Report

A work capacity evaluation report is an essential part of work rehabilitation. The following items are recommended to be included in a work capacity evaluation report:
 	
(1) Client's background: diagnosis, post-injury, or surgery time
(2) Purposes of work capacity report:
   ■ Baseline evaluation
   ■ Determining capability of returning to previous job
   ■ Exploring potential in returning to a specified job
(3) Summary of assessment:
   ■ Work history, job analyses, including critical job demand
   ■ Client's work capacity, including physical, cognitive, work behaviors, and performance in simulated work
(4) Major assets and limitations on returning to work
(5) Alignment between client's work capacity and job demand:
   ■ Aligned without significant limitations
   ■ Marginally aligned with a certain degree of limitation
   ■ Unaligned, with a high degree of limitation
(6) Current recommendations on returning to work:
   ■ Ready to return to previous job
   ■ Ready to return to previous job with modification(s)
   ■ Cannot resume previous job, but ready to take up a new one
   ■ Not ready for any paid job, but able to perform some productive work
   ■ Not recommended for work
(7) Recommendations on further management:
   ■ Discharge from work rehabilitation and follow the above recommendation on returning to work
   ■ Continue work rehabilitation with duration and reassessment plan
(8) Signature and credentials

Appendix 2.3 Example of a progress note in table format in OT practice

Occupational Therapy Progress Report				
Room/Bed no.: Name: Gender/Age: Date of birth: Diagnosis: Medical history: Insurance: Patient class: Name of occupational therapist:				
Treatment activities (procedures and requirements)	Date: (1st session)	Date: (2nd session)	Date: (3rd session)	Date: (4th session)
(1)				
(2)				
(3)				
(4)				
(5)				
(6)				
Signature of occupational therapist:				

Appendix 2.4 Examples of the official websites of public bodies and regulatory boards of OT in Asian countries

- Hong Kong Occupational Therapy Association: https://hkota.org.hk/
- Occupational Therapists Board Hong Kong: https://www.smp-council.org.hk/ot/en/intro.php
- China Occupational Therapy Association (in mainland China): https://wfot.org/member-organisations/china-china-occupational-therapy-association
- Malaysian Occupational Therapy Association: https://ot-malaysia.my/
- Singapore Association of Occupational Therapists: https://wfot.org/member-organisations/singapore-singapore-association-of-occupational-therapists
- Occupational Therapists Association of Thailand: https://wfot.org/member-organisations/thailand-occupational-therapists-association-of-thailand-otat
- Taiwan Occupational Therapy Association: https://www.ot.org.tw/

References

American Occupational Therapy Association. (2005). Occupational therapy code of ethics (2005). *American Journal of Occupational Therapy, 59*(6), 639–642.

American Occupational Therapy Association. (2006). Guidelines to the occupational therapy code of ethics. *American Journal of Occupational Therapy, 60*(6), 652–658.

American Occupational Therapy Association. (2014). *Occupational therapy practice framework: Domain and process* (3rd ed.). AOTA Press.

American Occupational Therapy Association. (2015a). Occupational therapy code of ethics (2015). *American Journal of Occupational Therapy, 69*(Suppl. 3), 6913410030p1–6913410030p8. https://doi.org/10.5014/ajot.2015.696S03

American Occupational Therapy Association. (2015b). Standards of practice for occupational therapy. *American Journal of Occupational Therapy, 69*(Suppl. 3), 6913410057p1–6913410057p6. https://doi.org/10.5014/ajot.2015.696S06

American Occupational Therapy Association. (2018). Guidelines for documentation of occupational therapy. *American Journal of Occupational Therapy, 72*(Suppl. 2), 7212410010p1–7212410010p7.

American Occupational Therapy Association. (2020). AOTA 2020 occupational therapy code of ethics. *American Journal of Occupational Therapy, 74*(Suppl. 3), 7413410005p1–7413410005p13. https://doi.org/10.5014/ajot.2020.74S3006

American Occupational Therapy Association. (2021). Standards of practice for occupational therapy. *American Journal of Occupational Therapy, 75*(Suppl. 3), 7513410030. https://doi.org/10.5014/ajot.2021.75S3004

Occupational Therapists Board Hong Kong. (2023). *Code of practice of the Occupational Therapists Board Hong Kong.* https://www.smp-council.org.hk/ot/file/pdf/Code_of_Practice_for_OT_e.pdf

Occupational Therapists Union of The Republic of China 中華民國職能治療師公會全國聯合會. (n.d.). *Occupational therapy professional ethics* 職能治療專業倫理. Retrieved December 28, 2021, from https://www.oturoc.org.tw/index.php?action=about&id=12

WHO Regional Office for Europe. (2020). *Screening programmes: A short guide. Increase effectiveness, maximize benefits and minimize harm.* World Health Organization.

World Federation of Occupational Therapists. (2016). *Code of ethics.* Retrieved December 28, 2021, from https://www.wfot.org/resources/code-of-ethics

World Health Organization. (n.d.). *International classification of functioning, disability and health (ICF).* https://www.who.int/standards/classifications/international-classification-of-functioning-disability-and-health

Assessment, evaluation, and intervention

Sensorimotor functions

Sam Chi Chung Chan, Josephine Man-Wah Wong, and Seiji Nishimura

Principles of sensory and motor assessments

When managing clients with acute or chronic orthopedic injuries, occupational therapists first conduct a series of assessments on sensory and motor functions to understand both the problems and assets of clients. These assessments help prioritize and implement physical and occupation-based treatments. Assessments can be divided into three stages: (1) a review of the client's medical history and records (Box 3.1), (2) an interview (Box 3.2), and (3) physical and functional examinations (Amini et al., 2018).

The following section outlines what an occupational therapist will go through when conducting organized and systematic sensorimotor assessments. The primary goal of

---

Box 3.1 Review of the client's medical history

Upon referral from a doctor or self-referral from a client:

- Review medical records and clinical notes prepared by the doctor and other professionals.
- Focus on any history of the medical condition(s), any medical intervention experienced by the client, and personal information.
- Identify or speculate on the cause(s) of the sensorimotor dysfunctions reported by the client at the onset of the injury.
- Examine the results of the radiographic or imaging examination to reveal the location and severity of bone or soft tissue injuries.
- Inspect the results of laboratory tests, which may also be a helpful indicator of any musculoskeletal conditions. This medical-related information helps the case occupational therapist determine the injury's location and severity, assess the rehabilitation prognosis, and develop an appropriate rehabilitation intervention plan while considering any contraindications or necessary precautions.

DOI: 10.4324/9781032721170-6

> **Box 3.2 Suggested aspects in an occupation-based interview**
> An interview covers the cause of the injury, the client's major physical complaints and psychological status, the time scale of the conditions, the client's occupational status, and other social factors.
>
> - Information can also be obtained about the client's medical history and symptoms that have been experienced.
> - For chronic conditions, any changes in symptoms in the past could be obtained from the client.
> - The nature of the pain or discomfort can also be identified. The pain interview will be discussed in the "Pain Assessments" subsection.
> - Preliminary occupation-based information about the client's current occupational status, life routine, home and work environment, and social support should also be collected (Table 3.1 illustrates some OT interview questions).

this process is to determine whether occupational therapy (OT) interventions would help the referred client improve their ability to perform daily activities.

A series of sensorimotor assessments need to be conducted in a sequential manner based on the "Look-Feel-Move" principles (Monrad et al., 2011). These principles recommend starting with passive assessments, such as observing joint alignment or palpating strained muscles, before progressing to active assessments, such as active range of motion (AROM) and manual muscle testing (MMT). AROM concerns a certain joint actively moving across the space. Goniometers of various sizes are commonly used as assessment tools. During MMT, a clinician uses his/her upper limb strength to assess the strength of the muscle contractions against gravity or on a gravity-eliminated plane. This approach is safer from the client's perspective as any discomfort or complaints can easily be expressed early on. This assessment allows the occupational therapist to determine whether to proceed with active tests, which require the client to move or apply force to the injured body part, e.g., contracting strained muscles or mobilizing misaligned joints. The main features of the Look-Feel-Move approach are outlined in Table 3.2.

Table 3.1 Overview of an OT interview with sample questions

Domain	Example
Cause of injury/physical condition	Could you describe how you got injured?
	How long did you have this physical condition? How did it occur?
Physical complaints	Could you describe the discomfort after the injury?
	Do you have any discomfort, such as pain, due to your physical condition?
Psychological status	How does your current injury affect your emotions?
Premorbid occupational status	What kind of job do you do?
	What was your daily routine before the injury?
Social factors	With whom do you live?
	What is your living setting – private flat or public housing estate?

Table 3.2 The Look-Feel-Move principles

Look	Clinical observations can begin during the interview and can be categorized as static or dynamic. Static observations include assessing a client's sitting or standing posture, joint alignment, and any swelling in the extremities. Dynamically, the client's gestures and facial expressions can also provide additional information about the client's mood and other psychological issues. This can help in planning subsequent physical assessments.
Feel	These assessments involve touching and feeling specific body parts to evaluate swelling, skin temperature, skin texture, and the size of bodily structures such as muscles. Force can also be exerted carefully on the client's body parts to induce localized tenderness or pain, and to feel if there is any tension or tight muscles due to inflammation. The bone structure and alignment of the joints can also be palpitated to detect any malalignment or subluxation. This examination can also include sensory tests (e.g., pinprick tests) and provocative tests, in which body parts are mobilized by the occupational therapist while the client remains relaxed (e.g., Phalen's test for carpal tunnel syndrome or the raised straight leg test for lumber radiculopathy).
Move	These assessments involve active client participation and include both physical and functional evaluations. Physical examinations assess specific aspects of musculoskeletal function, such as AROM and MMT. Functional assessments evaluate how integrated musculoskeletal functions impact the performance of meaningful activities.

Types of sensorimotor assessment

There are two types of "Move" assessment: standardized and non-standardized. Standardized assessments refer to evaluation tools that use common assessment tools and procedures, such as the Purdue Pegboard Test (PPT) (Causby et al., 2014), Jebsen-Taylor Hand Function Test (JTHFT) (Fabbri et al., 2021; Jebsen et al., 1969), and Minnesota Hand Function Test (Gloss & Wardle, 1982; Wang et al., 2018). The advantages to standardized tests are that the procedures are well known and studies have been conducted to demonstrate their psychometric properties. Standardized tests can be applied to specific client populations and used as outcome measures of rehabilitation programs.

In contrast, non-standardized assessments have not undergone the rigorous process of psychometric testing, and no extensive data has been collected to establish norms. The procedure and performance scoring can be modified for individual clients rather than larger populations. For example, an occupational therapist may assess a client's use of chopstick skills to evaluate fine hand coordination after a hand injury. Although the procedure is not standardized, such assessments are specifically designed to address the unique abilities and needs of a particular client.

Sensory-related assessments

Sensory function assessments

Occupational therapists should be aware of the normal sensory dermatomes[1] of the upper limb according to neurological levels, the distribution of cutaneous sensibility for the median, ulnar, and radial nerves in the hand, as well as the sensory signs and symptoms that result from various levels of injuries or compression along the nerve pathways. Sensibility testing can be conducted according to hierarchal levels, including autonomic/sympathetic response, detection of touch, touch discrimination, quantification, and identification as part of the rehabilitative process (Bell-Krotoski, 2011).

The motor and sensory functions of the hand are provided by three major peripheral nerves: the median, radial, and ulnar nerves located in the upper limb quadrant. These nerves are the peripheral branches of the brachial plexus, and the neurological levels are represented by the sensory distributions illustrated in Figure 3.1a and b. Nerve functions can be affected by traumatic injuries such as cuts or fractures to the upper arm, elbow, or wrist, entrapment or compression due to cumulative disorders, or other non-traumatic conditions. These injuries can result in a loss of movement and paresthesia in the areas supplied by the affected nerves. Figure 3.1c illustrates the sensory dermatome of the whole body, which would be used when the neural injuries involve the trunk and lower limbs.

Normal hand function requires normal sensibility. Tactile information from the hand is essential for the sense of touch during daily activities. The brain processes touch input and combines it with past experiences to help distinguish between objects of various shapes, thicknesses, temperatures, etc. There are four main types of somatic sensibility: touch, proprioception, pain, and temperature sense. In the later stages of sensory recovery, once protective sensation has returned, the final phase involves regaining discriminative touch and tactile sensation. This advanced level of recovery allows a person to identify shapes, textures, and thicknesses of objects without relying on visual input, an ability known as tactilegnosis.[2]

The physical examination of the hand is a crucial component of a comprehensive physical assessment. It provides valuable information about nerve function regeneration after surgery, recovery from nerve compression, progress in sensory and motor recovery, and the restoration of hand functionality. Sensibility assessments include provocative tests, threshold detection tests, discriminative tests, and functional tests (a summary of the sensory tests can be found in Table 3.3).

Provocative tests
Provocative tests include Tinel's sign test, with positive results indicating the location of nerve growth after surgery or nerve compression (Figure 3.2).

Threshold detection tests
Threshold detection tests include using cotton wool balls and neurotips to detect the early return of light touch and the protective sense of blunt and sharp sensations (Figures 3.3–3.6), a hot and cold discrimination kit to differentiate between hot and cold temperatures (Figure 3.7), and tuning forks (i.e., 30-Hz and 256-Hz) to test vibration responses (Figures 3.8 and 3.9).

Monofilament tests
The monofilament test is used to map the pattern of sensibility loss (Bell-Krotoski et al., 1993; Chen et al., 2021) (Figures 3.10 and 3.11).

Discriminative tests
Discriminative tests include the point of localization, which assesses the accuracy of identifying the location of a touch stimulus on the hand, and the two-point

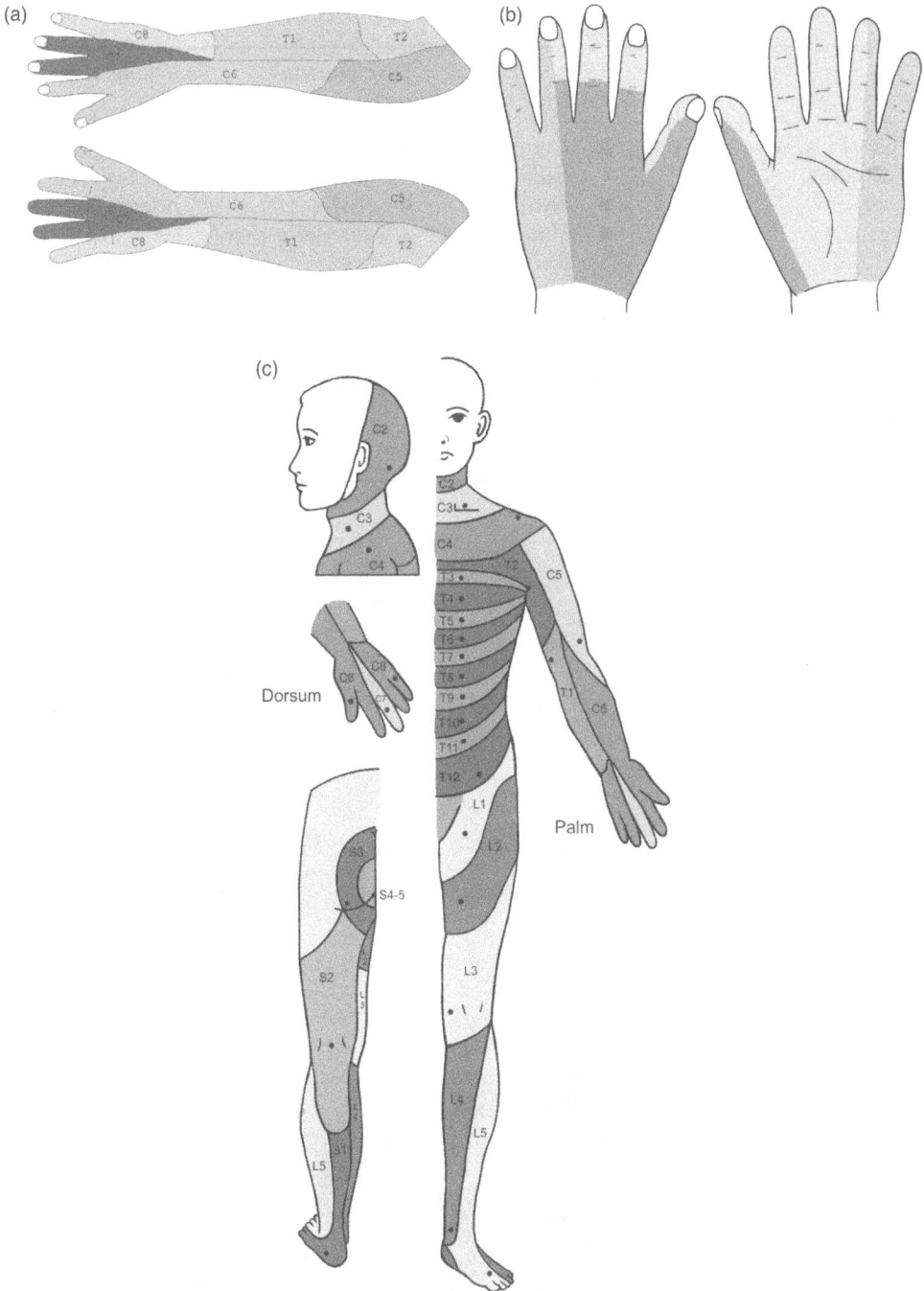

Figure 3.1 (a) Cutaneous dermatomes of the upper extremity. (b) Sensory distribution of the median (light gray, or pink in the e-book), radial (dark gray, or green in the e-book), and ulnar (medium gray, or blue in the e-book) nerves in the hand. (c) Sensory dermatomes of the body

Table 3.3 Summary of sensory assessments

	Provocative test	Threshold detection test	Discriminative test	Functional test
Types of sensation test	■ Tinel's sign test (Bell-Krotoski, 2011)	■ Cotton wool ball test ■ Neurotip test ■ Hot and cold discrimination test ■ Tuning fork test (Bell-Krotoski, 2011)	■ Monofilament test ■ Two-point discrimination test (Bell-Krotoski & Buford, 1997; Chen et al., 2021)	■ Moberg's Pick-up Test (Jerosch-Herold et al., 2016; Ng et al., 1999) ■ Nottingham Sensory Assessment (Borstad & Nichols-Larsen, 2014; Lincoln et al., 1998)

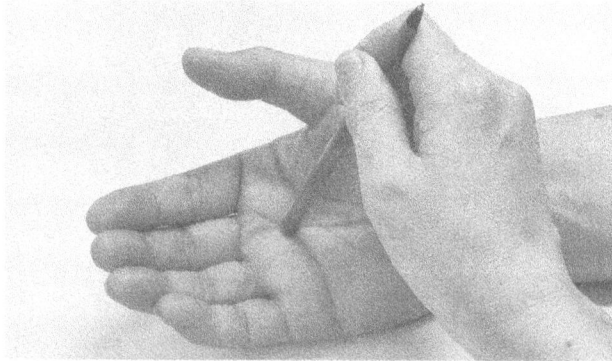

Figure 3.2 Tinel's sign test using a pen

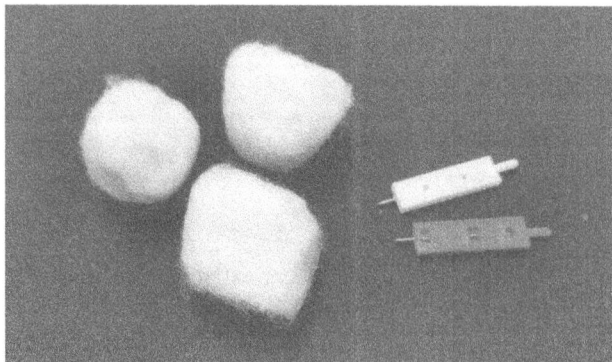

Figure 3.3 Cotton wool balls and neurotips

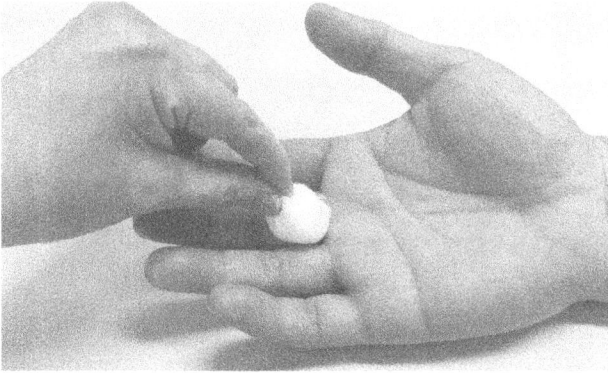

Figure 3.4 Cotton wool ball test for light touch

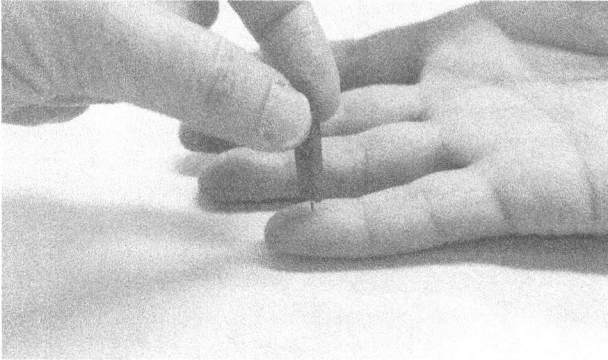

Figure 3.5 Neurotip test for sharp sensation

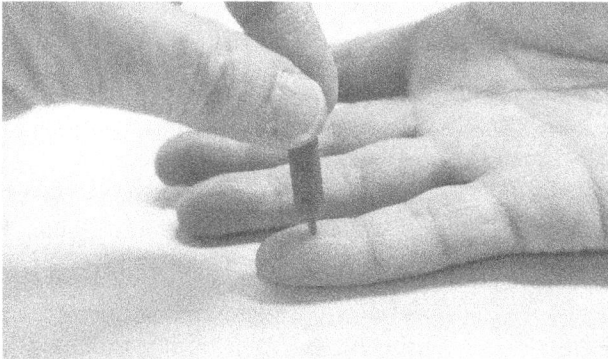

Figure 3.6 Neurotip test for blunt sensation

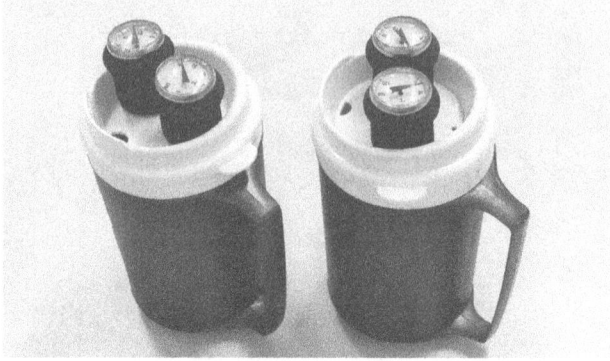

Figure 3.7 Hot and cold discrimination kit for hot and cold temperature differentiation

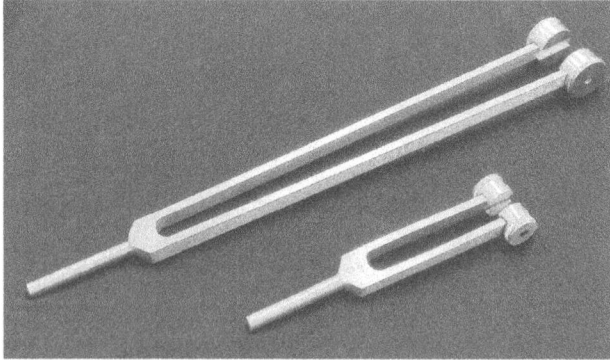

Figure 3.8 30-Hz (left) and 256-Hz (right) tuning forks

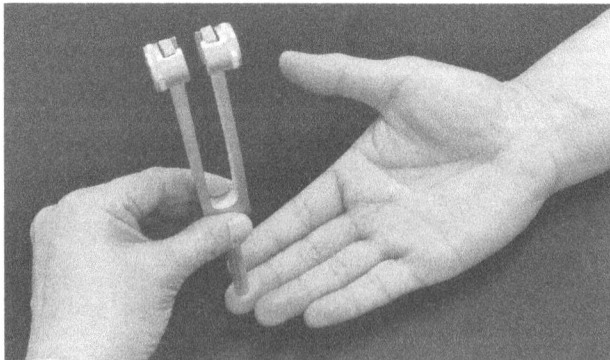

Figure 3.9 Tuning fork test for vibration sensation

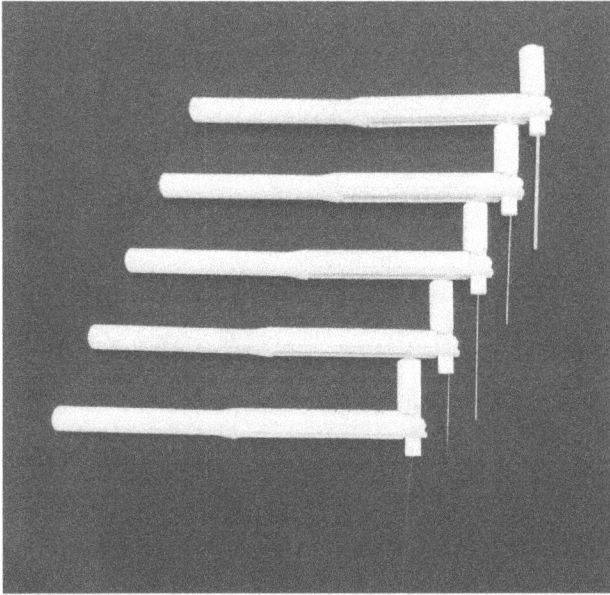

Figure 3.10 Monofilament test tools

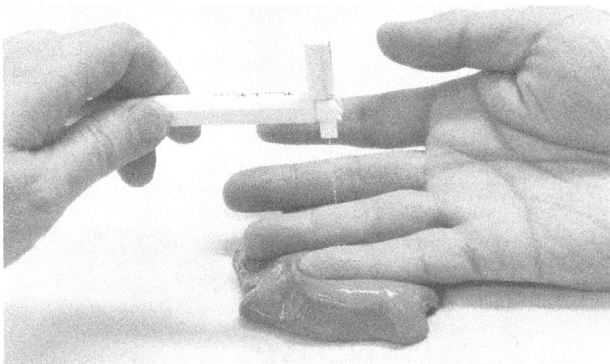

Figure 3.11 Monofilament test for cutaneous pressure sensation

discrimination test, which evaluates the return of discriminative sensibility in the fingertips (Bell-Krotoski & Buford, 1997; Chen et al., 2021) (Figures 3.12 and 3.13).

Functional tests
Functional tests use Moberg's Pick-up Test to evaluate the quality of functional pinching performance and recognition of various objects (Jerosch-Herold et al., 2016; Ng et al., 1999) (Figure 3.14).

Nottingham Sensory Assessment
The Nottingham Sensory Assessment is a standardized scale used to evaluate sensory impairments in stroke clients. It tests tactile sensation and kinesthetic sensation in

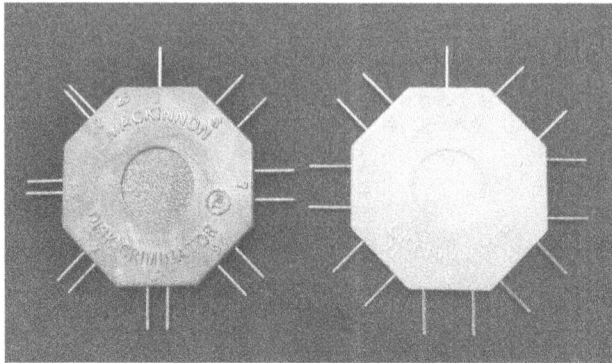

Figure 3.12 Two-point discrimination disks

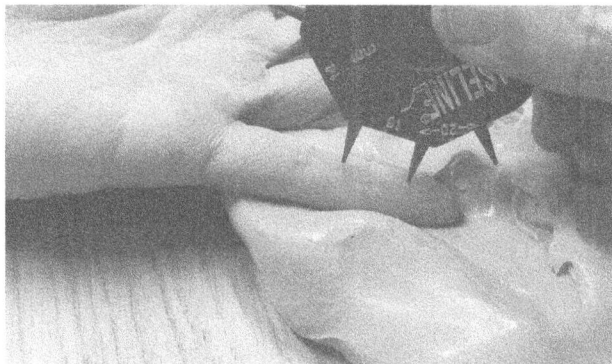

Figure 3.13 Two-point discrimination test for discriminative sensibility

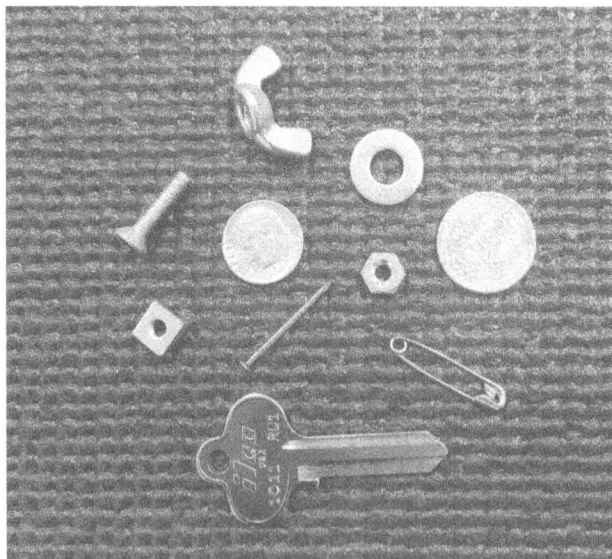

Figure 3.14 Moberg's Pick-up Test

various body parts, as well as stereognosis (Borstad & Nichols-Larsen, 2014; Lincoln et al., 1998).

Pain assessments

Clients with orthopedic conditions often experience pain after acute or chronic injuries. Clients with musculoskeletal conditions may generally experience two main types of pain: nociceptive and neuropathic. Nociceptive pain is a result of injuries to musculoskeletal tissues, including bones, muscles, tendons, and ligaments. Injured tissues cause inflammation and activate nociceptors, leading individuals to perceive unpleasant sensations. Nociceptive pain is characterized as focal, sharp, or aching and tends to be persistent, often worsening with movement. In contrast, neuropathic pain arises from injuries to impinged nerves. Clients experiencing neuropathic pain report radiating sensations along the nerve pathways, along with cutaneous numbness or tingling. The pattern of the pain tends to be more spontaneous and less related to body movement (Baron et al., 2010; Cavalli et al., 2019).

It is important for occupational therapists to understand the pain characteristics to have a better understanding of the etiology of musculoskeletal and neurological injuries. This can be done through a series of pain assessments, such as a pain interview, observation, and physical assessments based on Look-Feel-Move, to define the nociceptive, neuropathic, or mixed nature of the pain. An occupational therapist may hold a pain interview based on the "OLDCART formula", namely onset ("When and how did the pain occur?"), location ("Which part of the body does the pain bother you?"), duration ("How long does the pain last?"), characteristics ("How does the pain sensation feel — sharp or tingling?"), aggravating and relieving factors ("What kind of actions or activities do you do that worsen or alleviate your pain?"), and timing of pain ("Does your pain occur persistently or intermittently?").

For nociceptive pain, the location of the pain tends to be localized at the site of the injury, e.g., strained muscles and fractured bones. The characteristics of pain are often described by clients as clear and localized tenderness, aching, or sharp sensations. They may experience a dull ache or throbbing while at rest, and the pattern of pain tends to be persistent. The pain intensity is generally related to the anatomical characteristics of the injured area and the factors that aggravate or alleviate it. For example, nociceptive pain in the muscles may be worsened when a client with strained muscles contracts the injured muscle groups. This type of pain is likely to be relieved by simple analgesics, such as paracetamol, or non-steroid anti-inflammatory drugs, such as aspirin and ibuprofen.

For neuropathic pain, the location of pain or discomfort tends to be more diffuse or away from the site of neuropathy. A client with neuropathic pain might describe the abnormal sensation as shooting, moving, or radiating. It is also associated with other neurological symptoms, such as a cutaneous tingling sensation, numbness when sensory nerves are involved, and muscle weakness when motor nerves are injured. This type of pain typically follows a dermatomal distribution. The discomfort is often less related to movement and may occur more spontaneously or sporadically. Neuropathic pain is generally less responsive to standard analgesic medications and more responsive to anti-epileptic medications, such as Lyrica, or anti-depression medications, such as amitriptyline and nortriptyline.

The PainDETECT assessment is a validated clinical tool commonly used to determine whether a client's pain is neuropathic in nature. This questionnaire evaluates multiple aspects of pain (Freynhagen et al., 2006) and serves as a guideline for the pain interview and a better understanding of the client's pain condition. It covers intensity, location, and pattern of pain and contains seven questions (e.g., "Do you have a tingling or prickling sensation in the area of your pain [like crawling ants or electrical tingling]?") that are concerned with the clinical manifestations of the neuropathic pain on a six-point scale (from "Never" to "Very strong"). The total scores, ranging from 19 to 38, indicate a positive manifestation of neuropathic pain.

Occupational therapists need to conduct several pain assessments based on Look-Feel-Move to identify nociceptive or neuropathic types of pain. This helps to develop a better understanding of the severity and nature of the injury. During "Look" assessments, occupational therapists observe the client's static and dynamic posture during various functional movements. Clients with nociceptive pain may adopt a certain antalgic posture, such as uneven shoulder height or a slouched position, and may exhibit an antalgic gait to avoid exerting force on injured areas. Those with nociceptive pain may also show imbalances in movement or gait due to sensations such as cutaneous tingling or muscle weakness. During "Feel" assessments, occupational therapists conduct palpation tests on the injured body parts to assess nociceptive pain. This includes palpating contused bony prominences or strained muscles, as well as testing bony structures or soft tissues (e.g., ligaments and muscle bulges). Various types of palpation can be used; for example, point palpation helps detect localized tenderness, while cross-fiber palpation can identify edema or taut muscles. The intensity of pain reported by clients indicates the severity of the injury. For acute conditions, localized swelling and increased temperature may also be felt upon palpation. Provocative tests can reproduce the pain associated with the injured structure; for instance, muscle stretch tests can assess the severity of lateral epicondylitis (Soares et al., 2023) by passively stretching wrist extensors to induce pain at their common origin. In cases of neuropathic pain, occupational therapists use provocative tests to reproduce nerve impingement symptoms. A common test for lumbar sciatica involves having the client lie supine while the occupational therapist lifts one leg with a straight knee. Radiating neuropathic pain in the raised lower limb at hip angles of between 30 and 70 degrees indicates nerve impingement in the lumbar region. Other neurological tests, such as reflex testing, may also be included for clients with neurological injuries.

Finally, "Move" assessments evaluate active movement related to nociceptive or neuropathic etiology. These assessments examine the active function of the injured musculature or the function of the nerves that supply the muscles under examination. For nociceptive conditions, MMT is commonly used to assess muscle strength impacted by injuries (see the later section for details). Provocative tests can also replicate painful sensations or discomfort when injured muscles exert force; for example, Cozen's Test assesses inflammation in lateral epicondylitis by asking clients to perform wrist extension and radial deviation concurrently to induce nociceptive pain at the lateral epicondyle of the humerus. For neurological injuries, "Move" assessments aim to determine the extent of motor nerve injury by evaluating active control of muscles innervated by affected nerves, often referred to as myotome testing. For instance, to examine the nerve innervation of the sacral nerve, the power of the ankle plantarflexion is assessed (see the later section for details).

Motor-related assessments

Musculoskeletal motor tests

When evaluating a client's motor performance, assessments of the range of motion (ROM) of joints and conducting MMT are fundamental. Range of motion is the amount of movement that occurs at a joint to produce movement of a bone in space, while MMT is used to evaluate the function and strength of individual muscles and muscle groups based on the performance of movement in relation to the force of gravity and manual resistance.

Measurement of joint range of motion includes measuring the AROM and passive range of motion (PROM). AROM is the active muscle contraction to voluntarily move the body part through the range of motion without assistance. PROM is the therapist or other external force moving the body part through the range of motion. The range of motion produces an increase or decrease in the angle or rotation. Angular movement occurs within the range of 0 to 180 degrees between the adjacent bones, including flexion, extension, abduction, and adduction. Rotational movement, instead of angular movement, occurs around the longitudinal axis. Assessing the AROM can show a client's willingness to move, their ability to follow instructions, coordination, and whether the movement induces pain or is restricted by weakened muscles or limited joint mobility. Assessing PROM can show the maximum mobility of the joint that allows active joint movement or the factors that restrict movement or cause pain. Observing the measurement process is crucial to determine whether the range is full, limited, or exceeds what the joint structure can allow. By assessing the end-feel sensation, therapists can gauge feedback from the soft tissues around the joint during PROM, providing insight into the flexibility of these tissues (Clarkson, 2013).

Various sizes of universal goniometers are commonly used to measure joint angles. A large-sized goniometer is used for measuring shoulder, elbow, hip, and knee range of motion; a medium-sized goniometer is used for wrist and ankle measurement; and a small-sized goniometer is used for measuring finger movement.

Muscle strength is the maximum amount of force that a muscle or muscle group can voluntarily exert for maximum effort. The force results in the movement of the limb around the joint axis. Muscle force can result from various muscle contractions: isometric, isotonic (concentric or eccentric), and isokinetic. Conventional methods in MMT are based on three factors, including the evidence of muscle contraction, the influence of gravity, and the amount of manual resistance. After evaluation, a grade is given to quantify a client's performance. A grading system from 0 to 5, as shown in Table 3.4, evaluates whether a client's performance can be assessed in a gravity-resistive plane or gravity-free plane. It also indicates whether there is a positive change in joint range of motion due to muscle power, if no observable joint range of motion exists but muscle contraction can be palpated, or if there is no change of joint range of motion and no palpable muscle contraction. A more detailed grading of muscle strength is achieved by adding a plus or minus to the whole grade to indicate variations in the ROM or the ability to move against minimal resistance (Clarkson, 2013). Table 3.4 illustrates the conventional grading system used in MMT. Therapists should be aware of the correct positioning of clients in relation to the influence of gravity during the test, as well as the placement of resistance when assessing performance over grade 3. After implementing

Table 3.4 Conventional grading system used in MMT (Clarkson, 2013)

Numeral	Letter notation	Definition
Against gravity tests		
5	N (normal)	Full available range of motion (ROM) against maximal resistance.
4	G (good)	Full available ROM against moderate resistance.
4–	G–	Greater than one-half of the available ROM against gravity and against moderate resistance.
3+	F+	Full available ROM against gravity and against minimal resistance.
3	F (fair)	Full available ROM against gravity.
3–	F–	Greater than one-half of the available ROM against gravity.
2+	P+	Less than one-half of the available ROM against gravity.
Gravity eliminated tests		
2	P (poor)	Full available ROM with gravity eliminated.
2–	P–	Less than the full available ROM with gravity eliminated.
1	T (trace)	No observable ROM with gravity eliminated, but there is a palpable or observable flicker of a muscle contraction.
0	0 (zero)	No observable ROM with gravity eliminated, and there is no palpable or observable muscle contraction.

a joint range of motion and MMT assessments, the therapist should analyze how the limitations impact the client's daily living performance.

Motor tests for neurological conditions

For neurological conditions related to central nerve injury, such as spinal cord injury, several motor function aspects should be assessed, including reflexes, muscle tone, and myotome, to determine the severity and nature of the neurological injuries. A reflex test can be conducted to test the integrity of monosynaptic stretch reflexes. Reflex hammers can be used to apply percussion at a muscle tendon corresponding to a level of the spinal cord segment. For instance, biceps reflex (biceps jerk) represents the C5/C6 cord segment, while quadriceps reflex (knee jerk) represents the L3/L4 cord segment. Generally, a hyperreflexic reaction indicates an upper-motor neuron lesion (e.g., a cord injury), and a hyporeflexic reaction indicates a lower-motor neuron lesion (e.g., a peripheral nerve injury).

Muscle tone is defined as passive partial contraction of the muscles, or the muscle's resistance to passive stretching during rest. An occupational therapist must passively position a certain limb to pull or stretch certain muscle groups and then evaluate the resistance given by the muscles being tested. The Modified Ashworth Scale (Meseguer-Henarejos et al., 2018) is commonly used to rate the level of muscle tone based on the following Table 3.5.

Active muscle testing for neurological conditions involves assessing myotomes, which are groups of muscles innervated by specific spinal nerve roots. The primary purpose

Table 3.5 The Modified Ashworth Scale (Meseguer-Henarejos et al., 2018)

0	No increase in muscle tone.
1	Slight increase in muscle tone, with a catch and release or minimal resistance at the end of the range of motion when an affected part(s) is moved in flexion or extension.
1+	Slight increase in muscle tone, manifested as a catch, followed by minimal resistance through the remainder (less than half) of the range of motion.
2	A marked increase in muscle tone throughout most of the range of motion, but affected part(s) are still easily moved.
3	Considerable increase in muscle tone; passive movement difficult.
4	Affected part(s) rigid in flexion or extension.

of myotome testing is to evaluate the integrity of muscle innervation by measuring the strength of the corresponding muscle. As in MMT, a 5-point scale is used for myotome testing, where 0 = no contraction, 1 = trace contraction, 2 = active movement with gravity eliminated, 3 = active movement against gravity, 4 = active movement against slight to moderate resistance, and 5 = active movement against strong resistance regardless of the range of motion. The actions of the representative myotomes of the upper and lower extremities are shown in Table 3.6.

Upper limb and hand function tests

Upper limb functions include a client's ability to reach, support, push, pinch and grasp, release, and carry objects. Each joint of the upper limb contributes to the direction and support, reach, adjustment, and grip of the movement. Upper limb and hand function tests evaluate the ability to pinch, grasp, and carry objects.

For the upper limb function test, analyzing movement is crucial for understanding the function of the upper limbs and scoring results within the time available. It is also essential to understand the client's activities of daily living (ADLs) and work needs from an early stage, as well as to evaluate and treat upper limb function in relation to any activity limitations. In some cases, it is important to also assess trunk function and cognitive aspects. Additionally, if necessary, the use of assistive devices and special seating support should be considered.

During upper limb function tests, the range of motion and muscle strength of the upper limbs, thumbs, and fingers, sensory function, and hand coordination are also assessed. Trunk function, visual acuity/hearing function, and the presence of pain when sitting also affect the client's performance. It is important for occupational therapists to analyze movements during the upper limb and hand function tests. Since upper limb

Table 3.6 The actions of the representative myotomes of the upper and lower extremities

Upper extremity:	Lower extremity:
C5 – Shoulder abduction and elbow flexion	L2 – Hip flexion
C6 – Wrist extension	L3 – Knee extension
C7 – Elbow extension	L4 – Ankle dorsiflexion
C8 – Flexion of distal interphalangeal joints	L5 – Big toe extension
T1 – Finger abduction	S1 – Ankle plantarflexion

dysfunction is associated with activity limitations, motion analysis during the upper limb function tests can provide insights into clients' limitations in ADL performance. Prior to conducting the upper limb and hand function tests, occupational therapists must have a better understanding of the following functions:

(1) Cognitive and perceptual functions: The client must have the ability to comprehend and understand the contents and follow the instructions of the assessment.
(2) Visual and auditory functions: If the client has a visual impairment, he/she may not be able to perform the test. Written instructions or non-verbal gesturing will be necessary if the client has limited auditory function.
(3) Assessment environment: It is necessary to adjust the height of the desk and chair so that clients are seated comfortably when performing the assessment. Assistive devices and seat cushions are needed for clients with sitting problems, thereby facilitating their assessment performance.

The battery of upper limb and hand function assessments can be divided into two categories: (1) assessments using various test items to evaluate the upper limb and hand functions in manipulating various objects, and (2) assessments with identical testing items which evaluate the efficiency or speed of the upper limbs and hand coordination and precision (Poole, 2009). The standardized and non-standardized tests with norm- or criterion-reference characteristics are summarized in Table 3.7.

Assessments using various hand function test items

Jebsen-Taylor Hand Function Test (Fabbri et al., 2021; Jebsen et al., 1969; Li-Tsang et al., 2004)
The JTHFT was developed by Jebsen et al. in 1969 to enable objective and standardized assessment of the manual dexterity necessary for ADLs (Fabbri et al., 2021). It was translated into a Chinese version in 2004 for use in Hong Kong (Li-Tsang et al., 2004). As one of the most well-used upper limb function tests, JTHFT was designed to measure gross coordination and comprises seven subtests: writing, card turning, picking up small objects, simulated feeding, stacking, and picking up large, lightweight, and heavy

Table 3.7 Summary of various standardized and non-standardized upper limb and hand function tests

	Norm-reference test	*Criterion-reference test*
Standardized test	Motor assessments: ■ Nine-hole Peg Test ■ Purdue Pegboard Test ■ Moberg Pick-up Test ■ Jebsen-Taylor Hand Function Test	Motor assessments: ■ Minnesota Hand Function Test ■ Action Research Arm Test
Non-standardized test		Motor assessment: ■ Performance-based functional test

objects. The test evaluates the time needed to manipulate various objects using the non-dominant hand and the dominant hand. The US norms are categorized by maximum time, hand dominance, gender, and age.

Action Research Arm Test (Pike et al., 2018; Yozbatiran et al., 2008)

The Action Research Arm Test (ARAT) is recognized internationally as a standard evaluation method. It comprises 19 tests distributed across four subscales, with three to six tasks each, and assesses grasp, grip, pinch, and gross movement. The test materials include various-sized wooden blocks, a cricket ball, a sharpening stone, alloy tubes, a washer and bolt, two glasses, marbles, and ball bearings. Each task runs until the client completes the task or until reaching a time limit defined as 60 seconds. The quality of the task is rated on an ordinal four-point scale (i.e., from 0 to 3). The maximum score for the ARAT is 57 for each arm, with a higher score indicating better arm motor status. The standardized assessment aims to provide an efficient evaluation method for evaluating hand functions under the influence of neurological conditions such as cerebrovascular disease.

Simple Test for Evaluation of Hand Function (Kita et al., 2013; Yamakawa et al., 2023)

The Simple Test for Evaluation of Hand Function (STEF) is an upper limb function test developed in Japan for evaluating a client's ability to pinch, grasp, and transfer objects. The client is instructed to pick up items one by one from a storage space and move them into a target space as quickly as possible. The client performs the test using ten objects of varying shapes and sizes that need to be fitted into predetermined places. These objects include six small cubes, six middle-sized cubes, five large cuboids, six small balls, six middle-sized balls, five large balls, seven metallic circular disks, six wooden circular disks, eight pins, and six pieces of cloth. It is a highly reproducible evaluation tool for clients with cerebrovascular disease and cervical spine disease.

Moberg Pick-up Test (Jerosch-Herold et al., 2016; Ng et al., 1999)

The Moberg Pick-up Test (MPUT) is a functional sensibility test used for evaluating the sensory recovery of repaired nerves. Clients' precision sensory grip and the ability to perceive constant touch are required. The items in the test comprise 12 small, common metallic items, including a 50-cent coin, $2 coin, wing nut, key, key chain, nail, square nut, hexagon nut, washer, paper clip, safety pin, and press stud. The client is asked to pick up the items and place them into a small container. The left and right hands are assessed separately, and the client is tested without and with vision occluded.

Assessments using identical test items

Purdue Pegboard Test (Proud et al., 2020; Tiffin & Asher, 1948)

The PPT is a test of manipulative dexterity designed to assist in the selection of employees in industrial jobs such as assembly, packing, operation of certain machines, and other routine manual jobs of an exacting nature. This test evaluates a client's dexterity performance in manual assembly and packaging tasks, using metal pins and washers in five subtests: right hand only, left hand only, both hands, summation of left, right, and both hands, and assembly. The normative data are presented in categories according to gender: college men and women, male veterans, and male and female industrial applicants. The concurrent validity of the PPT scores with other objective measures and nerve conduction were found to be satisfactory (Amirjani et al., 2011).

O'Connor Finger Dexterity Test (Berger et al., 2009; Estorninho et al., 2022)

This test provides an evaluation of finger dexterity involving the insertion of three small pins per hole in a board. It has been used successfully as a predictor for rapid manipulation of small objects, such as in assembly line work. It has also been found to be useful in predicting success for instrument work, such as the assembling of armatures, miniature parts of clocks and watches, rapid hand and eye work, filling vials, and precision lathe work. A few recent studies have shown that the O'Connor Finger Dexterity Test is a reliable and valid hand assessment (Estorninho et al., 2022).

Box and Block Test (Mathiowetz et al., 1985; Solaro et al., 2020)

The Box and Block Test (BBT) is a hand function test that evaluates unilateral gross manual dexterity. The assessment comprises a wooden box with two compartments and 150 wooden blocks. The client is required to move the maximum number of blocks, one at a time, from one compartment of the box to another within 60 seconds. This is a simple test that can be performed in a short space of time. Its concurrent validity with other commonly used hand function assessments were found to be moderately correlated. Interrater reliability was revealed to be moderate, with an ICC of 0.67 ($P = .02$) (Prochaska & Ammenwerth, 2023).

Nine-hole Peg Test (Grice et al., 2003; Lindstrom-Hazel & Veenstra, 2015; Proud et al., 2020; Wang et al., 2015)

The Nine-hole Peg Test (NHPT) is a simple and validated test that requires a client to quickly pick up nine small pegs from a holding well, insert the pegs in nine holes in a 3 x 3 array, and then move them back to the well. The test is easy to administer for all age groups, particularly younger children. The time to administer the NHPT is brief (< 5 mins to measure for both hands). Literature supports this test as a reliable and valid measure of finger dexterity that is capable of assessing hand dexterity in various diagnostic groups (e.g., stroke, cerebral palsy, cerebellar impairment, Parkinson's disease, and multiple sclerosis). Norms are published for children at 5–10 years of age, 7–12 years of age, and 4–19 years of age, and for adults at 21–71 years of age and 20–75 years of age (Proud et al., 2020; Wang et al., 2015).

Functional Dexterity Test (Aaron & Jansen, 2003; Sartorio et al., 2020)

The Functional Dexterity Test (FDT) evaluates the gross prehension pattern and requires the client to flip over 16 pegs from a pegboard using a dynamic three-jaw chunk prehension pattern, starting from one corner of the hand being tested in a back-and-forth manner until all rows are turned over. Clients are required to complete the test as quickly as possible, and their finishing time is counted in seconds. A ten-second penalty time will be added if the client drops a peg during the test. The test is stopped at two minutes, and if the client exceeds 55 seconds, he/she receives a non-functional rating. Recent studies have shown that the FDT carries a moderate predictive validity with age, gender, and hand dominance among adult populations (Bachman et al., 2023).

A common caveat related to conducting upper limb and hand function tests is the focus on the test results only without analyzing the quality of the client's performance, which is affected by physical impairment. It is important to relate impairment and activity limitation to understand the disorder of upper limb function. For example, the cause of upper limb dysfunction may be a limitation of the range of motion in the proximal or distal part of the upper limb, or a decrease in muscle strength. As mentioned, cognitive impairment also has an effect. In other words, observing and analyzing the work and activities of the client throughout the upper limb function test is crucial for the evaluation and planning of rehabilitative treatments. The results of various upper limb and hand assessments can also be indicators for functional changes after OT interventions.

Technology-based methods for assessing sensory and motor functions

Other than conventional means of assessing sensory and motor functions, more advanced methods are also available for occupational therapists to quantifiably evaluate them. For sensory function assessment, there is the battery of quantitative sensory testing (QST) (Magerl et al., 2010; Rolke et al., 2006). This is a systematic test method to measure the sensory thresholds of tactile, pain, vibratory, and thermal sensations. The standardized procedure covers thermal testing, mechanical tactile detection, pain threshold and sensitivity, vibration detection threshold, pressure pain threshold, and temporal summation and is used to determine the levels of neuropathic pain experienced by clients with polyneuropathy or chronic osteoarthritis, for example.

More advanced motion systems, such as the VICON Motion Capture System (http://www.vicon.com/), are used to measure clients' range of motion, speed, and coordination in a three-dimensional space. Several video cameras are set up around the body parts in question to capture the client's movement during simple linear tasks (e.g., shoulder flexion) or complex tasks (e.g., picking up a cup from a table). Joint markers are placed on critical joints to measure the kinematics and kinetic data of the movements, with the motion-related data used to determine treatment effects across time.

Sensory interventions

Perception of sensation is the outcome of a sophisticated functional unit formed by the human hand and the brain. The hand is represented in the somatosensory cortex of the brain, with territorial divisions to receive impulses from specific areas of the hand. The results of numerous studies have shown that the territorial divisions can be changed by brain plasticity when prerequisites and demands for sensory input are changed, inducing functional reorganization. Various studies in monkeys have shown that direct recordings from the somatosensory cortex indicate experience-induced cortical remodeling following increased tactile stimulation of separate fingers. Additionally, rapid cortical reorganization in the somatosensory cortex was observed in adult primates as a result of altered sensory experiences and hand performance. Enlargement of the cortical areas of adult rats was shown after simultaneous tactile stimulation over the areas around the receptive fields of their paws. Similar results were also demonstrated in human subjects. Based on these results, it is believed that substantial functional reorganization changes occur in the brain immediately after a nerve injury in the upper extremity. The surrounding cortical areas will expand and invade the area that lacks sensory input, resulting in a distorted pattern. On the other hand, disorientation of regenerating axons at the repair site is often found after microsurgical nerve repair. This suggests that the skin areas of the hand lacking sensation will not be totally reinnervated by the original axons. Analogous findings have been observed in human subjects through investigation using functional magnetic resonance imaging (MRI) techniques. Hence, relearning is a crucial process in sensory re-education training (Rosén & Lundborg, 2011).

Phase 1 of sensory re-education training should start immediately after surgery on the nerve injury when there is no protective sensibility. Phase 2 should take place when the axons reach the area of the hand commonly characterized by hypersensitivity to normal touch. In Phase 1, there should be no sensation recovery in the hand. Sensory relearning is usually implemented together with mobilization training of the hand. Training focuses on maintaining the cortical representation of the hand in the somatosensory cortex of the brain by sensory imagery as well as visual-guided tactile stimulation, activating and maintaining the hand map in the brain.

Sensory imagery activates the sensory cortical areas. For instance, auditory cortical areas are activated when imagining music, while the visual cortex is active during visual imagery. Moreover, the activation of the somatosensory cortex during motor imagery is similar to the pattern observed during real movement. For example, thinking about stroking the fingertips activates the sensory cortex.

Another form of training is visual-guided tactile stimulation. This method stems from the known phenomenon that observing hand activity activates motor neurons, which may also serve as mirror neurons in the premotor cortex. The somatosensory cortical areas, SI and SII cortex, are related to the mirror neuron system; hence, observing a hand being touched can activate the somatosensory cortex. Parallel to these findings, it is suggested that a client's observation of his/her hand being touched is a significant form of early sensory training during the acute phase, facilitated through visual-tactile interaction. This method can be enhanced by using a mirror in the sensory training setup, where the injured hand is positioned behind the mirror, reflecting the image of the unaffected hand in the place of the injured one. When the client touches the unaffected hand, it creates an illusion of touching the injured hand as seen in the mirror, providing a perception of tactile stimuli in the insensate hand through the combined effects of the mirror illusion and the actual touch of the unaffected hand (Figure 3.15). This learning process should continue for three to four months following nerve repair surgery until measurable sensibility in the palm is detected (Rosén & Lundborg, 2011).

Phase 2 can begin when there is measurable sensibility recovered over the palmar area and some protective sensation with correct localization over the fingertip areas. Using objects of various shapes, textures, and thicknesses, clients can learn to identify with or without visual input. Examples of objects include fabrics of various textures, such as cotton, velvet, and hessian; various types of pasta; and coins of varying thicknesses and shapes. The aim of this exercise is to stimulate clients to identify objects with different characteristics at varying levels of difficulty. Using vision can aid training by providing visual guidance and gradually improving the impaired sensory perception in the hand and finger areas. Once a diminished protective sensation can be measured in the palmar area, training for touch localization (Figure 3.16a and b) can begin. Correctly localizing touch is essential for identifying objects without visual input, which is a crucial prerequisite for performing daily functions.

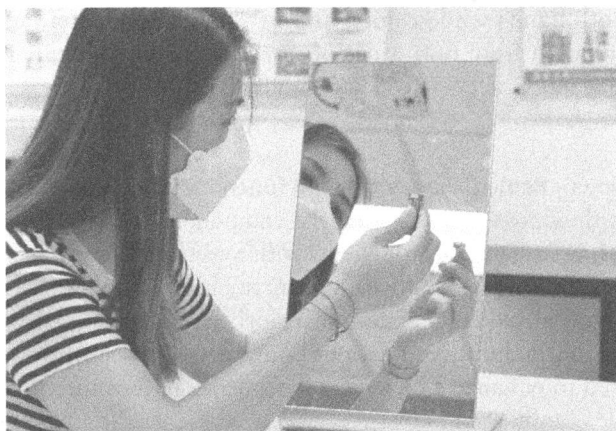

Figure 3.15 The unaffected hand touching a screw in front of a mirror, which gives the illusion of the injured hand behind the mirror touching the screw

Once touch localization improves, sensory relearning can be enhanced by incorporating familiar objects that clients use in their daily lives, thereby integrating the relearning process into their daily activities. For example, items such as door keys, earrings, and paper clips can be used in the relearning process. As clients regain moving and constant touch sensation in their fingers, training for object identification without visual input can be introduced to progressively increase the difficulty and effectiveness of the relearning progress. Furthermore, tactile stimulation can be applied to both hands simultaneously, as research has shown that improved tactile performance can transfer from a sensory-trained finger to the contralateral hand in humans. Sensory discrimination can occur across various skin locations, hemispheres, and modalities. To enhance the effectiveness of sensory re-education, actively using the hand in meaningful daily activities within an enriched environment can significantly benefit clients' relearning progress (Rosén & Lundborg, 2011). Examples of these meaningful daily activities include using both the affected and unaffected hands to wring out a towel dry during cleaning tasks, using forks and knives with both hands while eating, controlling

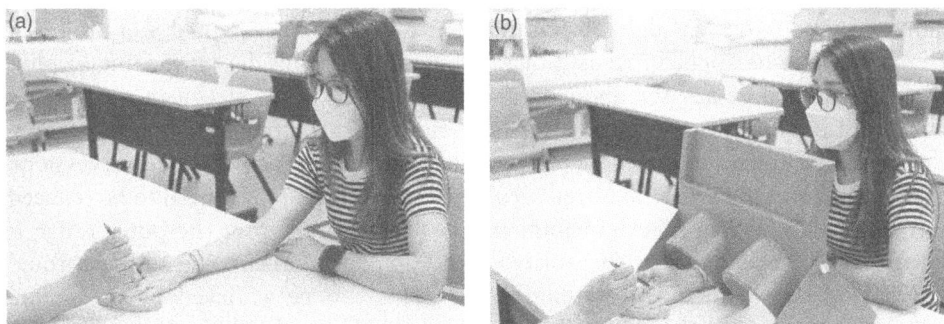

Figure 3.16 Localization training starts by allowing a client to visualize the location of the touch, trying to memorize the location assisted by visualization (a), and then identifying the location of the touch without visualization (b)

a bicycle with both hands while riding, and petting a furry puppy with both hands. This tactile stimulation from both sides of the hand during daily living activities can facilitate the relearning process (Rosén & Lundborg, 2011).

Motor interventions – Remedial activities and functional training

In accordance with approaches assessing the componential aspects of function before activity functions, OT treatments for clients with musculoskeletal conditions start with remedial activities, followed by a focus on functional mobility. These remedial activities aim to optimize specific aspects of musculoskeletal function, such as PROM and AROM, strength, and endurance in various body parts. Subsequently, functional training is implemented to enhance a client's independence in meaningful activities related to his/her life role (Amini et al., 2018).

Musculoskeletal training is based on a biomechanical frame of reference (Poole, 2009). Biomechanical approaches focus on the sequential training of four key aspects of function: maintaining joint range of motion, increasing joint range of motion, enhancing muscle strength, and improving muscle endurance. This means that the joint range of motion must be preserved before implementing treatments aimed at increasing it. Similarly, the joint range of motion should be maximized before considering muscle strengthening, followed by endurance training.

The aim of maintaining joint range of motion is to reduce pain, edema, and effusion related to the limitation of joint movement, and to prevent or minimize joint stiffness or muscle shortening. This helps to avoid contractures and deformities. When a client is unable to mobilize certain body parts, occupational therapists need to find ways to compensate for the lost functions of body parts to maximize the client's engagement in ADLs. If there is edema in the extremities, therapists should reduce it by elevating the affected areas and gently mobilizing the body parts to facilitate venous return. If the conditions allow, pressure should be applied manually, or a pressure garment can be used to reduce the diffused edema (Midgley & Pisano, 2020).

When the edema is under control, the joint with limited PROM should be mobilized passively to reach a maximum available length. Ballistic or so-called jerky stretching techniques should be avoided at all times as they may result in tissue damage. A prolonged hold will allow the motion to be repeated actively and is more effective than many repeated moves (Midgley & Pisano, 2020). If a more sustained and prolonged stretch needs to be applied, occupational therapists may consider fabricating a splint. The client should be advised about the concurrent pain in the stretched muscles and joints, and he/she will need to monitor the pain intensity after stretching has ceased. The stretching angle and time are optimal if the residual pain subsides one to two hours after treatment. Otherwise, the stretching range and duration may need to be reduced.

After the PROM of a certain joint has been increased from the outer range to the full range, occupational therapists should apply mobilization training through AROM together with muscle strengthening. This can be achieved by prescribing remedial activities for the client. Occupational therapists should implement motion analysis of specific movements in functional mobility to identify the primary joints and muscles, called prime movers, that clients need to enhance for specific ADLs. Two key concepts of dynamic movements are important when performing motion analysis: kinematics and the kinetics of movements (American Occupational Therapy Association, 2020):

- Kinematics refers to the study of motion in terms of displacement, velocity, and acceleration.
- Kinetics refers to the study of the direction and magnitude of force that generates the motion.

To maximize the AROM associated with kinematics, a remedial activity is needed to facilitate mobilization through the maximized joint range of motion. As for muscle strengthening associated with kinetics, the direction and magnitude of the muscle contraction of the prime mover(s) involved and the types of muscle contraction, in terms of isometric, isotonic concentric, isotonic eccentric, and isokinetic contractions, are outlined below:

- Isometric contraction occurs when the muscle contraction force is equal to the external force, resulting in an unchanged joint angle.
- Isotonic concentric contraction occurs when the magnitude of the muscle contraction is larger than the external force, leading to a decrease in the range of motion.
- Isotonic eccentric contraction occurs when the magnitude of the muscle contraction is less than the external force, resulting in an increase in the range of motion.

To promote muscle strength, the magnitude of the force the muscles need to exert should be at least 70–80% of the maximum muscle contraction, which is defined as the magnitude of force a muscle group could counteract not more than 10 times. The isometric contraction mode can be implemented for joint-related injuries (e.g., elbow joint dislocation) before advancing to the isotonic contraction mode. For the two types of isotonic contraction, concentric contraction is more intuitive for clients to increase their muscle strength. This mode of contraction is also relatively safer for the muscles as the direction of the muscle fiber shortening and the joint movement are the same. In contrast, eccentric contraction would need to be performed with control and attention as the muscle fibers elongate while the joint opens up due to the larger external force. Thus, muscles are more prone to injury if the action is not performed in a controlled and slower manner. The advantage of eccentric contraction is that it can induce better muscle tone and muscle bulge growth (Roig et al., 2009). When a client needs to enhance endurance, the magnitude of the force could be brought down to 50–60% of the maximum muscle contraction so that the motion could be performed continuously for 15 minutes or more to have a therapeutic endurance effect.

For example, when a client requires moderate assistance in self-feeding, the occupational therapist needs to apply motion analysis to identify whether the functional impairment is due to the limited active range of shoulder flexion and muscle weakness. The therapist will prescribe a remedial activity called "shoulder board" to promote an AROM (kinetics) of the flexion and extension of muscle prime movers, i.e., anterior deltoid and pectoralis major. When the shoulder joint moves in the shoulder flexion direction, this is known as muscle contraction. When the shoulder joint moves in the extension direction, this is known as eccentric contraction. Since the feeding activity requires the client to mobilize the upper extremity for a prolonged period of time, the weight for the client to counteract during the shoulder board remedial activity could be adjusted to 50% of the maximum muscle contraction. This will help to enhance the endurance of the muscles involved.

After the range of motion, strength, and endurance have been optimized through remediation training, functional training could be implemented for clients with musculoskeletal conditions. Similar to the ADL assessments, occupational therapists must provide training environments that are as close to the real-life situation as possible. The choice of the ADL tasks should also be specific to the needs of the client's life role. Basic ADL training would be done first at the bedside, including feeding, grooming, and upper and lower dressing, as the client can be positioned relatively safely on the bed or in a chair. The occupational therapist can create a safe and simulated environment for the client before initiating the training session. This includes applying a splint or prosthesis to ensure proper positioning for the client. If the joint range of motion or muscle strength is not fully functioning, various levels of physical assistance will need to be provided by the occupational therapist. A proper seating system may be required for those who are not independent sitters. If residual physical impairments remain after a reasonable period of functional training, occupational therapists may consider taking a compensatory approach to optimize the client's independence in ADLs. Various assistive devices can be used to maximize the client's engagement and independence during ADL training, such as plate guards and universal cuffed utensils for feeding, enlarged-handled toothbrushes for grooming, and long-handled reachers for lower garment dressing.

Transfer training for bed mobility and transitions between surfaces, such as from bed to chair, toilet, or bathtub, can be conducted after ADL training. The selection of transfer training types is based on the client's muscle strength, as shown in Table 3.8. Prior to transfer training, the occupational therapist must prepare the environment for a particular transfer type, including the height of the transfer and sufficient space for lower limb positioning. Additionally, any necessary assistive devices, such as a wheelchair and transfer board, should be ready before the transfer is performed. The therapist may need to provide physical support to various parts of the client's body, such as the pelvis and shoulders, while positioning himself/herself optimally in relation to the client's movements. For instance, when assisting with a front transfer where the client is in a long-seat posture, the therapist should stand behind the client. On the other hand, during a side transfer with the client in a short-seat position, the therapist should stand in front of the client. During transfer training, occupational therapists should minimize the distance between themselves and the client to avoid overloading their back muscles while keeping a professional distance (Johansson & Chinworth, 2018a, 2018b).

Table 3.8 Types of transfer method in relation to the relative muscle strength of various parts of the body

	UL	Trunk	LL
Dependent transfer using mobile hoist	0–2	0–2	0–2
Front transfer	4–5	0–3	0–2
Side transfer without lower limb strength	4–5	3–4	0–2
Side transfer with lower limb strength	3–5	3–4	3–4
Pivot transfer	2–5	3–4	4

Abbreviations: UL = upper extremity; LL = lower extremity.

After maximizing a client's functional mobility performance related to musculo-skeletal conditions, the therapist should apply these skills to daily living activities. The occupational therapist should implement occupation-based practice by identifying the significant daily activities related to the client's life role. For example, an elderly client with muscle strength of 3+ may need to use the pivot transfer technique for bed-to-chair transfer and toilet transfer with assistance from his/her carer to maintain his/her daily routine as a self-maintainer. As a part of the daily routine, he/she would also need to apply the pivot transfer technique when getting into the backseat of a taxi to visit family or when going on a day out to the countryside. Thus, an occupational therapist's role is to understand the functional recovery potential of a client with sensorimotor impairments through organized assessments in order to provide sensorimotor training to maximize sensorimotor recovery. Functional and occupation-based interventions need to be provided for clients so that they can fulfill their daily life roles.

Case study of a client with median nerve and wrist flexor injuries

Ms. X, aged 18, is a right-handed secondary school student. She cut her left wrist using her right hand after a quarrel with her boyfriend. She was transferred to the Accident and Emergency Department of a regional hospital and was diagnosed to have lacer-ated her wrist flexor tendons, including the flexor carpi radialis, palmaris longus, and median nerve of her left wrist. Surgical repair was done to the lacerated tendons and nerves. Ms. X was referred to the Occupational Therapy Department for splinting and a three-day rehabilitation program after the surgery. The OT assessments and treatments during the acute phase are illustrated in Table 3.9. Examples of information to be written down in the clinical record are also illustrated.

Upon completion of the assessment, Ms. X reported that she did not perceive any touch sensation stimulated by either of the four assessment items. The reported results were expected since the regeneration of the nerve would only start three weeks after repair. Yet, the assessment results provided the baseline information for comparison with the results of subsequent assessments. Apart from the threshold detection test, Tinel's sign was elicited by the therapist gently tapping his finger from the distal to the proximal direction within the insensate area. Ms. X reported a tingling sensation shoot-ing towards the index and middle fingers when the therapist tapped over the sutured site of the wrist region, corresponding to the repaired nerve site. All the assessment results were documented in the client's record for future reference.

Regular motor-sensory assessments can be done once every two to three weeks dur-ing the splinting and mobilization program. The same sensory assessment items were used until Ms. X could perceive the minimal threshold (= 6.65) of the monofilament.

Quiz 1

Which kind of splinting regime is best for Ms. X?

What is the advice for splint care, safety precautions, and adaptive measures in ADLs?

What kind of active and passive finger mobilization should Ms. X perform?

When should Ms. X start sensory relearning activities?

Table 3.9 OT assessments and treatments for Ms. X during the acute phase

Timeline of OT process	OT process	Rehabilitation process
Before the initial assessment after the surgery.	Retrieve basic information related to the surgery.	Details of the surgery records include: ■ clinical diagnosis, ■ date of surgery, ■ bodily structures repaired/fixated, ■ suturing/fixation techniques, and ■ any special attention/precaution remarked by doctors in charge.
Acute phase During the first assessment session around three to four days post flexor tendon and median nerve repair.	(1) Conduct interview: collect basic information related to the client's premorbid background.	Premorbid information includes: ■ job background (e.g., secondary school student), ■ life roles (e.g., student role), ■ leisure pursuits (e.g., playing computer games, shopping, etc.), and ■ peer and family support (e.g., whether Ms. X is staying with her family or elsewhere).
	(2) Assess the wound: describe the observed wound conditions (e.g., wound clean with stitches in-situ, mild clear oozing from wound), swelling status (e.g., generalized swelling over the whole hand, localized swelling over the wrist region), etc.	Change wound dressing from bulky to light dressing if client's boxing glove is kept in-situ, a necessary preparation for the consequent splint fabrication process. Remarks: Check if there are abnormal signs over the surgical wound, such as bad odor, yellowish oozing, etc. Inform ward nurse for instant follow-up.
	(3) Fabricate a splint for commencing the tendon and nerve rehabilitation program.	(1) Follow the tendon and nerve rehabilitation program protocol to fabricate a dorsal-blocked splint for early finger motion. (For example, a cock-down splint with wrist immobilized at 20-degree flexion is provided.) (2) Give advice on finger passive and active mobilization regime within splint, splinting regime, splint care, safety precautions, and adaptive measures in daily living task performance. (For example, a 24-hour splinting regime is suggested. Maintain elevation. Do not take out splint during shower/ bath. Mobilize the shoulder on the ipsilateral side to prevent potential stiffness formation.)

Table 3.9 OT assessments and treatments for Ms. X during the acute phase (*continued*)

Timeline of OT process	OT process	Rehabilitation process
	(4) Briefly assess active finger motion and advise on gentle passive finger flexion within splint.	(1) Assess active finger motion within splint, tracing the gliding action of the repaired tendon of the involved fingers by observing the change in range of motion of the interphalangeal joints.
		(2) Advise on gentle passive finger flexion of the involved fingers within the splint to maintain joint flexibility. (For example, advise to keep active mobilization of fingers with splint on. Passive motion over the finger joints is required to maintain suppleness of the finger joints.)
	(5) Briefly assess sensibility over the median nerve dermatome distal to the sutured area.	Sensibility assessment items include: ■ Tinel's sign test, ■ cotton wool ball, ■ neurotip, and ■ monofilament (threshold 6.65). Remarks: Demonstration of the assessment process is done over another of Ms. X's fingers with normal sensation to allow Ms. X to observe the assessment process and to perceive the normal sensation input she is expected to feel over the insensate area. (For example, Tinel's sign test: examined right over the sutured line area; unable to perceive a cotton wool ball, nor hot/cold temperature.)

Two months (or eight weeks) after the surgery, Ms. X confidently reported that she perceived the pressure stimulated by the monofilament over the proximal part of her right thenar eminence area, and the Tinel's sign migrated one centimeter distally. Yet, weak thumb abduction and opposition, as well as poor finger flexion over the radial three fingers, were reported. Ms. X reported that she struggled to make a full fist and was unable to abduct and oppose her thumb. She was barely able to hold a water bottle tightly or turn the key when opening the door of her residential flat. She was then prescribed graded strengthening activities to enhance her hand function strength and Phase 2 of sensory relearning process was started.

Quiz 2

During week 4 to week 6:

Which kinds of gentle non-resistive remedial activities can you prescribe to Ms. X?
What is the appropriate tendon gliding exercise that Ms. X should perform?

During week 7 to week 9:

Which kinds of graded strengthening remedial activities can you prescribe to Ms. X?
What are the items that you can use in Phase 2 of the sensory relearning process?

From post-surgery week 8 onwards, steady progress was noted, and the strengthening activities and sensory relearning process continued with graded enhancement. Thumb abduction and opposition strength gradually improved. A full fist was observed, and Ms. X was able to hold a lightweight water bottle tightly. Repeated sensation assessment results showed an improving trend with Tinel's sign migrating three centimeters distally to the wrist crease. The OT assessments and treatments during the subacute phase are illustrated in Table 3.10.

Quiz 3

During the pre-discharge phase:

What are the most appropriate items you can use for object recognition training?
How can you determine the correct timing of Ms. X's discharge from the rehabilitation program?

During the pre-discharge phase of Ms. X's rehabilitation, the sensibility assessment results showed that a diminished light touch sensation (monofilament threshold 3.22) was found over Ms. X's proximal half of the radial palm as well as the radial half of her ring finger, whereas a diminished protective sensation (monofilament threshold 4.08) was detected over the thumb, index, and middle fingers. Tinel's sign faded out and was undetectable. In view of this improving sensation status, a two-point discrimination was performed over Ms. X's thumb, index, and middle fingers, starting from 8 mm in width. After assessment, Ms. X confidently reported that she could discriminate between one point and two points ranging from 11 to 13 mm in width over the affected fingers, indicating a good sign of recovery of discriminative sensibility over the involved fingertips. By the time Ms. X could recognize all the familiar items she used daily, together with the competent performances she demonstrated in other hand function tests and work capacity evaluation, she was discharged from the rehabilitation program. Periodic follow-up appointments were arranged to continue monitoring Ms. X's progress. The OT assessments and treatments during the pre-discharge phase are shown in Table 3.11.

Table 3.10 OT assessments and treatments for Ms. X during the subacute phase

Timeline of OT process	OT process	Rehabilitation process
Subacute phase Around four to six weeks post flexor tendon and median nerve repair.	(1) Start gentle active finger mobilization and wrist motion at week 5. (2) Continue Phase 1 sensory relearning process.	(1) Start gentle active finger mobilization and educate on tendon gliding exercise. (2) Start gentle non-resistive wrist motion at week 5 through remedial activities. (3) Design gentle non-resistive remedial activities to enhance functional pinch performance. (4) Continue sensory relearning activities through imagery and with various tactile items.
Around seven to nine weeks until 12 weeks post flexor tendon and median nerve repair.	(1) Start graded strengthening of finger and wrist motion. (2) Start Phase 2 sensory relearning process.	(1) Prescribe graded strengthening remedial activities to improve strength of thumb abduction/opposition, finger flexion, and wrist motion. (2) Start Phase 2 sensory relearning when deep pressure sensation is assessed. (3) Start desensitization if hypersensitivity over the affected sensory areas is reported.

Table 3.11 OT assessments and treatments for Ms. X during the pre-discharge phase

Timeline of OT process	OT process	Rehabilitation process
Pre-discharge phase Around 12 weeks post flexor tendon and median nerve repair.	(1) Start work evaluation and hardening program to facilitate resumption of previous work. (2) Progress to Phase 3 of the sensory relearning process, i.e., object recognition.	(1) Conduct job analysis and design simulated work capacity evaluation and hardening program according to the problems identified. (2) Start object recognition training once the touch location ability recovers, with improving results of discriminative sensibility assessments.

Answers for Quiz 1

By the end of the first rehabilitation session, advice has been provided on the gentle mobilization of the involved fingers as well as the proximal uninvolved joints, special splint care, and adaptive measures in self-care. In addition, Ms. X was advised to start Phase 1 of the sensory relearning process. It was suggested that she observe and touch her right fingers and thumb with her left hand at least five to six times a day to provide tactile stimulation to the area. Moreover, she was advised to imagine the daily living tasks performed by her right hand, including the way she held a pen to do homework or held chopsticks during meals. Integrating a mirror in her home exercise was another home activity for Ms. X. By looking in the mirror, with or without putting a functional item in her hand, the image of the unaffected hand became an illusion for the affected hand to enhance the reorganization of the somatosensory cortex in the brain. She was also advised to keep her right hand away from extreme temperatures and sharp objects to avoid unnecessary injuries.

Answers for Quiz 2

Along with the favorable progress, Ms. X was given objects of various shapes and textures to start Phase 2 of the sensory relearning process for object recognition. For instance, materials such as fabrics of various textures and shapes were provided. She was advised to observe and touch the textures and identify the various shapes and thicknesses of the objects. She was told to use both her right and left hands to touch the materials during home training. A gradual increase in the level of difficulty required her to name the texture and shape of the fabrics without visual input. Regular assessment results showed a steady improvement from unrecognizable or false locations to correct locations.

Answers for Quiz 3

At this stage, training on object recognition continued with the items changed to those Ms. X felt familiar with in her daily living, such as her door keys, paper clips used during homework, earrings, rings, etc. The difficulty level was raised when Ms. X was instructed to repeat her training without visual input at a later stage. Her ability at object recognition was timed without visual input during the assessment to monitor her progress.

Conclusion

This chapter outlines the principles and skills involved in sensorimotor assessments and treatments for occupational therapists to use when prescribing interventions for clients with related dysfunctions. It begins by reviewing the client's medical history, followed by an interview and physical and functional examinations. The "Look-Feel-Move" principles are introduced to guide an organized and systematic assessment approach.

Several commonly used sensory-related and motor-related assessments are presented, along with discussions of up-to-date assessment methods, such as the motion system. In the section on Sensory Interventions, a variety of sensory training approaches and assessment methods aimed at optimizing sensory functions in clients with musculoskeletal and neurological conditions are described. For motor interventions, the concepts of remedial activities and functional training are explained. To illustrate how different assessments and intervention approaches can be applied in clinical settings, a case study of a client with nerve and tendon injuries is included, consolidating the assessment and intervention strategies for clients with sensorimotor dysfunctions.

Notes

1 A dermatome is the cutaneous area, an area of skin supplied by one spinal nerve, through both rami, or by a single posterior nerve root and its ganglion or one spinal cord segment, or the tissue within a somite that forms part of the dermis (Lee et al., 2008).
2 Tactilegnosis refers to the sensibility present in the fingertip being sufficient to permit the perception of neural impulses as a meaningful conscious perception, i.e., functional sensation, or the ability to discriminate the qualities of texture (King, 1997).

References

Aaron, D. H., & Jansen, C. W. (2003). Development of the Functional Dexterity Test (FDT): Construction, validity, reliability, and normative data. *Journal of Hand Therapy*, 16(1), 12–21. https://doi.org/10.1016/s0894-1130(03)80019-4

American Occupational Therapy Association (2008). Occupational therapy practice framework: Domain & process 2nd edition. *American Journal of Occupational Therapy*, 62(6), 625–683.

American Occupational Therapy Association. (2020). Occupational therapy practice framework: Domain and process, 4th edition. *American Journal of Occupational Therapy*, 74(Suppl. 2), 7412410010p1–7412410010p87.

American Society of Hand Therapists. (1992). *Clinical assessment recommendations* (2nd ed.). American Society of Hand Therapists.

Amini, D., Lieberman, D., & Hunter, E. (2018). Occupational therapy interventions for adults with musculoskeletal conditions. *American Journal of Occupational Therapy*, 72(4), 7204390010p1–7204390010p5. https://doi.org/10.5014/ajot.2018.724001

Amirjani, N., Ashworth, N. L., Olson, J. L., Morhart, M., & Chan, K. M. (2011). Validity and reliability of the Purdue Pegboard Test in carpal tunnel syndrome. *Muscle & Nerve*, 43(2), 171–177. https://doi.org/10.1002/mus.21856

Bachman, G., Ivy, C., Wright, D., Hightower, T., Welsh, A., Velleman, P., & Gray, S. (2023). The Functional Dexterity Test in adult populations: An exploration of a simplified test protocol and parameters guided by statistical outcomes. *Journal of Hand Therapy*, S0894-1130(23)00128-X. Advance online publication. https://doi.org/10.1016/j.jht.2023.09.001

Baron, R., Binder, A., & Wasner, G. (2010). Neuropathic pain: Diagnosis, pathophysiological mechanisms, and treatment. *The Lancet. Neurology*, 9(8), 807–819. https://doi.org/10.1016/S1474-4422(10)70143-5

Bell-Krotoski, J. (2011). Sensibility testing: History, instrumentation, and clinical procedures. In T. M. Skirven, A. L. Osterman, J. M. Fedorczyk, & P. C. Amadio (Eds.), *Rehabilitation of the hand and upper extremity* (6th ed., pp. 132–151). Elsevier Mosby.

Bell-Krotoski, J., Weinstein, S., & Weinstein, C. (1993). Testing sensibility, including touch-pressure, two-point discrimination, point localization, and vibration. *Journal of Hand Therapy*, 6(2), 114–123. https://doi.org/10.1016/S0894-1130(12)80292-4

Bell-Krotoski, J. A., & Buford, W. L. Jr (1997). The force/time relationship of clinically used sensory testing instruments. *Journal of Hand Therapy*, 10(4), 297–309. https://doi.org/10.1016/s0894-1130(97)80045-2

Berger, M. A. M., Krul, A. J., & Daanen, H. A. M. (2009). Task specificity of finger dexterity tests. *Applied Ergonomics*, 40(1), 145–147. https://doi.org/10.1016/j.apergo.2008.01.014

Borstad, A. L., & Nichols-Larsen, D. S. (2014). Assessing and treating higher level somatosensory impairments post stroke. *Topics in Stroke Rehabilitation*, 21(4), 290–295. https://doi.org/10.1310/tsr2104-290

Causby, R., Reed, L., McDonnell, M., & Hillier, S. (2014). Use of objective psychomotor tests in health professionals. *Perceptual & Motor Skills*, 118(3), 765–804. https://doi.org/10.2466/25.27.PMS.118k27w2

Cavalli, E., Mammana, S., Nicoletti, F., Bramanti, P., & Mazzon, E. (2019). The neuropathic pain: An overview of the current treatment and future therapeutic approaches. *International Journal of Immunopathology and Pharmacology*, 33, 2058738419838383. https://doi.org/10.1177/2058738419838383

Chen, L., Ogalo, E., Haldane, C., Bristol, S. G., & Berger, M. J. (2021). Relationship between sensibility tests and functional outcomes in patients with traumatic upper limb nerve injuries: A systematic review. *Archives of Rehabilitation Research and Clinical Translation*, 3(4), 100159. https://doi.org/10.1016/j.arrct.2021.100159

Clarkson, H. M. (2013). *Musculoskeletal assessment: Joint motion and muscle testing* (3rd ed.). Wolters Kluwer/Lippincott Williams & Wilkins.

Estorninho, M., Cheang, S. K., Chan, S. I., Ieong, K. I., Lam, C. U., & Liu, K. P. Y. (2022). Finger dexterity in well-functioning cohort of office workers in Macau. *Hong Kong Journal of Occupational Therapy*, 35(2), 154–158. https://doi.org/10.1177/15691861221114258

Fabbri, B., Berardi, A., Tofani, M., Panuccio, F., Ruotolo, I., Sellitto, G., & Galeoto, G. (2021). A systematic review of the psychometric properties of the Jebsen-Taylor Hand Function Test (JTHFT). *Hand Surgery and Rehabilitation*, 40(5), 560–567. https://doi.org/10.1016/j.hansur.2021.05.004

Freynhagen, R., Baron, R., Gockel, U., & Tölle, T. R. (2006). painDETECT: A new screening questionnaire to identify neuropathic components in patients with back pain. *Current Medical Research and Opinion*, 22(10), 1911–1920. https://doi.org/10.1185/030079906X132488

Gloss, D. S., & Wardle, M. G. (1982). Use of the Minnesota Rate of Manipulation Test for disability evaluation. *Perceptual and Motor Skills*, 55(2), 527–532. https://doi.org/10.2466/pms.1982.55.2.527

Grice, K. O., Vogel, K. A., Le, V., Mitchell, A., Muniz, S., & Vollmer, M. A. (2003). Adult norms for a commercially available Nine Hole Peg Test for finger dexterity. *American Journal of Occupational Therapy*, 57(5), 570–573.

Jebsen, R. H., Taylor, N., Trieschmann, R. B., Trotter, M. J., & Howard, L. A. (1969). An objective and standardized test of hand function. *Archives of Physical Medicine and Rehabilitation*, 50(6), 311–319.

Jerosch-Herold, C., Houghton, J., Miller, L., & Shepstone, L. (2016). A pragmatic, assessor-blinded, randomized trial of the clinical effectiveness of a 6-week sensory relearning home program on tactile function of the hand after carpal tunnel decompression. *Hand*, 11(1 Suppl.), 132S–133S. https://doi.org/10.1177/1558944716660555je

Johansson, C., & Chinworth, S. A. (2018a). Bed mobility. In C. Johansson, & S. A. Chinworth (Eds.), *Mobility in context: Principles of patient care skills* (2nd ed., pp. 263–284). F.A. Davis Company.

Johansson, C., & Chinworth, S. A. (2018b). Manual lateral transfers: Seated and pivot. In C. Johansson, & S. A. Chinworth (Eds.), *Mobility in context: Principles of patient care skills* (2nd ed., pp. 285–334). F.A. Davis Company.

King, P. M. (1997). Sensory function assessment: A pilot comparison study of touch pressure threshold with texture and tactile discrimination. *Journal of Hand Therapy*, 10(1), 24–28. https://doi.org/10.1016/S0894-1130(97)80007-5

Kita, K., Otaka, Y., Takeda, K., Sakata, S., Ushiba, J., Kondo, K., Liu, M., & Osu, R. (2013). A pilot study of sensory feedback by transcutaneous electrical nerve stimulation to improve manipulation deficit caused by severe sensory loss after stroke. *Journal of NeuroEngineering and Rehabilitation*, 10, 55. https://doi.org/10.1186/1743-0003-10-55

Lee, M. W. L., McPhee, R. W., & Stringer, M. D. (2008). An evidence-based approach to human dermatomes. *Clinical Anatomy*, 21(5), 363–373. https://doi.org/10.1002/ca.20636

Lincoln, N. B., Jackson, J. M., & Adams, S. A. (1998). Reliability and revision of the Nottingham Sensory Assessment for stroke patients. *Physiotherapy, 84*(8), 358–365. https://doi.org/10.1016/S0031-9406(05)61454-X

Lindstrom-Hazel, D. K., & Veenstra, N. V. (2015). Examining the Purdue Pegboard Test for occupational therapy practice. *The Open Journal of Occupational Therapy, 3*(3), 5. https://doi.org/10.15453/2168-6408.1178

Li-Tsang, C. W. P., Chan, S. C. C., Chan, S. Y. Y., & Soo, A. K. W. (2004). The Hong Kong Chinese version of the Jebsen Hand Function Test: Inter-rater and test-retest reliabilities. *Hong Kong Journal of Occupational Therapy, 14*(1), 12–20. https://doi.org/10.1016/S1569-1861(09)70024-5

Magerl, W., Krumova, E. K., Baron, R., Tölle, T., Treede, R.-D., & Maier, C. (2010). Reference data for quantitative sensory testing (QST): Refined stratification for age and a novel method for statistical comparison of group data. *Pain, 151*(3), 598–605. https://doi.org/10.1016/j.pain.2010.07.026

Mathiowetz, V., Volland, G., Kashman, N., & Weber, K. (1985). Adult norms for the Box and Block Test of manual dexterity. *American Journal of Occupational Therapy, 39*(6), 386–391.

Meseguer-Henarejos, A. B., Sánchez-Meca, J., López-Pina, J. A., & Carles-Hernández, R. (2018). Inter- and intra-rater reliability of the Modified Ashworth Scale: A systematic review and meta-analysis. *European Journal of Physical and Rehabilitation Medicine, 54*(4), 576–590. https://doi.org/10.23736/S1973-9087.17.04796-7

Midgley, R., & Pisano, K. (2020). Therapist's management of the stiff hand. In T. M. Skirven, A. L. Osterman, J. M. Fedorczyk, P. C. Amadio, S. B. Feldscher, & E. K. Shin (Eds.), *Rehabilitation of the hand and upper extremity* (7th ed., pp. 372–392). Elsevier.

Monrad, S. U., Zeller, J. L., Craig, C. L., & DiPonio, L. A. (2011). Musculoskeletal education in US medical schools: Lessons from the past and suggestions for the future. *Current Reviews in Musculoskeletal Medicine, 4*(3), 91–98. https://doi.org/10.1007/s12178-011-9083-x

Ng, C. L., Ho, D. D., & Chow, S. P. (1999). The Moberg pickup test: Results of testing with a standard protocol. *Journal of Hand Therapy, 12*(4), 309–312. https://doi.org/10.1016/s0894-1130(99)80069-6

Pike, S., Lannin, N. A., Wales, K., & Cusick, A. (2018). A systematic review of the psychometric properties of the Action Research Arm Test in neurorehabilitation. *Australian Occupational Therapy Journal, 65*(5), 449–471. https://doi.org/10.1111/1440-1630.12527

Poole, J. L. (2009). Musculoskeletal factors. In E. B. Crepeau, E. S. Cohn, & B. A. B. Schell (Eds.), *Willard & Spackman's occupational therapy* (11th ed., pp. 658–680). Lippincott Williams & Wilkins.

Prochaska, E., & Ammenwerth, E. (2023). A digital Box and Block Test for hand dexterity measurement: Instrument validation study. *JMIR Rehabilitation and Assistive Technologies, 10*, e50474. https://doi.org/10.2196/50474

Proud, E. L., Miller, K. J., Bilney, B., Morris, M. E., & McGinley, J. L. (2020). Construct validity of the 9-Hole Peg Test and Purdue Pegboard Test in people with mild to moderately severe Parkinson's disease. *Physiotherapy, 107*, 202–208. https://doi.org/10.1016/j.physio.2019.12.002

Roig, M., O'Brien, K., Kirk, G., Murray, R., McKinnon, P., Shadgan, B., & Reid, W. D. (2009). The effects of eccentric versus concentric resistance training on muscle strength and mass in healthy adults: A systematic review with meta-analysis. *British Journal of Sports Medicine, 43*(8), 556–568. https://doi.org/10.1136/bjsm.2008.051417

Rolke, R., Magerl, W., Campbell, K. A., Schalber, C., Caspari, S., Birklein, F., & Treede, R.-D. (2006). Quantitative sensory testing: A comprehensive protocol for clinical trials. *European Journal of Pain, 10*(1), 77–88. https://doi.org/10.1016/j.ejpain.2005.02.003

Rosén, B., & Lundborg, G. (2011). Sensory reeducation. In T. M. Skirven, A. L. Osterman, J. M. Fedorczyk, & P. C. Amadio (Eds.), *Rehabilitation of the hand and upper extremity* (6th ed., pp. 634–645). Elsevier Mosby.

Sartorio, F., Negro, F. D., Bravini, E., Ferriero, G., Corna, S., Invernizzi, M., & Vercelli, S. (2020). Relationship between nerve conduction studies and the Functional Dexterity Test in workers with carpal tunnel syndrome. *BMC Musculoskeletal Disorders, 21*(1), 679. https://doi.org/10.1186/s12891-020-03651-1

Soares, M. M., Souza, P. C., & Ribeiro, A. P. (2023). Differences in clinical tests for assessing lateral epicondylitis elbow in adults concerning their physical activity level: Test reliability, accuracy of ultrasound imaging, and relationship with energy expenditure. *International Journal of Environmental Research and Public Health*, 20(3), 1794. https://doi.org/10.3390/ijerph20031794

Solaro, C., Di Giovanni, R., Grange, E., Mueller, M., Messmer Uccelli, M., Bertoni, R., Brichetto, G., Tacchino, A., Patti, F., Pappalardo, A., Prosperini, L., Castelli, L., Rosato, R., Cattaneo, D., & Marengo, D. (2020). Box and block test, hand grip strength and nine-hole peg test: Correlations between three upper limb objective measures in multiple sclerosis. *European Journal of Neurology*, 27(12), 2523–2530. https://doi.org/10.1111/ene.14427

Tiffin, J., & Asher, E. J. (1948). The Purdue Pegboard: Norms and studies of reliability and validity. *Journal of Applied Psychology*, 32(3), 234–247. https://doi.org/10.1037/h0061266

Wang, Y. C., Bohannon, R. W., Kapellusch, J., Garg, A., & Gershon, R. C. (2015). Dexterity as measured with the 9-Hole Peg Test (9-HPT) across the age span. *Journal of Hand Therapy*, 28(1), 53–60. http://dx.doi.org/10.1016/j.jht.2014.09.002

Wang, Y. C., Wickstrom, R., Yen, S. C., Kapellusch, J., & Grogan, K. A. (2018). Assessing manual dexterity: Comparing the WorkAbility Rate of Manipulation Test with the Minnesota Manual Dexterity Test. *Journal of Hand Therapy*, 31(3), 339–347. https://doi.org/10.1016/j.jht.2017.03.009

Yamakawa, I., Yamada, A., Sonoda, Y., Wakita, K., Nishioka, T., Harada, Y., Ogawa, N., Kitamura, A., Sanada, M., Tani, T., Imai, S., & Urushitani, M. (2023). Occupational therapy using a robotic-assisted glove ameliorates finger dexterity and modulates functional connectivity in amyotrophic lateral sclerosis. *Journal of Clinical Neuroscience*, 107, 144–149. https://doi.org/10.1016/j.jocn.2022.11.004

Yozbatiran, N., Der-Yeghiaian, L., & Cramer, S. C. (2008). A standardized approach to performing the Action Research Arm Test. *Neurorehabilitation and Neural Repair*, 22(1), 78–90. https://doi.org/10.1177/1545968307305353

CHAPTER 4

Cognitive perceptual functioning

David Wai Kwong Man, Frank Ho-Yin Lai,
and Kenneth Nai-Kuen Fong

Effects of cognitive challenges from acquired brain injury on daily functioning

Acquired brain injury (ABI) refers to any brain injury that occurs after birth and can be caused by various factors such as traumatic brain injury, stroke, brain tumors, or infections. Individuals with ABI often experience a wide range of cognitive and perceptual challenges that significantly affect their daily functioning, limit their activities, and reduce their participation in various aspects of life.

Cognitive perceptual problems encompass challenges in areas such as visual perception, spatial awareness, attention, memory, and problem-solving. These difficulties greatly affect an individual's ability to perform everyday tasks and engage in meaningful activities, leading to limitations in activities and reduced participation (Brown & Gordon, 2013; Dawson & Chipchase, 2015).

Activity limitations refer to difficulties or restrictions in performing specific tasks or actions, while participation restrictions refer to limitations in engaging in life situations and fulfilling societal roles. For example, individuals with ABI may struggle to recognize objects or faces, judge distances, maintain focus, remember important information, or solve problems in complex situations. These cognitive perceptual problems can lead to challenges in self-care, work, leisure activities, and social participation, ultimately affecting overall occupational performance (Radomski & Trombly Latham, 2014; Schaber & Lieberman, 2010).

However, by addressing these challenges and implementing appropriate strategies and interventions, occupational therapists can play a crucial role in helping individuals with cognitive perceptual problems regain independence, enhance their participation in daily activities, and improve their overall quality of life.

Enhancing assessment and evaluation of cognitive and perceptual functioning

Assessment is the process of gathering information, while evaluation involves interpreting and making judgments based on that information. Both assessment and evaluation are crucial for understanding cognitive and perceptual functioning in individuals with ABI, identifying areas of difficulty, and determining appropriate interventions or support strategies. When assessing and evaluating an individual's cognitive and perceptual status, occupational therapists should demonstrate good observational skills and take a holistic approach. The process begins with a comprehensive review of the individual's medical history, including the location of the brain injury, pre-existing conditions, and discharge plans. Chart information and interviews provide initial personal, medical, mental status, and psychosocial data. These factors help determine the individual's age, educational background, work history, and orientation responses, which guide the selection of appropriate tests and evaluation activities.

Cognitive assessment can be categorized as either formal, standardized, or non-flexible tests or informal, non-standardized, or flexible tests (Coelho et al., 2005; Uomoto, 1992). Formal or standardized tests are valuable for identifying problems and evaluating treatment effectiveness at various stages of recovery/rehabilitation. Commonly used formal tests include paper-and-pencil tests, criterion-referenced tests, and standardized cognitive-perceptual tests such as the Rivermead Perceptual Assessment Battery (RPAB), Rivermead Behavioural Memory Test (RBMT), Mini-Mental State Examination (MMSE), and Montreal Cognitive Assessment (MoCA). Additionally, digital testing or computerized assessment, such as the Vienna Test System (VTS online or offline mode; www.schuhfried.com/vienna-test-system/), can be employed for cognitive and perceptual assessment. Informal or flexible tests complement formal tests by allowing therapists to adapt tasks and procedures based on available information and their own expertise. This approach focuses on how an individual performs a task instead of just measuring success or failure, facilitating ongoing evaluation and personalized intervention. Simulation tasks can also be developed to target an individual's specific cognitive and perceptual deficits.

In addition to cognitive and perceptual factors, occupational therapists need to consider the interplay between sensorimotor, psychosocial, and environmental aspects when observing and evaluating individuals with ABI. For example, before administering a cognitive and perceptual evaluation, it is important to assess the individual's visual, tactile, and auditory abilities. Visual field, acuity, and range of motion should be examined to rule out any visual impairments before conducting visual perceptual tests. Motor performance demands, such as upper extremity strength and functional mobility, should also be taken into account to ensure accurate and safe measurements. The impact of poor postural control and balance on cognitive-perceptual evaluation should not be overlooked. Observing an individual's psychosocial behavior in a home or work environment during a task can provide insights into their cognitive and perceptual functioning. Furthermore, personal factors such as fatigue, depression, anxiety, and pain can significantly affect cognitive test performance.

In summary, occupational therapists should consider individuals' primary senses before conducting cognitive and perceptual assessments. The combined use of standardized and non-flexible tests, as well as non-standardized and flexible tests, along with tailored behavioral and situational assessments, greatly enhances the validity and reliability of the evaluation process. When evaluating functional skills, it is essential to holistically consider the impact of sensorimotor and psychosocial changes on cognitive-perceptual deficits. This approach ensures proficiency in testing procedures and enables valid problem identification for efficient goal setting.

Perceptual evaluation in acquired brain injury

Perception refers to the meaningful interpretation of external stimuli. When assessing individuals with high-level functioning in order to determine their ability to live independently or return to work or school, standardized perceptual tests can be useful. Occupational therapists may administer assessments such as the widely used RPAB (Jesshope et al., 1991). The RPAB evaluates individuals' visual perceptual deficits across 16 different functions, including form constancy, figure-ground discrimination, body image, and spatial awareness. It also helps assess changes in perception over time. In addition to standardized tests, occupational therapists should also consider other evaluation methods based on direct observations of the individual during functional activities. For example, therapists may note if an individual tends to ignore items on the left or right side while feeding, dressing, or reading a menu. Tests such as the Behavioral Inattention Test (BIT; Halligan et al., 1991; Wilson et al., 1987) (Figure 4.1), Albert's Test (Fullerton et al., 1986), or the Letter Cancellation Task (Diller et al., 1974) can be administered to assess unilateral visual inattention.

If individuals with ABI experience difficulties in sequencing routine tasks, such as feeding, grooming, or dressing, therapists can further look for signs of perseveration (e.g., continuously combing one section of hair), inappropriate use of objects (e.g., using a spoon as a comb), or ineffective motor patterns (e.g., difficulty initiating or following cues or demonstrations). These observations can provide insights into motor planning problems, such as:

(1) Ideational apraxia, which involves a disruption in the concept formation of action planning, selecting, and organizing movements, resulting in difficulty performing a skilled activity. Signs of ideational apraxia may include incorrect use of objects.
(2) Ideomotor apraxia, which refers to the inability to produce individual task elements in the correct sequence, even when the individual retains the concept or idea of the task. Signs of ideomotor apraxia may include incorrect movement patterns and perseveration.

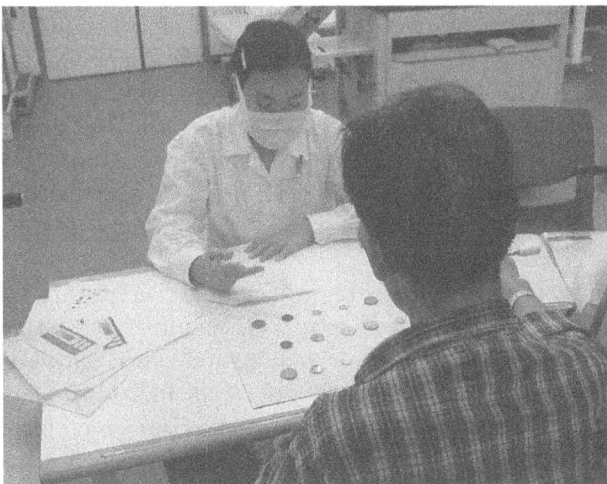

Figure 4.1 Behavioral Inattention Test

Occupational therapists also incorporate functional tasks such as personal hygiene and dressing into perceptual evaluations. Analyzing the performance of specific tasks provides information about attention to the task, the ability to cross the midline, motor planning, sequencing, spatial awareness, and visual processing. In assessing tactile processing, therapists observe finger identification, sensitivity to touch, stereognosis, and kinesthesia. For visual perception, therapists assess color and shape recognition, depth perception, visual pursuit, fixation, and scanning.

Two assessment tools commonly used by occupational therapists to evaluate cognitive-perceptual difficulties in the context of activities of daily living (ADL) are the Arnadottir OT-ADL Neurobehavioural Evaluation (A-ONE) and Perceive, Recall, Plan, Perform (PRPP). The A-ONE is a standardized assessment that involves clinical observation of ADL tasks and evaluates the level of assistance required for performance. It assesses ADL independence, the need for assistance, and the severity of neurobehavioral impairment that limits function, providing guidance for goal setting and treatment planning (Arnadottir et al., 2009; Gardarsdottir & Kaplan, 2002). The PRPP is a cognitive-perceptual assessment tool that aims to identify and analyze the cognitive processes underlying functional performance. It focuses on perceiving relevant information, recalling task steps, planning actions, and executing the task. The PRPP assessment involves observing and rating performance on specific ADL tasks, considering factors such as attention, problem-solving, sequencing, and organization (Chapparo & Ranka, 2013). It provides detailed information about the cognitive processes involved in task performance and helps in developing targeted intervention strategies.

Cognitive evaluation in acquired brain injury
Standardized tests provide a higher degree of cognitive challenges and include norms for the diagnosis of cognitive deficits. Occupational therapists often use micro-batteries to screen cognition in multiple cognitive domains. A commonly used screening test for ABI can be MoCA (Chiti & Pantoni, 2014; Nasreddine et al., 2005), which evaluates visuospatial functions, naming, attention and working memory, language, abstraction, and orientation. Occupational therapists assess global cognitive function using standardized test batteries such as the Neurobehavioral Cognitive Status Examination (NCSE or Cognistat; Kiernan et al., 1987). This is a screening test of cognitive functions in three general domains (consciousness, orientation, and simple attention) and five major domains (language, spatial skills, memory, calculations, and reasoning). A profile of cognitive performance, instead of a figure or aggregated score, can identify impaired domain(s), and performance can be monitored over time upon repeated measurement.

Short flexible tests offer advantages to occupational therapists as they allow for the observation of an individual's approach to specific cognitive tasks. When assessing sustained attention, therapists observe how well an individual with an ABI attends to relevant information during task performance. If an individual shows no difficulty in simple routine tasks, such as basic memory exercises or problem-solving activities, in a quiet and controlled environment, it is recommended to increase the level of challenge. This can be achieved by introducing tasks with greater complexity, such as puzzles, memory games with larger sets of information, or multitasking activities.

Additionally, therapists can modify the environment to provide additional stimulation. This may involve introducing distractions or background noise that simulate real-life situations where the individual needs to focus amid external stimuli. Examples include playing soft background music, having conversations nearby, or incorporating visual distractions. Gradually increasing the task difficulty and environmental stimulation challenges the individual to enhance their cognitive abilities, including attention span, working memory, and executive functions. The goal is to simulate real-world scenarios and equip the individual with the skills needed to successfully manage complex cognitive demands in their daily life.

Occupational therapists can also employ simple and relevant standardized tests to assess attention. Tests such as Digit Span, Serial 7, the Letter Cancellation Test, and the Visual Vigilance Test can provide insights into an individual's selective attention. The ability to remain focused on functional activities, such as reading, playing a game, or performing simulated work tasks, reflects their selective attention. Therapists can evaluate whether the individual can effectively filter out distractions. The selective attention can be further assessed in a distracting environment. Additionally, the therapist can evaluate the individual's performance in tasks that require attention to multiple stimuli simultaneously, such as setting a table while observing cooking or writing a record while listening to a meeting. Standardized tests specifically designed to assess attention deficits, such as the Trail Making Test (TMT) or its language-free version, the Color Trails Test (CTT), can also be utilized.

Memory function in ABI can be assessed in terms of various sensory channels, duration of memory recall, and types of memory (short-term or working memory, long-term memory, and prospective memory). For auditory short-term or working memory, therapists can take note of an individual's ability to recall relevant new information for about one minute, such as recalling the therapist's name or instructions given. An individual is asked to point to describe a person or object seen before in order to test visual working memory. Alternatively, the individual is given photographs of functional objects to memorize and recall later. Similarly, a person's tactile or kinetic memory can be tested by being asked to repeat an action that was just demonstrated. To test long-term memory, occupational therapists need to lengthen the time that memory is required. For instance, at the end of the treatment hour, the occupational therapist can ask the individual to demonstrate or describe a few of the activities in the therapy session. Again, standardized assessment tools such as the RBMT (Wilson et al., 1985) can also assess everyday memory functions by testing items such as remembering to deliver a message or to retrieve a personal belonging after an interval. The Cambridge Prospective Memory Test (CAMPROMT; Wilson et al., 2005) can measure specific prospective memory failures using three time-based tasks and three event-based tasks. Memory complaints can be reflected by self-report questionnaires, such as the Everyday Memory Questionnaire (EMQ; Sunderland et al., 1983), which tests retrospective memory problems. The Comprehensive Prospective Memory Questionnaire (CAPM; Fleming et al., 2009; Man et al., 2015) or its short-form, the Brief Assessment of Prospective Memory (BAPM; Man et al., 2011), can identify prospective memory failures, which are also found to be associated with an individual's BADL and IADL independence. The Contextual Memory Test (CMT; Turner & Levine, 2008) is an assessment tool that was developed by occupational therapists specifically for individuals with ABI.

The test focuses on evaluating contextual memory, which refers to the ability to recall and use information within a specific context or environment. During the test, the occupational therapist presents the participant with various contextual cues or stimuli and then assesses their ability to recall the associated information. The CMT evaluates the individual's memory performance, including their ability to encode, store, and retrieve contextual information. The test provides valuable insights into the individual's contextual memory abilities and helps identify any deficits or difficulties they may have. The results of the CMT can guide occupational therapists in developing targeted interventions and strategies to improve the individual's contextual memory skills and enhance their overall functional independence in daily life activities.

Occupational therapists often use functional observation to assess a person's problem-solving ability and executive function. Verbal problem-solving tasks are commonly employed, where individuals are asked to verbally solve functional problems. For example, they may be presented with a situation like being locked out of their house and asked to describe how they would handle it. Occupational therapists may also assign tasks such as planning and executing community trips or engaging in meal planning, grocery shopping, and cooking.

However, it is crucial to recognize that verbal problem-solving and planning have limitations for individuals with ABI. These limitations stem from language and communication impairments, cognitive deficits, reduced processing speed, difficulties with abstract thinking, and the potential for fatigue and mental exhaustion.

In assessing problem-solving abilities, occupational therapists observe several components. First, they observe whether the individual can identify problems in the environment or during activities as they arise. Second, they evaluate the individual's ability to generate solutions by drawing from their experience or trying novel approaches to accomplish tasks. The individual's planning skills are assessed by determining if they can independently implement plans or if they consistently require guidance. The therapist also estimates the individual's self-monitoring abilities by gauging their awareness of changes in the activity or environment and their ability to adapt their plans accordingly. Finally, both the therapist and the individual collaboratively evaluate the outcomes to assess their effectiveness, safety, and whether the set goals were achieved in a timely manner.

Executive function encompasses a range of cognitive processes involved in goal-directed behavior, including planning, problem-solving, decision-making, working memory, cognitive flexibility, and inhibition. Occupational therapists commonly use standardized tests to assess executive function, which includes components such as inhibition, working memory, cognitive flexibility, planning and organization, problem-solving, and decision-making. Examples of standardized tests for assessing executive function or frontal lobe function include the Wisconsin Card Sorting Test (WCST), available in both the paper-and-pencil version (Drewe, 1974; Mountain & Snow, 1993) and the Computer Version 4 Research Edition WCSTCV4 (available at https://paa.com.au/product/wcstcv4/). Other options include The Stroop Color and Word Test (Scarpina & Tagini, 2017), One Minute Animal Naming Test (OMAT; Cummings, 2004), The Frontal Assessment Battery (FAB; Dubois et al., 2000), and The Behavioral Assessment of the Dysexecutive Syndrome Test (BADS; Wilson et al., 1996). In assessing individuals' occupational functioning, The Multiple Errands Test (MET; Burns et al., 2019) is an assessment that examines how executive dysfunction manifests in individuals' everyday lives. Various location-specific versions of the MET, including a Chinese version (Lai et al., 2020a; Lai et al., 2020b), have been developed over the past few decades.

Specifically, in the context of ABI, self-awareness problems refer to difficulties an individual may face in recognizing and understanding their own cognitive, physical, and emotional deficits resulting from the injury. These deficits can manifest as a lack of insight, limited self-monitoring and self-reflection, impaired self-identity, and reduced awareness of social impacts. Addressing self-awareness is crucial for effective rehabilitation (Fleming et al., 2019) and has numerous benefits, including maximizing functional outcomes, promoting safety and risk management, supporting emotional well-being, improving social integration, facilitating long-term adjustment, and providing guidance to families and caregivers. Examples of self-awareness tests include the Self-Awareness of Deficits Interview (SADI; Toglia et al., 2010) and the Self-Awareness Deficit (SAD) interview (Cheng & Man, 2006).

General principles for cognitive and perceptual treatment in acquired brain injury

Treatment approaches for individuals with ABI who have cognitive and perceptual impairments can vary, but several general principles can guide therapy. These principles aim to improve cognitive and perceptual skills, promote functional independence, and enhance the individual's overall quality of life.

One treatment model commonly used is the sensorimotor approach, which focuses on restoring normal motor function. This approach encourages the individual to actively explore and interact with their environment, thereby promoting improved cognitive and perceptual skills. By engaging in sensorimotor activities, the individual can regain or enhance their ability to perceive and process sensory information, leading to improved motor function.

Another approach is the skill training approach, which focuses on teaching specific component skills that contribute to cognitive and perceptual functioning. For example, visual-spatial awareness may be targeted to improve the individual's ability to navigate their environment effectively. The goal of this approach is to facilitate the transfer of these component skills to functional tasks, enabling the individual to perform daily activities more independently.

Cognitive training is another important aspect of treatment. It involves targeting specific cognitive skills such as computation, time management, and telephone use through practical training exercises. Repetition of these activities is crucial until the individual can incorporate the strategies spontaneously into their daily life. The aim is to enhance their cognitive abilities and promote independence in everyday tasks.

The functional approach to treatment emphasizes repetition, compensation, and practice in a specific skill area. While it does not directly address the underlying cause of cognitive or perceptual dysfunction, it offers immediate benefits to the individual. ADL training is an example of this approach, where occupational therapists structure activities to maximize individuals' participation and encourage their independence. Additionally, modifying the environment can also play a significant role in promoting cognitive and perceptual functioning. Simple changes such as clear road signage and distinct color contrast can be helpful for individuals with visual limitations. Minimizing auditory distractions by using sound-absorbing materials can also improve focus and attention. Furthermore, adaptive equipment or methods can assist in compensating for cognitive or perceptual loss. Examples of adaptive equipment include pill organizers, adapted cutting boards, and prepared food, all of which promote safety and independence in daily tasks. By utilizing these treatment principles and tailoring interventions to the specific needs of individuals with ABI, occupational therapists can help optimize their cognitive and perceptual abilities, enhance their functional performance, and support their overall rehabilitation and recovery process.

Perceptual rehabilitation

There are several main types of perceptual disorders: visual perceptual disorder, agnosia, topographic disorientation, and apraxia. A summary of training examples can be found in Table 4.1.

Cognitive rehabilitation: Restorative and functional adaptive approaches

Cognitive rehabilitation can be categorized into two main approaches: restorative and functional adaptive/compensatory approaches (Neistadt, 1990). Whether utilizing one approach or a combination of both, the overarching objective is to support individuals in their reintegration into their daily lives.

Restorative approach

The restorative approach aims to improve functioning or re-train specific cognitive domains, with the ultimate goal of restoring functioning in those domains to pre-morbid levels. It involves the use of cognitive training and cognitive stimulation techniques. Cognitive stimulation refers to engaging in non-regimented activities that require mental functioning. It is less structured than cognitive training and may include activities such as computer games without active therapist involvement, fun or leisure activities, hobbies, and more. On the other hand, cognitive training focuses on improving cognitive functioning regardless of the specific mechanism of action. It can target cognitive domains such as memory, attention, and problem-solving, as well as task domains such as paper-and-pencil tasks, computer tasks, basic activities of daily living (BADL), and instrumental activities of daily living (IADL). A combination of domain-specific and task-specific activities can be carefully chosen for delivering cognitive training.

Cognitive training that targets the various cognitive domains is discussed below.

Cognitive training in arousal and attention

Treatment for decreased arousal often begins with stimulating the vestibular system through whole-body movement. Additional sensory stimulation can enhance alertness by using novel stimuli through various sensory channels. Meaningful activities such as self-care tasks can be attempted to further promote arousal. For sustained attention, the individual can engage in activities that match their skills and interests before gradually increasing the duration and complexity of the tasks. Creating a distracting environment can also help improve attention. To enhance selective attention, occupational

Table 4.1 Perceptual training examples

Visual perceptual functioning	Agnosia	Topographic disorientation	Apraxia			
			Constructional	Dressing	Ideomotor	Ideational
■ Spatial relationship: computer remediation, copying, or reading exercise. ■ Figure-ground impairment: look for objects inside a cupboard or drawer. ■ Depth perception impairment: strengthen depth judgment by training to go up and down stairs. ■ Spatial relationship impairment: build blocks, find routes, or read maps.	■ Somatoagnosia: encourage combining various input senses at the same time, including visual and tactile senses, or say the names of objects. ■ Gerstmann syndrome: use calculators and word-processing software to cope with the disorder, such as using computers, including those with voice-recognition capability. ■ Spatial neglect: encourage visual scanning, trunk rotation, limb activation, constraint-induced movement therapy (CIMT), mental imagery; use half-field eye-patch glasses or special lenses that induce a deviation of the whole visual field toward the lesion side.	■ Follow directional instructions (verbal cues) initially and then draw the path on a map or simple floor plan. ■ Withdraw the verbal cues and use of the map accordingly.	■ Duplicate a 2D or 3D figure with demonstration. ■ Offer hints or remind initially, but gradually reduce hints after making progress while also increasing the complexity of the figure or composition.	■ Break down the task step by step to practice (forward chaining); may give verbal cues if needed. ■ Make obvious marks or use labels to arouse attention on the left and right sides of clothes when putting on either upper or lower garments.	■ Use a general statement of "let's get ready" instead of giving step-by-step instructions for each task. ■ Imitate movements, such as lifting hands, clapping hands, and stretching out the tongue.	■ Try to kick off unconscious or spontaneous actions, e.g., put a toothbrush in his/her hand for he/she to brush teeth automatically. ■ Give step-by-step commands for each task so as to execute the appropriate movements.

therapists can manipulate the complexity of materials, the individual's motivation, and the level of distraction. Once selective attention is established, the individual can work on alternating attention, such as participating in two activities simultaneously, e.g., answering the telephone and taking messages in a work simulation task.

Cognitive training in memory
Cognitive training approaches for memory include the following strategies.

Effortful learning
Individuals are taught to use various strategies intentionally to improve their performance in valued tasks. Effortful learning involves conscious effort and mental activity. Examples of effortful learning techniques include spaced retrieval (recalling information over longer periods) and vanishing cues (repeatedly presenting information with diminishing intensity). Vanishing cues utilize priming effects observed in severely amnesic individuals, gradually reducing cues across trials. Memory mnemonics are internal strategies used to improve prospective memory (remembering to do something in the future) and retrospective memory (recalling past events). Internal strategies help encode, store, organize, and understand information, reduce errors, and promote deep thinking. They can involve simplifying, reducing, organizing, linking, or associating with other information, using visual imagery, repetition, categorization, and visualization techniques, among others.

General internal strategies for memory improvement include organizing information through categorization or chunking, using association techniques such as linking information to a story or context, employing visualization techniques such as creating diagrams or mind maps, utilizing multiple sensory channels for encoding, and using repetition, questioning, and paraphrasing during learning.

It is important to note that these approaches and techniques are not exhaustive, and the specific treatment methods used may vary depending on individual needs, clinical judgment, and therapeutic goals. The examples are further elaborated in Table 4.2.

Errorless learning
The errorless learning technique emphasizes learning without errors or mistakes, as it is believed to be more effective than the trial-and-error approach (Baddeley, 1992). This technique can be particularly beneficial for individuals with severe memory deficits who learn better when prevented from making mistakes during the learning process.

Reality orientation
Reality orientation (RO) involves continually presenting information and current events to help individuals maintain orientation to time and place. In a classroom setting, RO can be implemented through various themes, such as means of transportation, public places, personal events such as birthdays and wedding anniversaries, cultural events, and the use of updated technology, among others.

Memory group
Memory group training is often conducted for economic reasons, social engagement, enjoyment through memory games, and sometimes to benefit relatives. Memory group

Table 4.2 Examples of specific internal strategy techniques

Method	Strategies
First letter cuing	When trying to remember new facts or a list of words, remember the first letter of each item to be remembered. The first letter may facilitate retrieval.
Rhymes	Recall a fact by changing the fact into a rhyme or tune.
Story method	Elaborate on new information. Link a series of facts into a story.
Retracing events	Reconstruct environment in which information was received.
Chunking	Organize information in associations and groups.
Visual imagery	Visualize verbal information in graphs, pictures, cartoons, or action-based imagery.
Face	Name association.
Verbalization/talking aloud	Verbalizing visual-spatial information or talking aloud each step of the task assists in focusing attention on the task.
Rehearsal	Overt or covert; auditory-vocal or motor.
PQRST strategy	Preview/Question/Read-reread/State answer/Test (works well as a study guide).
	Self-questioning: Do I understand? Do I need to ask a question? Periodically look for gaps, misconceptions, or confusions.
Memory practice, exercises, and drills	Computer remediation or paper-and-pencil tasks.

training often starts with an introductory session to increase participants' knowledge about memory processes and factors that impede or improve memory functioning. This is followed by a series of sessions that introduce memory aids or mnemonic strategies, providing sufficient time for clients to discover their own coping methods for memory difficulties (Figure 4.2).

Cognitive training in problem-solving
Problem-solving is a complex activity that relies on basic cognitive and perceptual skills. For example, memory difficulty will impair an individual's ability to learn from their mistakes, and poor alternative attention will interfere with their awareness of relevant factors in the environment. When a component skill deficit limits problem-solving, it must be addressed separately. Individuals who may directly benefit from focusing on one or more problem-solving steps can follow this procedure: problem identification, solution generation, planning, implementation, self-monitoring, and outcome.

(1) Identification of a problem is the first step in the problem-solving process. An individual who is unaware of the nature of the deficit may benefit from being allowed to make mistakes. When difficulties are experienced, the therapist can ask the individual to define the problem. Reasons for the problem and possible solutions might be discussed. Selection of a solution and its implementation can then be facilitated.
(2) Some individuals may recognize problems when they occur but are unable to anticipate them. They may try generating solutions using a trial-and-error approach but may not be able to plan ahead. The methods used could be minimizing

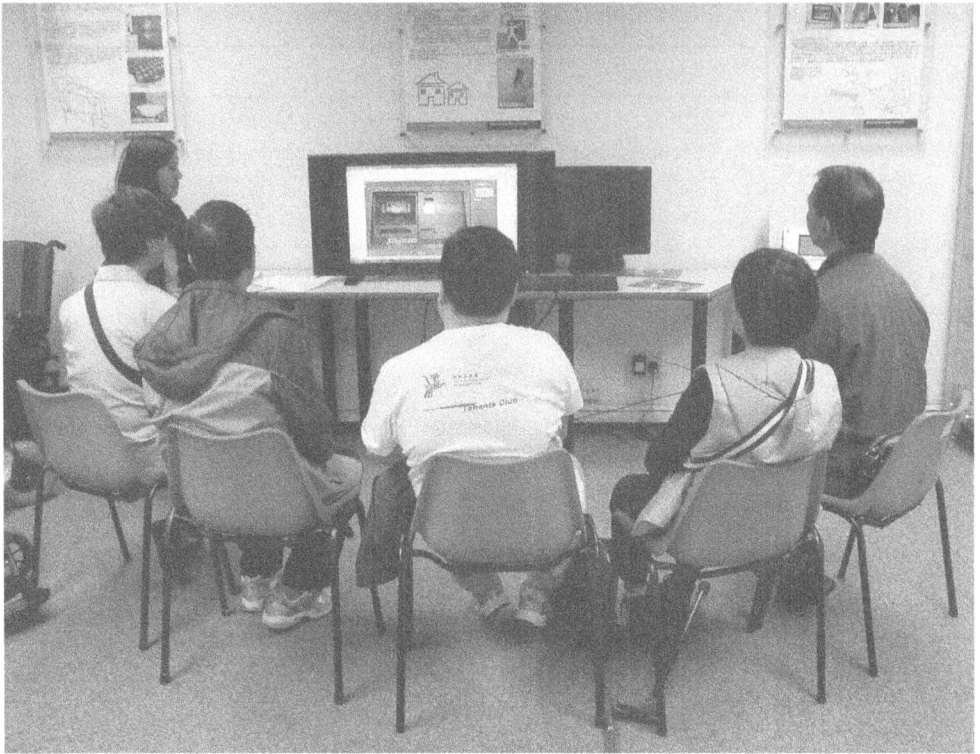

Figure 4.2 Group cognitive skills training

distractions to allow the individual to focus on the relevant aspects of the task, cuing the individual to slow down and think about alternatives and the consequences of the intended actions. The individual should be encouraged to generate several solutions to each problem and evaluate the effectiveness of the various solutions.

(3) Planning skills can be promoted by offering opportunities to plan and carry out multistep tasks. The amount of material, number of steps, and complexity of the task can be graded to increase the challenge (e.g., planning a simple meal first and then a community trip). Once a plan has been devised, the individual can write down the sequence of the activity to facilitate task completion. Pictorial cues can sometimes assist an individual in organizing a task. Gradually, the individual should be given more responsibility to plan and carry out tasks without the therapist's intervention.

(4) The therapist can provide a graded structure and cueing during implementation while gradually allowing the individual to make their own decisions. Alternative actions can be suggested to maximize problem-solving, such as any safety issues.

(5) The individual must learn to evaluate their own performance independently to promote self-monitoring. The occupational therapist can encourage the individual to evaluate their own actions and provide cues to attend to relevant information in the environment. Gradually, the difficulty of the task should increase. Ongoing decision-making and the creation of alternate plans based on environmental factors should be encouraged.

(6) The outcome of the individual's action should be reviewed with the individual in terms of safety, efficiency, goal accomplishment, problems, and alternative actions. Finally, the individual should be able to analyze problems independently, thereby achieving true independence.

In addition, using the problem-solving mode, social problem-solving skills (D'Zurilla et al., 2004) are outlined in Table 4.3.

Table 4.3 Social problem-solving skills

Domain	High-level thought processes	Examples
Problem identification	*Convergent thinking*: recognition and analysis of relevant information to identify the problem.	Ask the individual to read some information and verbally identify what the paragraph describes, e.g., Jack opened the door and was greeted by a house full of people. The room is decorated, and there is a cake with candles on the table. What is this story about?
Problem representation	*Deductive reasoning*: drawing conclusions based on premises or general principles in a step-by-step manner regarding a given situation.	Ask the individual to identify the correct item after reading the clues, e.g., ruler, hammer, or watch. Is it a tool? Yes. Does it contain numbers? Yes. Is it round in shape? No.
	Inductive reasoning: formulation of solutions based on details that lead to but do not necessarily support a standard conclusion.	Ask the individual to find the opposites of words or situations in pictures.
Planning	*Divergent thinking*: generation of unique abstract concepts or hypotheses that deviate from standard concepts or ideas.	Ask the individual to construct a sentence using the words provided by you and write it down; explain a phrase or sentence.
	Multi-process reasoning: task-specific, i.e., a particular situation.	What will you do when your stove is on fire?
	Multi-process reasoning: domain-specific, i.e., a particular cognitive problem.	Jack's age was two times his sister's age two years before. His sister is eight years old; how old is Jack now?
Monitoring	*Time estimation*	How long will it take to travel from Hung Hom East Rail Station to Sheung Shui, New Territories?
	Error estimation	Ask the individual to predict the number of errors when doing a math exercise.
	Self-evaluation/grading	Ask the individual to rate his/her performance before and after a cooking task.

Compensatory approach

The compensatory approach teaches new ways of performing cognitive tasks by passing by or working around cognitive deficits. External aids and devices help the client to memorize past activities, remember future events or appointments, and organize his/her daily activity schedule. Examples of environmental adaptation include the use of environmental cues, calendars and daily reminders, and ambient environmental devices, all of which provide automatic detection of movement activity and assistance. Common external devices include organizational ones such as notebooks and timetables, prospective memory devices such as pagers, alarms, calendars, watches, and smartphones, as well as environmental modifications such as reminders and labeling.

Environmental adaptation reduces external demands from the environment so that an individual can cope with his/her existing ability. It can usually be done by adapting the work or home environment or by simplifying the work routine. It seldom makes the individual adapt to new environments or suggests ways of performing tasks that may cause interference. It is relatively suitable for individuals who are slower learners and who have inadequate metacognitive ability.

The use of aids and devices involves active learning. There are a number of compensatory strategies that simplify information and tasks and aid in the organization of time. For example, notebook training is not simply about asking clients to use notebooks to write things down or record information, it involves various stages of compensatory training, otherwise known as the 3As.

Acquisition

- Becoming familiar with the purpose.
- Learning how to perform the strategy.
- Repetitive administration of questions regarding the use of the strategy.
- Ensuring the notebook is carried at all times.
- Learning names, the purpose, and to use each notebook section via question-and-answer exercises.

Application

- Learning when and where to use the strategy.
- Role-playing the use of the strategy.
- Learning appropriate methods for recording in the notebook via role-play.

Adaptation

- Learning the ability to adapt and modify skill use to accommodate novel situations.
- Practicing using the strategy in a variety of natural settings.
- Demonstrating appropriate notebook use in natural settings via home exercises and community training.
- Pairing the use of the notebook with reminders, i.e., checking the notebook when the alarm sounds, and fading this out upon getting used to checking.

Efficient use of the notebook will not occur naturally. Training the individual to know their notebook and how to use it is crucial. This can be achieved in the following ways:

- Question and answer exercises regarding the notebook's purpose and contents.
- Practice note writing so that information can be recorded in an accurate and concise manner.
- Discourage one-word entries or copious amounts of notes.
- Include photographs, maps, and diagrams to reinforce written words.
- Start with one or two sections; once learned, gradually add more sections one at a time.

Some individuals may not be able to write and may need help from another person. All entries must be dated, and a tick should be used to indicate that something has been completed.

Cultural factors in cognitive and perceptual assessment and intervention

When conducting cognitive and perceptual assessments and interventions, it is crucial to consider cultural factors and ensure the assessments are culturally relevant and ecologically valid. This practice ensures that the assessments accurately detect the individual's problems and effectively monitor the treatment progress. Although there are cognitive and perceptual assessment tools that claim to be culture-free or language-free, occupational therapists need to be cautious and select tools that are appropriate to the individual's cultural background.

In Western cultures, many standardized perceptual and cognitive assessment tools have been developed. However, before applying these tools in various other cultural contexts, it is essential to validate them both psychometrically and linguistically. This validation process ensures that the assessments are appropriate and effective for specific cultural populations. For example, when working with Chinese-speaking populations in Hong Kong, China, and Taiwan, it is crucial to adapt and validate assessment tools to ensure their cultural relevance and accuracy.

Innovative and technology-driven approaches have been developed and validated for cognitive and perceptual assessments in local practices, particularly in places such as Hong Kong. These approaches aim to provide culturally relevant and validated assessment and treatment packages that cater to the specific cognitive and perceptual needs of the local population. While it is not possible to provide an exhaustive list of these assessment and treatment packages, ongoing efforts are being made to develop and refine these tools to enhance their cultural relevance and effectiveness.

By considering cultural factors and utilizing culturally relevant assessment and treatment approaches, occupational therapists can ensure that their interventions are tailored to the unique cognitive and perceptual needs of each individual, regardless of their cultural background. This approach promotes accurate assessment, effective intervention, and improved overall outcomes for individuals.

The following are examples of locally validated or developed assessment tools:

- Behavioral Inattention Test (BIT), Hong Kong version (Fong et al., 2007)
- Mini-Mental State Examination (MMSE), Cantonese version (Chiu et al., 1998)

- Hong Kong Brief Cognitive Test (HKBC; Chiu et al., 2018)
- Montreal Cognitive Assessment, Hong Kong Chinese version (MoCA-CV; Wong et al., 2009; Wong et al., 2015)
- Neurobehavioral Cognitive Status Examination, Chinese version (NCSE-CV; Chan et al., 1999; Chan et al., 2002)
- Rivermead Behavioural Memory Test, Chinese version (RBMT-CV; Man & Li, 2001) and the online version of the RBMT-CV (Man et al., 2009) for stroke survivors. Rivermead Behavioural Memory Test – Third Edition (RBMT-3) has also been validated for local application (Figure 4.3) (Fong et al., 2017).
- Cambridge Prospective Memory Test, Chinese version (CAMPROMPT-CV; Man et al., 2015)
- Brief Assessment of Prospective Memory (BAPM; Man et al., 2011)

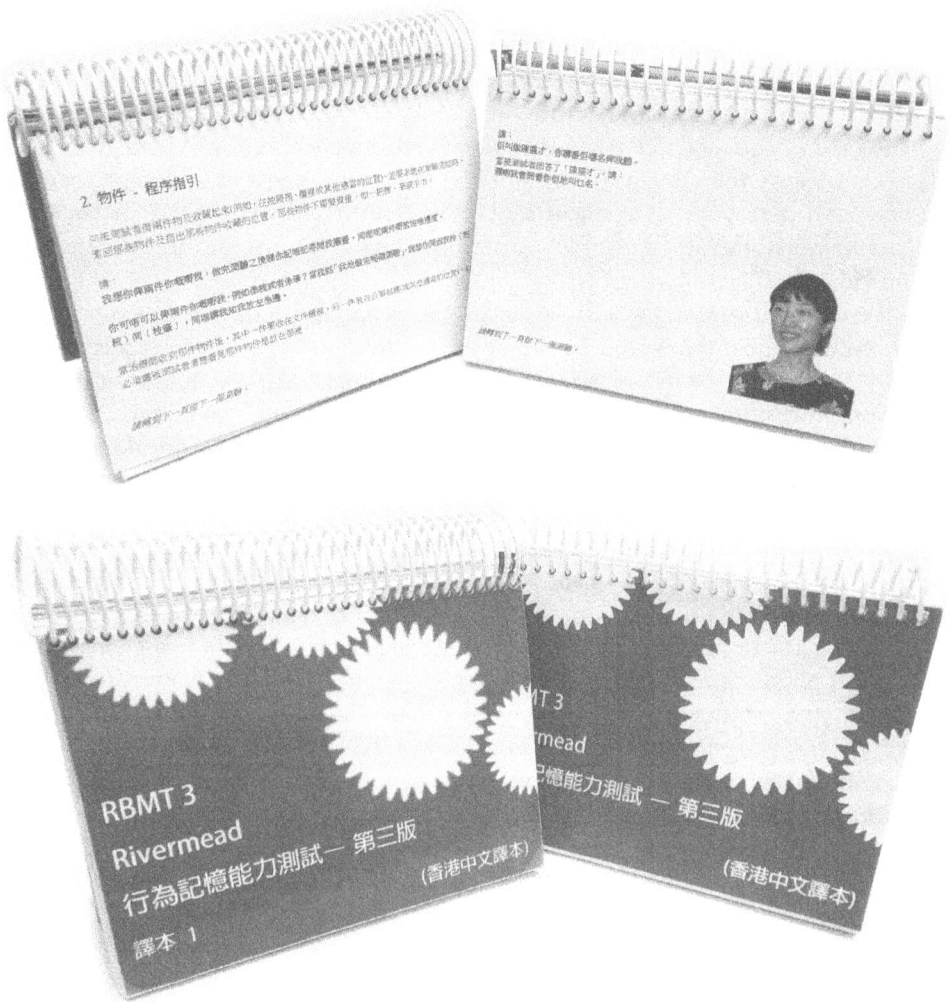

Figure 4.3 Rivermead Behavioural Memory Test – Third Edition (RBMT-3)

- A virtual reality-based system assessing prospective memory in traumatic brain injury (Canty et al., 2014)
- An intelligent cognitive assessment system adopting a computerized adaptive testing approach in traumatic brain injury (Yip & Man, 2010)
- Home-based evaluation of executive function is an ecologically valid assessment that characterizes how executive dysfunction manifests in individuals' everyday activities within their living environment (Lai et al., 2020b)

Training packages have also been developed to suit local individuals' needs. Below are some examples:

- CogniPlus® is a software package developed by SCHUFRIED, offering training of scientifically proven trainable cognitive functions. It has various language versions including Chinese.
- Compensatory cognitive training (CCT), Hong Kong version (https://cogsmart. s3.amazonaws.com/CogSMART-C_Participant_Manual(A4).pdf)
- Computerized training package in memory (Dou et al., 2006) and community living skills (Lam et al., 2006)
- Tele-cognitive rehabilitation for individuals with brain injuries (Man et al., 2006)
- Cultural-based cognitive intervention of traditional Cantonese opera songs on community-dwelling older adults' cognitive and psychological function, well-being, and health (Man et al., 2022)
- Virtual reality-based ATM machine training for ABI (Fong et al., 2010)
- Examples of internet resources:
  - C-Rehab platform (http://crehab.hk/)
  - The e123 website (https://game.e123.hk/)
  - Hong Kong Alzheimer's Disease Association (https://apps.apple.com/hk/developer/hong-kong-alzheimers-disease-association/id455899709)

Summary

This chapter aims to provide structured and practical information to assist students and occupational therapists in addressing the evaluation and treatment challenges associated with cognition and perception. It serves as a valuable guide for conducting evaluations, writing goals, and implementing treatments in clinical settings. By gaining a deeper understanding of this information, occupational therapists can develop realistic goals, help individuals with ABI and caregivers understand the impact of cognitive and perceptual deficits on daily functioning, and deliver optimal treatment.

During the treatment process, occupational therapists should be mindful that individuals may present a diverse range of problem areas, strengths, and interests. Therefore, it is crucial to select cognitive and perceptual treatments that address various issues and are personally motivating to each individual. The therapist's creativity, knowledge of the individuals, awareness of general treatment principles, and understanding of the interplay among various factors (such as sensorimotor, perceptual, cognitive, psychosocial, family, and environmental) all contribute to the selection of appropriate therapeutic activities.

By considering these factors and tailoring treatments accordingly, occupational therapists can effectively address cognitive and perceptual challenges and facilitate meaningful improvements in their individuals' daily lives. The chapter serves as a valuable resource to guide therapists in their clinical practice, enabling them to provide comprehensive and individualized care.

References

Arnadottir, G., Fisher, A. G., & Löfgren, B. (2009). Dimensionality of nonmotor neurobehavioral impairments when observed in the natural contexts of ADL task performance. *Neurorehabilitation and Neural Repair*, 23(6), 579–586. https://doi.org/10.1177/1545968308324223

Baddeley, A. D. (1992). Implicit memory and errorless learning: A link between cognitive theory and neuropsychological rehabilitation? In L. R. Squire, & N. Butters (Eds.), *Neuropsychology of memory* (pp. 309–313). The Guilford Press.

Brown, M., & Gordon, W. A. (2013). Impact of cognitive impairments on functional outcome in individuals with traumatic brain injury. *Journal of Head Trauma Rehabilitation*, 28(4), 270–279.

Burns, S. P., Dawson, D. R., Perea, J. D., Vas, A., Pickens, N. D., & Neville, M. (2019). Development, reliability, and validity of the Multiple Errands Test Home Version (MET-Home) in adults with stroke. *American Journal of Occupational Therapy*, 73(3), 7303205030p1–7303205030p10.

Canty, A. L., Fleming, J., Patterson, F., Green, H. J., Man, D., & Shum, D. H. K. (2014). Evaluation of a virtual reality prospective memory task for use with individuals with severe traumatic brain injury. *Neuropsychological Rehabilitation*, 24(2), 238–265.

Chan, C. C. H., Lee, T. M. C., Fong, K. N. K., Lee, C., & Wong, V. (2002). Cognitive profile for Chinese patients with stroke. *Brain Injury*, 16(10), 873–884. https://doi.org/10.1080/02699050210131975

Chan, C. H. C., Lee, T. M. C., Wong, V., Fong, K., & Lee, C. (1999). Validation of the Chinese version of Neurobehavioral Cognitive Status Examination. *Archives of Clinical Neuropsychology*, 14(1), 71.

Chapparo, C., & Ranka, J. (2013, December 10). *The perceive: recall: plan: perform (PRPP) system of task analysis*. Occupational Performance Model (Australia). Retrieved December 27, 2023, from http://www.occupationalperformance.com/category/assessments/prpp/

Cheng, S. K. W., & Man, D. W. K. (2006). Management of impaired self-awareness in persons with traumatic brain injury. *Brain Injury*, 20(6), 621–628. https://doi.org/10.1080/02699050600677196

Chiti, G., & Pantoni, L. (2014). Use of Montreal Cognitive Assessment in patients with stroke. *Stroke*, 45(10), 3135–3140. http://doi.org/10.1161/STROKEAHA.114.004590

Chiu, H. F. K., Lam, L. C. W., Chi, I., Leung, T., Li, S. W., Law, W. T., Chung, D. W. S., Fung, H. H. L., Kan, P. S., Lum, C. M., Ng, J., & Lau, J. (1998). Prevalence of dementia in Chinese elderly in Hong Kong. *Neurology*, 50(4), 1002–1009. https://doi.org/10.1212/WNL.50.4.1002

Chiu, H. F. K., Zhong, B. L., Leung, T., Li, S. W., Chow, P., Tsoh, J., Yan, C., Xiang, Y. T., & Wong, M. (2018). Development and validation of a new cognitive screening test: The Hong Kong Brief Cognitive Test (HKBC). *International Journal of Geriatric Psychiatry*, 33(7), 994–999. https://doi.org/10.1002/gps.4883

Coelho, C., Ylvisaker, M., & Turkstra, L. S. (2005). Nonstandardized assessment approaches for individuals with traumatic brain injuries. *Seminars in Speech and Language*, 26(4), 223–241.

Cummings, J. L. (2004). The one-minute mental status examination. *Neurology*, 62(4), 534–535. https://doi.org/10.1212/WNL.62.4.534

D'Zurilla, T. J., Nezu, A. M., & Maydeu-Olivares, A. (2004). Social problem solving: Theory and assessment. In E. C. Chang, T. J. D'Zurilla, & L. J. Sanna (Eds.), *Social problem solving: Theory, research, and training* (pp. 11–27). American Psychological Association. https://doi.org/10.1037/10805-001

Dawson, D. R., & Chipchase, S. (2015). Cognitive rehabilitation in occupational therapy. In J. Case-Smith, & J. C. O'Brien (Eds.), *Occupational therapy for children and adolescents* (7th ed., pp. 923–945). Elsevier.

Diller, L., Weinberg, J., Gordon, W., Goodkin, R., Gerstman, L. J., & Ben-Yishay, Y. (1974). *Studies in cognition and rehabilitation in hemiplegia (rehabilitation monograph no. 50).* Institute of Rehabilitation Medicine, New York University Medical Center.

Dou, Z. L., Man, D. W. K., Ou, H. N., Zheng, J. L., & Tam, S. F. (2006). Computerized error-less learning-based memory rehabilitation for Chinese patients with brain injury: A preliminary quasi-experimental clinical design study. *Brain Injury, 20*(3), 219–225. https://doi.org/10.1080/02699050500488215

Drewe, E. A. (1974). The effect of type and area of brain lesion on Wisconsin Card Sorting Test Performance. *Cortex, 10*(2), 159–170. https://doi.org/10.1016/S0010-9452(74)80006-7

Dubois, B., Slachevsky, A., Litvan, I., & Pillon, B. (2000). The FAB: A Frontal Assessment Battery at bedside. *Neurology, 55*(11), 1621–1626. https://doi.org/10.1212/WNL.55.11.1621

Fleming, J., Kennedy, S., Fisher, R., Gill, H., Gullo, M., & Shum, D. (2009). Validity of the Comprehensive Assessment of Prospective Memory (CAPM) for use with adults with traumatic brain injury. *Brain Impairment, 10*(1), 34–44. https://doi.org/10.1375/brim.10.1.34.

Fleming, J., Strong, J., & Gracey, F. (2019). The relationship between self-awareness and participation after traumatic brain injury: A systematic review. *Neuropsychological Rehabilitation, 29*(10), 1589–1611.

Fong, K. N. K., Chan, M. K. L., Chan, B. Y. B., Ng, P. P. K., Fung, M. L., Tsang, M. H. M., & Chow, K. K. Y. (2007). Reliability and validity of the Chinese Behavioural Inattention Test–Hong Kong version (CBIT-HK) for patients with stroke and unilateral neglect. *Hong Kong Journal of Occupational Therapy, 17*(1), 23–33. https://doi.org/10.1016/S1569-1861(07)70004-9

Fong, K. N. K., Chow, K. Y. Y., Chan, B. C. H., Lam, K. C. K., Lee, J. C. K., Li, T. H. Y., Yan, E. W. H., & Wong, A. T. Y. (2010). Usability of a virtual reality environment simulating an automated teller machine for assessing and training persons with acquired brain injury. *Journal of NeuroEngineering and Rehabilitation, 7*, 19. https://doi.org/10.1186/1743-0003-7-19

Fong, K. N. K., Lee, K. K. L., Tsang, Z. P. Y., Wan, J. Y. H., Zhang, Y. Y., & Lau, A. F. C. (2017). The clinical utility, reliability and validity of the Rivermead Behavioural Memory Test-Third Edition (RBMT-3) in Hong Kong older adults with or without cognitive impairments. *Neuropsychological Rehabilitation, 29*(1), 144–159. https://doi.org/10.1080/09602011.2016.1272467

Fullerton, K. J., Mcsherry, D., & Stout, R. W. (1986). Albert's Test: A neglected test of perceptual neglect. *The Lancet, 327*(8478), 430–432. https://doi.org/10.1016/S0140-6736(86)92381-0

Gardarsdottir, S., & Kaplan, S. (2002). Validity of the Árnadottir OT-ADL Neurobehavioral Evaluation (A-ONE): Performance in activities of daily living and neurobehavioral impairments of persons with left and right hemisphere damage. *American Journal of Occupational Therapy, 56*(5), 499–508.

Halligan, P. W., Cockburn, J., & Wilson, B. A. (1991). The behavioural assessment of visual neglect. *Neuropsychological Rehabilitation, 1*(1), 5–32. https://doi.org/10.1080/09602019108401377

Jesshope, H. J., Clark, M. S., & Smith, D. S. (1991). The Rivermead Perceptual Assessment Battery: Its application to stroke patients and relationship with function. *Clinical Rehabilitation, 5*(2), 115–122. https://doi.org/10.1177/026921559100500205

Kiernan, R. J., Mueller, J., & Langston, J. W. (1987). The Neurobehavioral Cognitive Status Examination: A brief but differentiated approach to cognitive assessment. *Annals of Internal Medicine, 107*(4), 481–485.

Lai, F. H., Dawson, D., Yan, E. W., Ho, E. C., Tsui, J. W., Fan, S. H., & Lee, A. T. (2020a). The validity, reliability and clinical utility of a performance-based executive function assessment in people with mild to moderate dementia. *Aging & Mental Health, 24*(9), 1496–1504. https://doi.org/10.1080/13607863.2019.1599818

Lai, F. H., Yan, E. W., & Yu, K. K. (2020b). Home-based evaluation of executive function (Home-MET) for older adults with mild cognitive impairment. *Archives of Gerontology and Geriatrics, 87*, 104012. https://doi.org/10.1016/j.archger.2020.104012

Lam, Y. S., Man, D. W. K., Tam, S. F., & Weiss, P. L. (2006). Virtual reality training for stroke rehabilitation. *NeuroRehabilitation, 21*(3), 245–253.

Man, D. W. K., Chan, M. K. L., & Yip, C. C. K. (2015). Validation of the Cambridge Prospective Memory Test (Hong Kong Chinese version) for people with stroke. *Neuropsychological Rehabilitation, 25*(6), 895–912. https://doi.org/10.1080/09602011.2014.997253

Man, D. W. K., Chung, J. C. C., & Mak, M. K. Y. (2009). Development and validation of the Online Rivermead Behavioral Memory Test (OL-RBMT) for people with stroke. *NeuroRehabilitation, 24*(3), 231–236.

Man, D. W. K., Fleming, J., Hohaus, L., & Shum, D. (2011). Development of the Brief Assessment of Prospective Memory (BAPM) for use with traumatic brain injury populations. *Neuropsychological Rehabilitation, 21*(6), 884–898. https://doi.org/10.1080/09602011.2011.627270

Man, D. W. K., Lai, F. H. Y., Yu, E. C. S., & Lee, G. Y. Y. (2022). Effects of traditional Cantonese opera songs on Cantonese-speaking, community-dwelling older adults' cognitive and psychological function, well-being, and health. *Aging & Mental Health, 26*(5), 958–970. https://doi.org/10.1080/13607863.2021.1871880

Man, D. W. K., & Li, R. (2001). Assessing Chinese adults' memory abilities: Validation of the Chinese version of the Rivermead Behavioral Memory Test. *Clinical Gerontologist, 24*(3/4), 27–36. https://doi.org/10.1300/J018v24n03_04

Man, D. W. K., Soong, W. Y. L., Tam, S. F., & Hui-Chan, C. W. Y. (2006). A randomized clinical trial study on the effectiveness of a tele-analogy-based problem-solving programme for people with acquired brain injury (ABI). *NeuroRehabilitation, 21*(3), 205–217.

Mountain, M. A., & Snow, W. G. (1993). Wisconsin Card Sorting Test as a measure of frontal pathology: A review. *Clinical Neuropsychologist, 7*(1), 108–118. https://doi.org/10.1080/13854049308401893

Nasreddine, Z. S., Phillips, N. A., Bédirian, V., Charbonneau, S., Whitehead, V., Collin, I., Cummings, J. L., & Chertkow, H. (2005). The Montreal Cognitive Assessment, MoCA: A brief screening tool for mild cognitive impairment. *Journal of the American Geriatrics Society, 53*(4), 695–699. https://doi.org/10.1111/j.1532-5415.2005.53221.x

Neistadt, M. E. (1990). A critical analysis of occupational therapy approaches for perceptual deficits in adults with brain injury. *American Journal of Occupational Therapy, 44*(4), 299–304.

Radomski, M. V., & Trombly Latham, C. A. (2014). *Occupational therapy for physical dysfunction* (7th ed.). Lippincott Williams & Wilkins.

Scarpina, F., & Tagini, S. (2017). The Stroop Color and Word Test. *Frontiers in Psychology, 8*, 557.

Schaber, P., & Lieberman, D. (2010). *Occupational therapy for physical dysfunction*. Lippincott Williams & Wilkins.

Sunderland, A., Harris, J. E., & Baddeley, A. D. (1983). Do laboratory tests predict everyday memory? A neuropsychological study. *Journal of Verbal Learning and Verbal Behavior, 22*(3), 341–357. https://doi.org/10.1016/S0022-5371(83)90229-3

Toglia, J. P., Kirk, U., & James, R. A. (2010). The Self-Awareness of Deficits Interview: A new measure of insight in acquired brain injury. *Journal of Head Trauma Rehabilitation, 25*(5), 402–411.

Turner, G. R., & Levine, B. (2008). The functional neuroanatomy of episodic and semantic autobiographical remembering: A prospective functional MRI study. *Journal of Cognitive Neuroscience, 20*(11), 2178–2189.

Uomoto, J. M. (1992). Neuropsychological assessment and cognitive rehabilitation after brain injury. *Physical Medicine and Rehabilitation Clinics of North America, 3*(2), 291–318.

Wilson, B. A., Alderman, N., Burgess, P. W., Emslie, H., & Evans, J. J. (1996). *Behavioural assessment of the dysexecutive syndrome (BADS)*. Thames Valley Test Company.

Wilson, B. A., Cockburn, J., & Baddeley, A. D. (1985). *The Rivermead behavioural memory test*. Thames Valley Test Company.

Wilson, B. A., Cockburn, J., & Halligan, P. W. (1987). *The behavioral inattention test*. Thames Valley Test Company.

Wilson, B. A., Emslie, H., Foley, J., Shiel, A., Watson, P., Hawkins, K., Groot, Y., & Evans, J. J. (2005). *The Cambridge prospective memory test*. Harcourt Assessment.

Wong, A., Nyenhuis, D., Black, S. E., Law, L. S. N., Lo, E. S. K., Kwan, P. W. L., Au, L., Chan, A. Y. Y., Wong, L. K. S., Nasreddine, Z., & Mok, V. (2015). Montreal Cognitive Assessment

5-minute protocol is a brief, valid, reliable, and feasible cognitive screen for telephone administration. *Stroke*, 46(4), 1059–1064. https://doi.org/10.1161/STROKEAHA.114.007253

Wong, A., Xiong, Y. Y., Kwan, P. W. L., Chan, A. Y. Y., Lam, W. W. M., Wang, K., Chu, W. C. W., Nyenhuis, D. L., Nasreddine, Z., Wong, L. K. S., & Mok, V. C. T. (2009). The validity, reliability and clinical utility of the Hong Kong Montreal Cognitive Assessment (HK-MoCA) in patients with cerebral small vessel disease. *Dementia and Geriatric Cognitive Disorders*, 28(1), 81–87. https://doi.org/10.1159/000232589

Yip, C. K., & Man, D. W. K. (2010). Validation of the Intelligent Cognitive Assessment System (ICAS) for stroke survivors. *Brain Injury*, 24(7-8), 1032–1038. https://doi.org/10.3109/026 99052.2010.490514

Additional reading

Cicerone, K. D., Goldin, Y., Ganci, K., Rosenbaum, A., Wethe, J. V., Langenbahn, D. M., Malec, J. F., Bergquist, T. F., Kingsley, K., Nagele, D., Trexler, L., Fraas, M., Bogdanova, Y., & Harley, J. P. (2019). Evidence-based cognitive rehabilitation: Systematic review of the literature from 2009 through 2014. *Archives of Physical Medicine and Rehabilitation*, 100(8), 1515–1533. https://doi.org/10.1016/j.apmr.2019.02.011

Giles, G. M., Radomski, M. V., Carroll, G., Anheluk, M., & Yunek, J. (2022). Cognitive interventions with occupational performance as a primary outcome for adults with TBI (June 2013–October 2020). *American Journal of Occupational Therapy*, 76(Suppl. 2), 7613393180. https://doi.org/10.5014/ajot.2022/76S2018

O'Donoghue, M., Leahy, S., Boland, P., Galvin, R., McManus, J., & Hayes, S. (2022). Rehabilitation of cognitive deficits poststroke: Systematic review and meta-analysis of randomized controlled trials. *Stroke*, 53(5), 1700–1710. https://doi.org/10.1161/STROKEAHA.121.034218

Radomski, M. V., Anheluk, M., Bartzen, M. P., & Zola, J. (2016). Effectiveness of interventions to address cognitive impairments and improve occupational performance after traumatic brain injury: A systematic review. *American Journal of Occupational Therapy*, 70(3), 7003180050p1–7003180050p9.

Radomski, M. V., Giles, G. M., Carroll, G., Anheluk, M., & Yunek, J. (2022). Cognitive interventions to improve a specific cognitive impairment for adults with TBI (June 2013–October 2020). *American Journal of Occupational Therapy*, 76(Suppl. 2), 7613393170.

CHAPTER 5

Psychosocial practice for Chinese population

Hector Wing Hong Tsang, Erin Yiqing Lu,
Wendy Wing Yan So, and Zoey Yutong Li

Introduction

All human occupations and functions are embedded in their psychosocial processes and contexts, and it is necessary to address these aspects in occupational therapy (OT). Psychosocial aspects in OT can be defined as all interactions and experiences at the intrapersonal, interpersonal, social, cultural, and spiritual levels that can influence occupational development and performance (Mosey, 1986). Psychosocial concepts such as belief, motivation, symbolic meaning, personality, and values are highly relevant to the OT process (American Occupational Therapy Association, 2020). Although the reasons for referral to OT may not be directly related to psychosocial issues, occupational therapists should address the psychological responses that arise from disruptions in occupations and work on the psychological factors that enhance engagement in meaningful occupations (Ramsey, 2004). This is in line with the principle of the International Classification of Functioning, Disability and Health (ICF), which adopts a biopsychosocial model to consider the roles of psychological, social, and cultural factors in viewing health and disability (World Health Organization, 2001).

The application of OT in the Chinese population inevitably must address Chinese cultural uniqueness and adapt to the Chinese context. Scholars in the past 30 years have observed and elaborated on several aspects of Chinese culture that deviate from the philosophy of OT. For example, traditional Chinese medicine (TCM) denotes the central health beliefs in Chinese culture, and there are TCM-based concepts such as *qi* (i.e., vital energy) that should be noted in Chinese approaches to rehabilitation (Hopton & Stoneley, 2006). Stress management is a common need among various groups of rehabilitation service users, and it is also an essential health promotion strategy for healthy populations. Throughout the long history of TCM, many culturally specific, non-pharmacological, and non-invasive bodywork techniques have emerged and been developed. These techniques are widely used by Chinese people for health promotion and relaxation. These bodyworks include *qigong, tai chi*, acupressure, etc., and they

DOI: 10.4324/9781032721170-8

can be effective complementary and alternative therapies for stress management in the Chinese population, given their high cultural relevance and the growing empirical support for their treatment benefits.

Another major difference is the understanding of mental illness. In Chinese culture, mind and body are viewed as closely connected entities, and mental conditions should be regarded as an extension of physiological dysfunction (Hopton & Stoneley, 2006). In addition, people with mental health rehabilitation needs can be seen as passive and dependent individuals who require the care of their families, and mental illness is believed to be a consequence of the family's sins (Jang, 1995). Public and self-stigma about mental illness is a significant obstacle to the rehabilitation of people with mental health conditions, and the issue of stigma is especially evident among Chinese populations. It is important to understand how Chinese sociocultural contexts cultivate the mental illness stigma, as well as to develop interventions to counteract these social and psychological phenomena.

As reflected in Confucianism, employment and productivity are valued in Chinese culture. Social skills and employment are common occupations to be cultivated in OT, and the training and maintenance of these occupations should be key areas to localize OT in Chinese communities (Yau, 2007). Behavioral training programs with adaptations to Chinese culture are essential to the psychosocial rehabilitation of people with mental illness.

Therefore, this chapter introduces the development of psychosocial rehabilitation in stress management, mental illness stigma, and social skills training over the past two decades as they reflect typical areas of OT in Chinese populations. The chapter aims to consolidate knowledge about these issues in China and to inspire the development of innovative and culturally grounded strategies and interventions in OT for Chinese people.

Stress management

Stress is a common issue for people with physical or mental conditions, and experiencing high-level or prolonged stress is also detrimental to healthy populations. Hence, occupational therapists regard stress management as an important skill for achieving mastery of daily living (Affleck et al., 1984). Various techniques for stress management, such as relaxation, breathing exercises, and cognitive-behavioral coping strategies, have been practiced by occupational therapists to alleviate psychological distress and promote physical and psychological well-being. TCM is a commonly practiced approach in Chinese communities, and there are several TCM-based non-pharmacological and non-invasive techniques that have been applied to stress management and tested for their effectiveness in the past two decades. Commonly practiced TCM-based techniques include *qigong*, *tai chi*, and acupressure. With principles embedded in TCM theories, growing scientific evidence on their effectiveness, and high cultural relevance to Chinese people, these techniques are promising complementary and alternative approaches to alleviate stress and promote mental health.

Understanding stress

Stress is defined as individual responses that include psychological distress, physiological reactions, and behavioral changes, which all occur after the experience of a stressor

(Baum, 1990; Selye, 1993). A stressor is any internal or external force that can result in emotional or physiological stress (American Psychological Association, n.d.). From the perspective of psychology, stress experience results from the (mis)fit between one person and his/her environment, and one's cognitive appraisal plays an important role in stress responses. Specifically, a person will assess the valence (positive, neutral, or negative) of a stressor; if it is perceived as negative, an estimation of its consequences and challenges will be performed; also, the person will need to assess his/her own capabilities, resources, and support to cope with the stressor. All the above appraisals will determine the emotional experience, physiological responses, and behavioral strategies that constitute the phenomenon of stress (Lazarus & Folkman, 1984). Multiple neurophysiological pathways have been discovered to be involved in stress responses. Physiologically, stress is recognized as the interplay among nervous, endocrine, and immune systems. Stress responses involve the activation of the sympathetic-adreno-medullar (SAM) axis and the hypothalamus-pituitary-adrenal (HPA) axis (Chu et al., 2023), and stress can also suppress hippocampal neurogenesis (Warner-Schmidt & Duman, 2006). Repeated response to acute or prolonged stress experiences can lead to physiological maladaptation, such as neurochemical imbalance, impaired immunity, and dysregulations in cardiovascular functions (Chu et al., 2023).

TCM theories adopt a holistic view of health, with emotion and physiology closely interconnected. *Qi*, as a key concept in TCM, is defined as the vital energy that flows in the human body, and optimal health comes from the balanced and harmonious flow of *qi*. Organs in TCM are functional terms that incorporate anatomy, physiology, and psychology. The flow of *qi* is regulated by organs, and impaired functions in organs can lead to imbalanced *qi*, which is expressed as emotional or physical distress (Sun et al., 2013). TCM treatments aim to restore *qi* balance through herbal medicine, body movement, and other non-pharmacological approaches. The liver in TCM is a functional system responsible for controlling the flow of *qi* throughout the body, processing nutrients, and regulating emotions such as anger, frustration, and bitterness. Dysregulation of liver *qi* is regarded as the cause of emotional distress and disorders, which is suggested to be related to the neuroendocrine system. Impaired liver functions have been proposed as being connected to dysregulations in the SAM axis and the HPA axis (Ye et al., 2019). It is plausible that stress management can be achieved through the regulation of *qi*.

TCM-based non-pharmacological and non-invasive techniques

TCM-based techniques such as *qigong*, *tai chi*, and acupressure were developed in ancient China and have been used by TCM practitioners for centuries. Scientific research on the effectiveness of these techniques and the exploration of their underlying treatment mechanisms began roughly three decades ago, and there is a growing international interest in their practical application (Hao & Mittelman, 2014; Yang et al., 2015).

Qigong is defined as the ancient Chinese system of exercise that regulates breathing, vital energy, and the mind to promote health. It also incorporates slow movements, breathing exercises, and meditation (Cohen, 1997; Dong & Esser, 1990) (Figure 5.1). It was developed based on the rationale that *qi* can be directed, strengthened, and regulated through breathing, postures, and body movements, with *qigong* practice

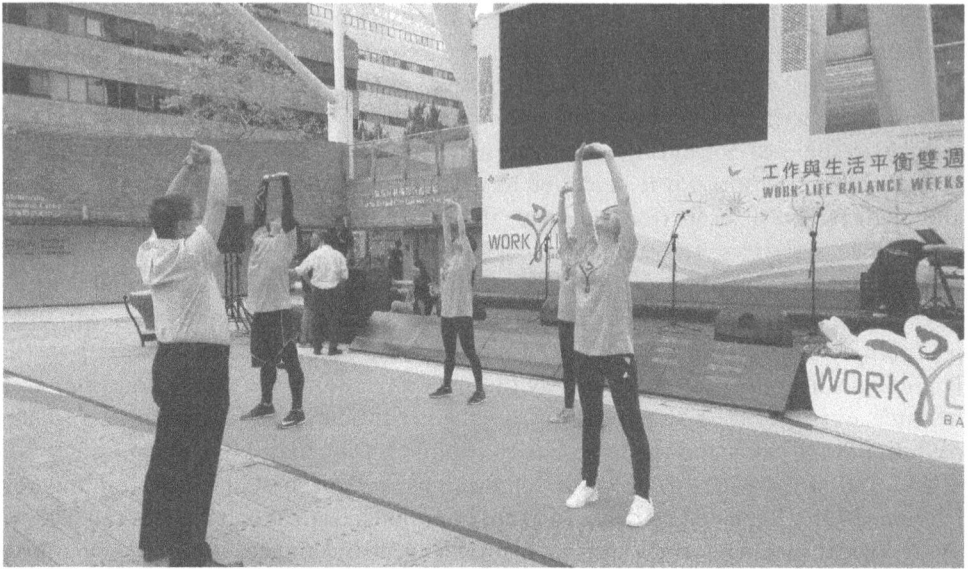

Figure 5.1 Prof. Hector Tsang, the first author, leading *qigong* practice in a health promotion program in Hong Kong

aiming to achieve a dynamic equilibrium of body function (Sun & Li, 1997). As such, *qigong* is seen as a type of mind-body exercise that can be classified into static *qigong* and dynamic *qigong*, with the former focusing on meditation and breathing in static positions and the latter emphasizing coordinated movement, breathing, and mindfulness (Chan & Tsang, 2019). Compared with static *qigong*, dynamic *qigong* is more frequently studied and practiced. Common forms of dynamic *qigong* include Eight-section Brocades (i.e., *Baduanjin*), *Wuqinxi*, *Yijinjing*, and *Liuzijue*, with most of the published studies on *qigong* being about Eight-section Brocades (Zhang et al., 2020).

Tai chi was developed as an ancient Chinese martial art based on the Taoist philosophy of *yin* and *yang*, which holds that seemingly opposite forces are interconnected and complementary to one another. Hence, it is essential to redirect the hardness (i.e., *yang*) in the force of an opponent with softness (i.e., *yin*). The movements of *tai chi* and the physical state required to perform this martial art were designed to embrace forces from opponents instead of direct resistance (Yeung et al., 2019). Despite the common principle derived from *yin* and *yang*, various types of traditional *tai chi* were developed in ancient China, such as the Chen, Yang, and Sun styles, among others. Today, *tai chi* is recognized more as a physical exercise for health promotion than as a martial art. Specifically, it is regarded as a mind-body exercise, similar to *qigong*, as it involves gentle and flowing movements and requires a meditative mind (Kong et al., 2019). To promote health in China, the Chinese Sports Commission developed several modern forms of *tai chi* with simplified movements based on traditional *tai chi* styles, such as the 24-form *tai chi chuan* (Liang & Wu, 2014).

Acupressure is closely related to the meridian system in TCM theory. Meridians are channels in the body where *qi* flows to regulate one's physical and psychological functions, with there being 12 standard meridians and eight extraordinary meridians

(Li et al., 2021). Acupoints are a set of special locations along the meridians, which are believed to be where life energies are exchanged (Zhang et al., 2015). Although the meridians and acupoints are not anatomical systems, both acupoints and non-acupoints have been found to exhibit different surface electric potentials (Li et al., 2021). Acupressure is a TCM-based bodywork technique that involves stimulating acupoints with the fingers, hands, or other tools, with finger-based acupressure being the most commonly used (Beal, 2000). Finger stimulation methods include pressing, kneading, and tapping, designed to achieve soreness, numbness, or distention at acupoints (Beal, 2000). Stimulation of these acupoints is believed to restore the balance of *qi* flow in the body and promote health (National Cancer Institute, n.d.). Acupressure commonly targets acupoints on the head, ears, neck, forearms, and legs.

Effectiveness and mechanisms in stress management

Qigong, *tai chi*, and acupressure have been used for rehabilitation and health promotion among the Chinese population for centuries, and scientific studies on their health benefits and underlying mechanisms have been increasing since the 2000s. There is accumulating documentation of the treatment effects of *qigong*, *tai chi*, and acupressure on the psychosocial outcomes of various healthy or client groups. Several systematic reviews have reported the synthesized benefits of *qigong*, *tai chi*, or acupressure on mental health, including stress. However, it is important to be aware of the high heterogeneities in treatment protocols, duration, clients, and outcomes in previous studies on *qigong*, *tai chi*, and acupressure.

Effectiveness in stress management

Based on a search for "[*qigong* OR *tai chi* OR acupressure] AND [stress]" in PubMed in February 2023, eight relevant systematic reviews published since 2010 were identified. Although these systematic reviews might evaluate the pooled effects on various psychosocial outcomes, findings about stress management elicited by *qigong*, *tai chi*, or acupressure are summarized in Table 5.1.

The meta-analysis by Wang et al. (2014) has shown the significant effect of *qigong* on alleviating perceived stress among healthy adults, whereas a marginally insignificant pooled effect was found by Zeng et al. (2019) in stress management for cancer patients. Since there were only two included studies in the analysis by Zeng et al. (2019), it may not be powerful enough to detect a significant pooled effect. Nonetheless, Zeng et al. (2019) acknowledged the positive trend that favored the stress management effect of *qigong* over the controls. In a systematic review by Churchill et al. (2022), significant treatment effects of *qigong* on the perceived stress of older adults with chronic health conditions were also recognized based on qualitative synthesis. It is notable that the *qigong* protocol of each included study in the above three systematic reviews was unique, making it unclear as to which active ingredient in *qigong* works on stress. Most of the included studies compared *qigong* to no intervention or standard care. Moreover, the *qigong* training duration for older adults (Churchill et al., 2022) was evidently longer than the training duration for healthy adults (Wang et al., 2014) and cancer patients (Zeng et al., 2019). It is plausible that older adults required longer training time given their impaired cognitive or physical functions compared with younger populations.

Table 5.1 Systematic reviews on *tai chi, qigong,* or acupressure for management of stress published in 2010–2023

Systematic review	Included studies	Population	Research design (number of included studies)	Intervention	Control	Main findings
Wang et al. (2014)	Chow et al. (2012) Griffith et al. (2008) Hwang et al. (2013)	Healthy adults	RCT (n = 3)	*Qigong* ■ Protocols: ■ *Chanmigong* (n = 1) ■ Basic Eight *Qigong* (n = 1) ■ Brief *Qigong*-based Stress Reduction Program (n = 1) ■ Duration: 4–12 weeks	Wait-list (n = 3)	*Qigong* could significantly reduce perceived stress in healthy adults at post-intervention, pooled SMD = -0.88, 95% CI $[-1.22, -0.55]$, $Z = 5.16$, $p < .001$, $I^2 = 0\%$.
Churchill et al. (2022)	Campo et al. (2014) Xiao et al. (2018) Zhang et al. (2016)	Older adults with chronic physical conditions	RCT (n = 3)	*Qigong* ■ Protocols: ■ General *qigong* (n = 1) ■ *Baduanjin* (n = 1) ■ *Yijinjing* (n = 1) ■ Duration: 3–6 months	Stretching (n = 1) Usual care (n = 2)	All three studies found significant stress reduction in *qigong* groups compared with control groups.
Zeng et al. (2019)	Loh et al. (2014) Oh et al. (2014)	Cancer survivors	RCT (n = 2)	*Qigong* ■ Protocols: ■ Internal *qigong* (n = 1) ■ Medical *qigong* (n = 1) ■ Duration: 8–10 weeks	Usual care (n = 1) Meditation (n = 1)	The pooled effects of *qigong* on stress at post-intervention were marginally insignificant, MD = -8.56, 95% CI $[-17.56, 0.44]$, $Z = 1.86$, $p = .06$, $I^2 = 74\%$.

Table 5.1 Systematic reviews on *tai chi*, *qigong*, or acupressure for management of stress published in 2010–2023 *(continued)*

Systematic review	Included studies	Population	Research design (number of included studies)	Intervention	Control	Main findings
Wang et al. (2010)	McCain et al. (2008), Fransen et al. (2007), Li et al. (2001), Sun et al. (1996)	Various populations, in general[a]	RCT (n = 4)	*Tai chi* ■ Protocols: ■ *Tai chi* with eight movements (n = 1) ■ Sun-style *Tai Chi* (n = 1) ■ Yang-style *Tai Chi* (n = 1) ■ *Tai chi* with an unspecified style (n = 1) ■ Duration: 10–24 weeks	Wait-list (n = 3), Routine physical activities (n = 1)	*Tai chi* could significantly reduce stress at post-intervention, SMD = 0.97, 95% CI [0.06, 1.87].[b]
Yang et al. (2022)	Chan et al. (2018), Liu et al. (2020)	Clients with cardiovascular disease or cardiovascular risk factors	RCT (n = 2)	*Tai chi* ■ Protocols: ■ 24 simplified *tai chi* (n = 1) ■ 24-form *tai chi* (n = 1) ■ Duration: 12–40 weeks	Usual care (n = 2)	Both studies found significant stress reduction in *tai chi* groups compared with control groups.
Webster et al. (2016)	Caldwell et al. (2011), Esch et al. (2007)	University students	Quasi-experiment (n = 1), Prospective study (n = 1)	*Tai chi* ■ Protocols: ■ Chen-style *Tai Chi* (n = 1) ■ Yang-style *Tai Chi* (n = 1) ■ Duration: 14–15 weeks	Recreational activities (n = 1)	Compared with the control group (recreational activities), the *tai chi* group had significantly more reduction in stress. Healthy adults who participated in the 15-week *tai chi* training had significant stress reduction compared with the baseline.

Table 5.1 Systematic reviews on *tai chi, qigong,* or acupressure for management of stress published in 2010–2023 *(continued)*

Systematic review	Included studies	Population	Research design (number of included studies)	Intervention	Control	Main findings
Song et al. (2015)	Honda et al. (2012)	University students	RCT (n = 1)	Acupressure ■ Protocol: Self-acupressure on three acupoints (*Wangu* GB12, *Tianrong* SI17, *Futu* LI18) during morning, mid-day, and night ■ Duration: 4 weeks	No intervention	University students who were in the acupressure group had significantly more stress reduction than the control group at mid-intervention and post-intervention.
Church et al. (2018)	Rogers & Scars (2015)	University students	RCT (n = 1)	Acupressure ■ Protocol: Emotional Freedom Techniques (EFT) with acupoint tapping ■ Duration: 15–20 minutes for each session	EFT with sham acupoint tapping	University students who were in the EFT group had significantly more stress reduction than the control group at post-intervention, implying that acupoint tapping was an effective treatment factor.

Notes:

a Populations included individuals with HIV, older adults with symptomatic hip or knee osteoarthritis, and healthy older adults.

b The meta-analysis result was extracted from a subgroup analysis in Wang et al. (2010), and the relevant Z score, *p*-value, and I^2 were not reported by the authors.

According to the meta-analysis by Wang et al. (2010), *tai chi* was, in general, an effective treatment for stress in various populations compared with no intervention or standard care. Similar findings supporting the treatment benefits of *tai chi* on stress management were reported by Webster et al. (2016) and Yang et al. (2022) based on qualitative synthesis. It is important to note the potential bias in the included studies of the review by Webster et al. (2016), given their research designs did not involve randomization or a control. However, Webster et al. (2016) also pointed out the limited number of available studies on *tai chi* for stress management among university students, particularly in the Chinese population. Similar to *qigong*, the previous studies on *tai chi* also tested various protocols in comparison with no intervention or usual care, leaving the active ingredients in *tai chi* unclear.

There were significantly fewer studies available on the effects of acupressure on stress compared with *qigong* and *tai chi*, and both focused on university students (Church et al., 2018; Song et al., 2015). Among the 10 studies included in the review by Song et al. (2015), only one study focused on stress management. This study supported the effectiveness of a four-week acupressure program involving daily self-practice on three acupoints on the neck (Honda et al., 2012). Acupoint tapping is a type of acupressure technique and is incorporated in a standardized protocol called Emotional Freedom Techniques (EFT) for the management of mental health conditions (Gallo, 2004). Church et al. (2018) reviewed clinical studies that compared standard EFTs with adjusted EFTs involving sham acupressure and confirmed acupressure as an active treatment element in EFTs. Among the six studies reviewed by Church et al. (2018), Rogers and Sears (2015) study was the only one to look at stress management. Despite the limited evidence, acupressure appeared to be an effective technique to manage stress in healthy adults.

Effectiveness in alleviating depression and anxiety
According to the systematic reviews summarized in Table 5.1, empirical studies testing the stress management effects of *qigong*, *tai chi*, or acupressure appear to be limited. More studies have been conducted to evaluate their treatment effects on depression and anxiety. This might be due to stronger rehabilitation needs in people suffering from depression and anxiety compared to those under stress. Chronic stress has been recognized as an etiological factor of depression and anxiety (Patriquin & Mathew, 2017; Tafet & Nemeroff, 2016). Hence, it is plausible to suggest the effectiveness of *qigong*, *tai chi*, and acupressure in reducing stress based on their treatment effects on depression and anxiety.

Two systematic reviews and meta-analyses have reported significant antidepressant effects of *qigong* in clients with depression and other adults with chronic physical conditions (Liu et al., 2015; So et al., 2019). Lin et al. (2022b) and Liu et al. (2021) both found significant pooled effects of *qigong* on depression and anxiety in student populations based on meta-analyses. All three systematic reviews about *tai chi* summarized in Table 5.1 synthesized the empirical findings on depression and anxiety. Webster et al. (2016) reviewed 76 studies on *tai chi* among university students, with the majority of studies having been conducted with Chinese participants. Significant reductions in depression and anxiety were reported in 19 and 17 relevant studies, respectively. Meta-analyses by Wang et al. (2010) and Yang et al. (2022) both demonstrated significant pooled effects of *tai chi* on depression and anxiety in healthy adults and clients. As for acupressure, Lin et al. (2022a) conducted a systematic review and meta-analysis, synthesizing 14 RCTs. They found significant pooled effects of acupressure on alleviating depressive symptoms and anxiety in clients with primary or secondary depression. Based on a systematic review and meta-analysis of seven RCTs, Au et al. (2015a) confirmed the superior effectiveness of acupressure over sham controls in managing anxiety. They also identified *Yintang* (EX-HN3) and *Shenmen* (HT7) as the commonly involved acupoints for the treatment of anxiety. The effectiveness of acupressure in alleviating anxiety was confirmed again based on a more recent systematic review and meta-analysis conducted by Chen et al. (2022).

Mechanisms underlying stress management

Activation of the SAM axis and the HPA axis are the two major components of the stress response system (Godoy et al., 2018). Hence, it is essential to manage stress through the regulation of physiological activities in these systems. According to previous studies on treatment-related changes in neurobiological outcomes after *qigong, tai chi*, or acupressure, it is plausible that they alleviate stress through activation of the parasympathetic nervous system (PNS) and regulation of the HPA axis, as shown in Figure 5.2.

As a mind-body exercise, both *qigong* and *tai chi* cultivate a mindful state that can enhance relaxation, counteracting stress responses in the body (Liu et al., 2021).

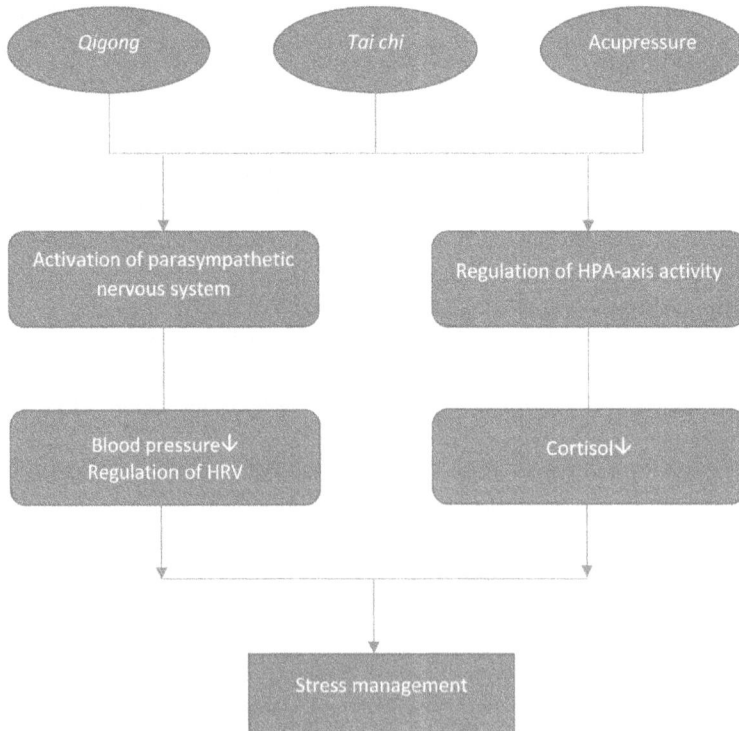

Figure 5.2 Mechanisms of stress management using *qigong, tai chi*, and acupressure

Acupressure on acupoints (e.g., *Yintang* [EX-HN3]) relevant to emotional regulation based on TCM theories is also expected to promote relaxation (Kwon & Lee, 2018). According to the systematic review and meta-analysis by So et al. (2019), *qigong* could significantly reduce blood pressure in people with depressive symptoms. Zou et al. (2017) synthesized various health benefits of *Baduanjin* (a form of health *qigong*) for both healthy adults and clients and also reported significant pooled effects on blood pressure. Similar synthesized effects of *tai chi* on blood pressure were reported by Guan et al. (2020) in their meta-analysis of RCTs. In addition, Zeng et al. (2014) have confirmed the significant pooled effects of *qigong* and *tai chi* on enhancing heart rate variability and reducing cortisol levels in cancer survivors. Other clinical studies and meta-analyses have also supported the regulation of the HPA axis as one of the treatment effects of *qigong* in adolescents (Liu et al., 2021) and depressed older adults (Lu et al., 2020). Similarly, *tai chi* was found to effectively reduce cortisol levels in healthy adults (Nedeljkovic et al., 2012) and people with severe mental illness (SMI) (Ho et al., 2016). As for acupressure, studies into its treatment effects on neurobiological outcomes about stress are relatively limited. There was an RCT that found a significant reduction in blood pressure among older adults with hypertension after acupressure (Kim & Park, 2023). Another two RCTs reported an acupressure-related significant reduction in the cortisol levels of healthy adults (McFadden et al., 2012) and older adults with dementia (Kwan et al., 2017). Ultimately, more evidence from systematic reviews and meta-analyses is warranted to confirm that acupressure can effectively regulate the automatic nervous system and HPA axis.

Mental illness and public stigma

Individuals suffering from mental illness are a highly stigmatized group. It is common for them to face public stigma of mental illness, which is defined as the negative perceptions, attitudes, and behaviors from the general public toward people with mental illness (Corrigan, 2018). Research over the past two decades has demonstrated mental illness stigma as a significant issue among the Chinese population despite the growing recognition of mental illness issues and the expansion of mental health services. Chinese people with mental illness are vulnerable to obstacles in help-seeking, education and employment, and other aspects of social life. It is important to understand the sociocultural roots of mental illness stigma in the Chinese population, assess the stigmatizing attitudes and behaviors from various groups, investigate the negative influences on people with mental illness, and explore interventions to overcome the public stigma of mental illness.

Understanding mental illness in Chinese culture

People's lay concepts and theories about mental illness are closely connected to public stigma. Research has revealed that traditional cultural values and orientations play an important role in Chinese people's understanding of mental illness. Based on a holistic view of health following the principles of Taoism, Chinese people tend to perceive no boundaries between physiological and mental illness. Influenced by Confucianism and Buddhism, having a mental illness is regarded as a punishment of one's wrongfulness or the failures of one's family or ancestors. In Chinese culture, which is strongly influenced by collectivistic values, particularly Confucian principles, people emphasize harmonious social relations and the core role of family. Having an individual with mental illness in the family is regarded as a threat to the "*mianzi*" (面子, i.e., face or reputation) of both the individual and the family. It will also harm the "*guanxi*" (關係, i.e., social network and relations) of all family members (Lam et al., 2010). Hence, empirical studies have demonstrated associations between mental illness and shame, negative perceptions, and negative attitudes in Chinese culture (Wu et al., 2020; Zhang et al., 2019). Additionally, Chinese people have shown a stronger endorsement of the sociological model of mental illness than Westerners (e.g., Furnham & Chan, 2004).

Apart from lay concepts and theories, people's mental health literacy, i.e., the knowledge and attitudes about mental illness (Jorm, 2000), is also an influential factor of public stigma. Empirical studies have consistently found low mental health literacy among Chinese people from various regions. A survey in Hong Kong found that people had difficulty correctly identifying most mental disorders, while depression and obsessive-compulsive disorder were relatively better recognized (Lui et al., 2016). Another study found that Chinese people in Shanghai had a lower awareness of professional support for mental illness compared with people in Hong Kong and Australia (Wong et al., 2012). A large-scale survey in Tianjin showed low health literacy about the causes, treatment, and prevention of mental disorders. It also demonstrated the negative association between mental health literacy and public stigma (Yin et al., 2020).

Public attitudes toward mental illness

Given the limitations of Chinese people's understanding of mental illness, high levels of public stigma have been found in recent studies. As shown in studies with explicit measures (e.g., psychological scales) and implicit measures (e.g., implicit association tests), Chinese people tend to endorse negative stereotypes about mental illness, such as the perception that people with mental illness are violent, aggressive, and incompetent (Wang et al., 2012; Zhang et al., 2019). In light of these negative attitudes toward people with mental illness, Chinese people show a tendency to socially avoid them and reject community-based measures for psychiatric rehabilitation (Tsang et al., 2003a; Yin et al., 2020). Public stigma in Hong Kong was found to be mostly salient in people with low educational attainment aged 50 or above (Lo et al., 2021).

In addition, studies have focused on specific groups' attitudes and behavioral tendencies toward people with mental illness. One frequently studied group includes health professionals, workers, and trainees. For instance, a group of community mental health staff in Guangzhou showed only a moderate level of willingness to contact people with mental illness (Li et al., 2014). Non-mental health professionals in Hunan also expressed reluctance to have people with mental illness marry into their families (Wu et al., 2020). Trainees of OT in Hong Kong preferred working with individuals with physical disabilities and no history of aggressive behaviors in placement training compared with other types of clients, including people with mental illness (Tsang et al., 2004).

Employers constitute another important group in research on the public stigma of mental illness because employment of ex-mentally ill persons is essential for their psychosocial rehabilitation and wellness. A qualitative interview study on the concerns of hiring people with psychotic disorders was carried out among 100 employers from various industries in Beijing, Hong Kong, and Chicago (Tsang et al., 2007). The study revealed that themes of stigma expressed by employers were generally common to all three groups; however, their degrees of endorsement varied across groups. Employers in Beijing and Hong Kong were mostly concerned about how coworkers might be affected, whereas employers in Chicago were mainly worried about compromised job performance. Variations in individualism were found to explain the cultural differences in employers' stigmatizing attitudes. Another large-scale survey of 300 employers from the same three cities explored their perspectives in hiring people with AIDS, or a history of drug abuse, alcohol abuse, or psychosis (Corrigan et al., 2010). The study showed that employers with a stronger perception of health conditions as behaviorally driven would hold more stigmatizing views; however, this association was weaker in employers from Chicago compared with the other two groups.

Consequences of public stigma

Living in a stigmatizing community or society poses great challenges to the rehabilitation and well-being of people with mental illness. It is common for Chinese people with mental illness to experience public stigma and discrimination (Lv et al., 2013), which can result in social isolation, limited support, lower help-seeking tendencies, and less use of mental health services (Sirey et al., 2001). In addition, people with mental illness can experience physical distress, such as sleep disturbance, which impairs their health-related quality of life (Chan & Fung, 2019). Due to the stigmatizing views of employers, it is difficult for people who used to have mental illness to obtain competitive employment (Tsang et al., 2010a). A core psychological manifestation of this consequence is the internalization of stigmatizing views from the public, which is detrimental to the self-efficacy and self-esteem of people with mental illness (Corrigan & Rao, 2012). This will be extensively introduced in the next section.

In addition, public stigma affects not only Chinese people with mental illness but also their caregivers. These caregivers face an objective burden due to social isolation and financial difficulties, partly caused by the low employment rates and poor job retention of their carees (Tsang et al., 2003b; Yin et al., 2014). Caregivers also experience subjective burdens such as frustration, anxiety, low self-esteem, and helplessness (Tsang et al., 2003b). Consequently, they express a strong need for services to obtain and secure employment with carees (Tsui & Tsang, 2017). Public stigma significantly increases the caregiving burden. In turn, caregivers' negative emotions and practical difficulties can lead to increased perceived stigma by their carees (Chien et al., 2014). This creates a vicious cycle of psychological distress for both people with mental illness and their caregivers.

Approaches to reduce public stigma

Confronting and reducing public stigma of mental illness have been conceptualized as multifaceted processes carried out through various methods (Corrigan, 2018). Specifically, common approaches to erase public stigma include protests, education, and interpersonal contact. Affirmative actions designed to recognize positive images of people with mental illness and develop positive attitudes and behaviors toward them are also important steps to combat public stigma. Changes in not only social interactions, but also in mass media and social policy, are needed to tackle the public stigma of mental illness. For example, there was a redefining of the Chinese translation of psychosis in Hong Kong, which replaced "*jingshen fen lie*" (精神分裂, meaning a split mind) with "*si jue shi tiao*" (思覺失調, meaning dysregulations in perceptions and thoughts). Furthermore, the correct media depiction of mental illness was made a requirement by the National Mental Health Work Plan (2015–2020) in mainland China (Zhang et al., 2019).

Studies on public stigma reduction interventions among Chinese populations have emerged in the past two decades, providing a preliminary understanding about the effectiveness of these interventions. A systematic review was conducted by Xu et al. (2017b) that synthesized nine studies published from 2002 to 2014 on anti-public stigma programs in samples from mainland China, Hong Kong, Macau, and Taiwan. Five of the studies adopted an educational approach (e.g., lectures, videos, and educational materials about scientific understanding and common myths of mental illness), while the remaining studies tested a combined approach with education and interpersonal contact (in-person or video-based). Taken together, a small effect on stereotype reduction and improvement in mental health literacy was found. Programs with the combined approach did not outperform those with education alone, as shown in the review by Xu et al. (2017b). However, this remains inconclusive given the limited number of included studies and their methodological limitation – most studies did not incorporate randomization. In summary, the majority of participants in the nine studies were Chinese students (adolescents or university students), and anti-public stigma programs appeared to be effective in this group; it remains unclear as to the effectiveness in other Chinese populations.

More recent studies have documented additional approaches or intervention programs to tackle the public stigma of mental illness among Chinese populations. For example, Li et al. (2019) conducted a randomized controlled trial to examine the effectiveness of anti-stigma training for care assistant workers for people with SMI in a hospital in Guangzhou, China. Both the intervention group and control group received three hours of training comprising three modules, including two common modules on financial assistance and mental health knowledge. In the third module, the intervention group learned about mental illness stigma, its consequences, and coping strategies, whereas the control group had training about insurance policies. While both groups showed an improvement in mental health knowledge, the intervention group showed a significantly enhanced positive attitude toward people with mental illness than the control group. In Yuen and Mak's (2021) study, an anti-public stigma strategy was combined with virtual reality (VR). Using a randomized controlled design, participants in the intervention group received an immersive VR experience on the daily life and perceived stigma from the subjective perspective of an animated character with mental illness (i.e., immersive group). Another group of participants received a mainly text-based and third-person narration of the same story of the animated character (i.e., text group), while the remaining participants watched a neutral VR video (i.e., control group). After ten minutes of the VR experience, both the immersive group and text group showed a significant reduction in public stigma, but not the control group. However, the changes in public stigma did not differ between the immersive group and the text group. More interactive VR components were suggested for the immersive group to boost its effectiveness.

Self-stigma of mental illness

Living with negative stereotypes, prejudice, and discrimination from the public, people with mental illness can internalize stigmatizing perceptions and attitudes and even self-discriminate. This is called self-stigma (Corrigan, 2018), and this psychological phenomenon is evident in the Chinese population. As mentioned earlier, self-stigma is the core psychological mechanism that processes the psychological distress and behavioral difficulties experienced by people with mental illness. The formation and negative outcomes of self-stigma have been investigated in the Chinese population, and efforts have also been made to develop and test strategies for self-stigma reduction.

Theoretical model and the cultural factor

Self-stigma is conceptualized as the aftermath of public stigma, and it evolves in stages. According to Corrigan and Rao (2012), a person with stigmatized condition is initially aware of public stigma; next, the person starts to agree that the negative stereotypes about his/her condition are true; third, the person endorses the negative stereotypes and applies them to himself/herself; lastly, the person's self-worth is significantly compromised. The above four stages constitute the factor structure of self-stigma, which includes stereotype awareness, stereotype agreement, self-concurrence, and self-esteem decrement (Corrigan et al., 2006). This factor structure has been validated in both Western and Chinese cultures (Corrigan et al., 2006; Fung et al., 2007). However, strong correlations between stereotype awareness and the other three factors were only found in the Chinese population (Fung et al., 2007), and the association between self-stigma and psychological distress was stronger in Chinese people with mental illness than in a Western group (Au et al., 2019; Li et al., 2022). Self-stigma of people with first-episode psychosis in Hong Kong was significantly correlated with their "face concern", which denotes concerns about violating social norms, losing others' respect, or making others disappointed (Chen et al., 2016). According to large-scale surveys by Young and Ng (2016), the prevalence rates of self-stigma among mental health service consumers in Hong Kong and Guangzhou were 38% and 50%, respectively.

The above findings suggest that Chinese people with mental illness are more vulnerable to self-stigma compared to Westerners. This can be explained by the collectivistic cultural orientation endorsed by Chinese people. The self-concept of Chinese people with mental illness was found to form a hierarchical and multidimensional model with five factors, namely interpersonal relationships, social integrity, personal competency, personal qualities, and external achievements; higher importance was placed on the first two factors, which represent the interpersonal dimension of the self (Tam et al., 2004). Influenced by the Confucian value of fate acceptance, Chinese people with mental illness are more ready than Westerners to justify the stigmatizing views of others (Fung et al., 2007). It is easier for Chinese people with mental illness to be aware of public stigma and agree with it. Given the importance of the interpersonal self (Markus & Kitayama, 1991), Chinese people with mental illness often base their self-concept and self-worth on public stigma. As a result, they may quickly internalize public stigma, leading to self-stigma. This process involves self-concurrence and decreased self-esteem, which can significantly harm the psychological well-being of Chinese people with mental illness.

Consequences of self-stigma

The consequences of self-stigma have been conceptualized as the "why try" effect, which captures the psychological phenomenon of people with mental illness who suffer from psychological distress due to the internalization of negative stereotypes about mental illness (Corrigan et al., 2009). "Why try" is defined as a sense of worthlessness about oneself, where the pursuit of life goals and engagement in meaningful activities seem to be pointless due to the negative expectation of any self-generated action (Corrigan et al., 2016). According to an online survey of more than 500 American adults with mental illness, Corrigan et al. (2016) found significant correlations between the "why try" phenomenon and depression and a lowered sense of recovery. Similar consequences of self-stigma were documented in the Chinese population, manifesting in terms of psychological well-being, help-seeking, and treatment compliance.

Apart from suffering due to their mental conditions, Chinese people with mental illness generally experience diminished global psychological well-being if they endorse self-stigma. According to a survey of 100 adults with schizophrenia in Taiwan, their global mental health was significantly and negatively correlated with four components of self-stigma: alienation, stereotype endorsement, discrimination experience, and social withdrawal (Tang & Wu, 2012). In addition, global mental health was not significantly associated with stigma resistance, the fifth component of self-stigma. This may be explained by the low awareness of the discourse on the human rights of people with mental illness in the Chinese context (Tang & Wu, 2012). Similarly, in a stratified sample of 602 people with chronic schizophrenia in Shanghai, high levels of self-stigma were significantly correlated with a low quality of life, particularly in the psychosocial aspect (Guo et al., 2018). Another survey of 282 people with mental illness in Hong Kong also confirmed the mediating role of sleep disturbance on the connection between self-stigma and diminished health-related quality of life in both the physical and mental aspects (Chan & Fung, 2019). In other words, the endorsement of self-stigma about mental illness can lead to significantly reduced sleep quality, which significantly compromises ones' physical and mental health.

Although the internalization of stigma about mental illness can worsen Chinese people's mental health, it can also hinder them from seeking professional help. The negative association between self-stigma and professional help-seeking has been consistently found in surveys of Chinese adolescents (Chen et al., 2014), Chinese international students studying in Western countries (Ma et al., 2022), Hong Kong Chinese adults (Chen et al., 2020), and Chinese immigrants in the United States (Yee et al., 2020). A meta-analysis of 94 studies showed that the negative effect of the self-stigma of mental illness on professional help-seeking was culturally universal (Yu et al., 2023). As an antecedent of self-stigma and a low intention to seek professional help, face concern was found to be significantly higher in Chinese samples than in European Americans (Chen et al., 2020). For Chinese adolescents with more self-reported mental health issues, they endorsed self-stigma more strongly and were less likely to seek help (Chen et al., 2014). However, Chinese females were less prone to self-stigma than males, which, in turn, resulted in relatively more willingness to seek professional help (Yee et al., 2020).

For Chinese people with diagnosed mental health conditions, the endorsement of self-stigma has been recognized as a significant barrier to treatment adherence. Despite the limited number of studies published, there is qualitative documentation showing that Chinese people with mental illness in rural areas were reluctant to take medication because of the stigma related to their illness (Chai et al., 2021). Specifically, drugs for mental conditions were regarded as a symbol of personal or family shame, and Chinese people intended to hide their mental illness through the avoidance of medication. Similarly, Chinese people with schizophrenia showed low adherence to psychosocial treatment. It was consistently demonstrated in previous studies that self-stigma negatively predicted psychosocial treatment participation (Fung et al., 2008; Fung et al., 2010; Tsang et al., 2010b). Even when taking self-esteem and global functioning into account, self-stigma remained a significant barrier to attendance and participation in psychosocial treatments for Chinese people with schizophrenia (Fung et al., 2008; Tsang et al., 2010b). In addition, clients suffering from schizophrenia with high self-stigma would lead to low awareness of treatment benefits and low readiness to deal with their mental health issues, which, in turn, would result in low adherence to psychosocial treatments (Fung et al., 2010).

Approaches to reduce self-stigma

Self-stigma is multifaceted and comprises multiple stages. Moreover, self-stigma experiences can vary among mental illnesses. Hence, numerous strategies have been developed and tested in Western countries to address the issues related to self-stigma about mental illness. According to a review by Yanos et al. (2015), psychoeducation, cognitive techniques, reflection on stigma-related experiences, and behavioral strategies for empowerment were common features observed in the interventions for mental health self-stigma; however, it is also important to acknowledge individual circumstances and the context surrounding self-stigma. Similar efforts to reduce self-stigma have also been implemented among Chinese people with mental illness, although these are less frequently documented in English-language academic papers.

The Self-stigma Reduction Program (Fung et al., 2011) was a pioneering intervention for addressing mental health self-stigma in the Chinese population. In several previous systematic reviews on interventions for self-stigma among mental health rehabilitation service users (Büchter & Messer, 2017; Tsang et al., 2016), only one of the included studies was conducted among Chinese people with SMI, and this study was about the Self-stigma Reduction Program. Developed based on experiences of self-stigma and its negative consequences for Hong Kong Chinese people with schizophrenia, the Self-stigma Reduction Program incorporates several modalities: (1) psychoeducation to acquire scientific understanding about mental illness, (2) cognitive behavioral therapy (CBT) to combat irrational self-concepts, (3) motivational interviewing to enhance readiness for change, (4) social skills training to handle difficult social situations, and (5) a goal attainment program to facilitate a sense of self-worth and hope. These modalities were developed based on the theoretical framework that self-stigma is detrimental to treatment adherence through diminished insights into treatment and readiness for change. The program is delivered in 12 group sessions, followed by four individual sessions. An overview of the program is presented in Figure 5.3. A randomized controlled trial compared 32 participants with schizophrenia in a Self-stigma Reduction Program group to 34 participants in a newspaper reading control group. The program significantly reduced self-esteem decline, enhanced readiness for change, and promoted treatment participation post-intervention. However, these benefits did

Psychoeducation
- Beginning the journey toward recovery
- Confronting the myths about schizophrenia

Cognitive behavioral therapy/ motivational interviewing
- Impact of social stigma on recovery
- Self-stigma as barriers to recovery
- Combating self-stigma I: Affirming personal worth
- Combating self-stigma II: Disputing by evidence
- Combating self-stigma III: The art of acceptance

Social skills training
- Social skills training I: Being assertive
- Social skills training II: Dealing with stigmatizing social situations

Goal attainment program
- Goal attainment I: Goal setting
- Goal attainment II: Action planning

Round-up/individual follow-up
- Round-up of group sessions
- Monitoring progress

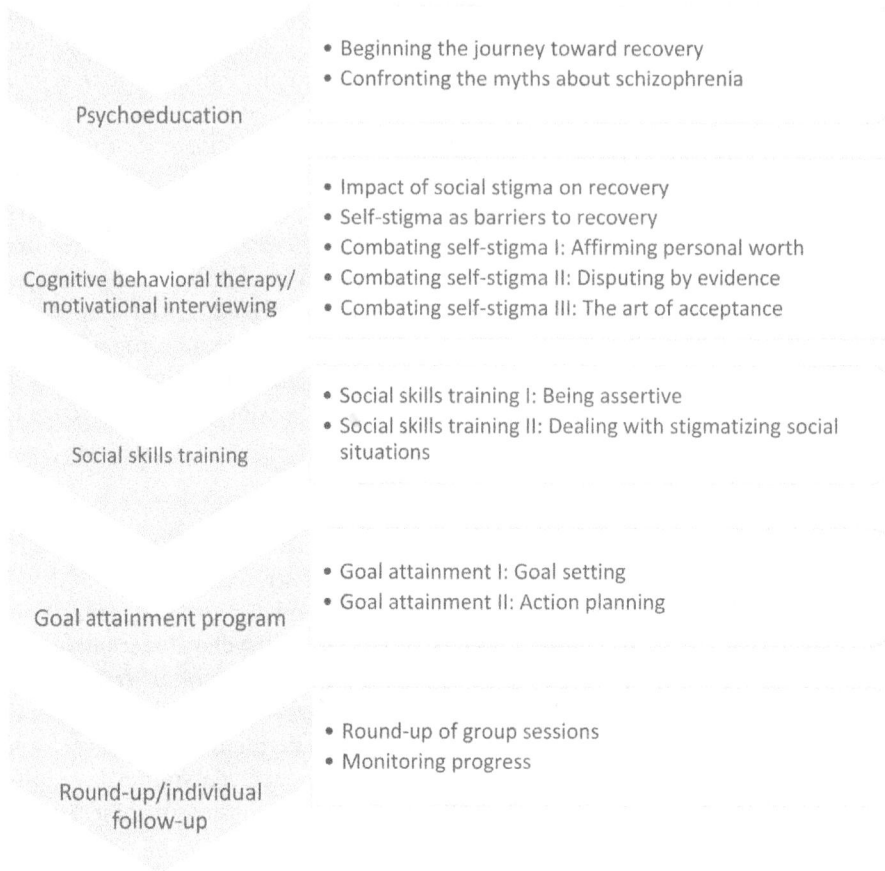

Figure 5.3 An overview of the Self-stigma Reduction Program for individuals with schizophrenia

not persist beyond six months after program completion (Fung et al., 2011). The Self-stigma Reduction Program provides a model for treating mental illness self-stigma and its related issues in the Chinese context.

Focusing on self-stigma among Chinese people with depression, Young et al. (2020) developed a CBT-based group intervention (CBT Group), which lasted for ten weeks with a 90-minute session per week. CBT Group includes a session on team building; a session of psychoeducation on the antecedents, beliefs, and consequences (ABC) model underlying CBT; five sessions on cognitive restructuring to change irrational beliefs and self-concepts related to mental illness stigma; a session on relaxation techniques to address stigma-related anxiety; a session on social skills to handle stigma-related social situations; and a round-up session. CBT Group was evaluated in comparison to standard treatment in a quasi-experiment (Young, 2018) and a randomized controlled trial (Young et al., 2020). Both studies found CBT Group to significantly alleviate self-stigma post-intervention. In addition, the reduction in self-stigma led to decreased depressive symptoms (Young et al., 2020). However, no follow-up assessment was performed, and it remains unclear whether the treatment benefits of CBT Group can be sustained upon completion of the intervention.

Both the Self-stigma Reduction Program and CBT Group are multi-component interventions. Both of which adopt approaches that include psychoeducation, CBT, and social skills training. Given the interconnected nature of self-stigma with the other psychosocial needs of people with mental illness, such as treatment adherence, social support, education, and employment, it is necessary to address self-stigma using multiple strategies. A highly comprehensive psychosocial intervention, known as Comprehensive Intervention, was developed for people with schizophrenia in Guangzhou, China. This intervention included: (1) psychoeducation on the basic understanding of schizophrenia, medication, side-effects, policies, and stigma about schizophrenia; (2) social skills training on communication, vocational performance, medication, self-management, and strategies to combat stigma and discrimination; and (3) CBT to overcome any misunderstandings or stigma attached to schizophrenia and to promote self-acceptance (Li et al., 2018). The intervention adopted a conventional framework of comprehensive psychosocial rehabilitation for people with schizophrenia, with the elements on stigma and discrimination being embedded in each of the three modules mentioned above. Comprehensive Intervention was delivered in eight 120-minute sessions over nine months. Based on a multicenter randomized controlled trial of 169 participants with schizophrenia in an intervention group and another 158 participants with schizophrenia in a control group, Comprehensive Intervention was found to significantly improve mental health service users' capability to overcome stigma and lower their anticipated discrimination upon completion of the nine-month training (Li et al., 2018). The maintenance effect of the intervention has yet to be tested.

While there are limited studies published in English-language academic journals on interventions for mental illness stigma among Chinese people, Xu et al. (2017a) conducted a systematic review and meta-analysis covering both English and Chinese journal articles on randomized and unrandomized controlled trials about anti-stigma interventions for Chinese people with mental illness, with 17 studies being included for synthesis. These studies evaluated the effectiveness of either psychoeducation or CBT in reducing perceived, experienced, or anticipated mental illness stigma by people with mental health conditions. The majority of the studies were conducted in mainland China, and a significant and large pooled effect on mental illness stigma reduction was found. However, caution must be taken when interpreting this finding given the generally moderate to high risk of bias in most of the studies.

Social skills and employment

Social skill as a cultural concept

Social skills are a group of skills, which can be verbal or non-verbal, that enable effective interaction and communication among people. Gestures, tones of voice, facial expressions, body language, etc. are all features of social skills. They allow us to identify other people's desires and emotions, as well as to exchange our ideas and thoughts (Tsang & Li, 2010). Social skills are not inherent but can be learned through formal or informal social interaction with other individuals. Social skills are complex, and it is difficult to adopt a generalized set of social skills for all situations. Rather, social skills are highly specific to cultures and situations (Bellack, 2004). When social skills are presented effectively during social interactions, there is a high probability of favorable outcomes for an individual, group, or community.

As mentioned above, social skills are culturally specific, meaning that acceptable social behaviors may vary across cultures. For instance, some foreign countries such as the United States may value people expressing their needs in a direct and polite manner, while this behavior may not be valued in Chinese culture (Cheung et al., 2017). Whether certain social behavior is adaptive or not depends on the culture. As a result, it is important to take culture into consideration to define what social skills are appropriate for a specific culture. Similarly, training or intervention that targets improving social skills should also be culturally applicable in order to maximize the effect.

Deficits in social skills and employment in Chinese people with mental illness

It is well documented that social skills play an important role in job searching and job retention. Social skills are essential in every workplace regardless of the job. Effective interactions with supervisors, coworkers, and customers are important qualities that employers look for during the recruitment process. Surprisingly, research shows that many people lose their jobs not because of poor job performance but because of having trouble fitting into the workplace socially (Agran et al., 2016). While this happens to people without mental illness, individuals with SMI encounter many difficulties in terms of social adjustment in the workplace. People with SMI are often characterized by poor social skills, which largely affect their employment outcome. This also explains the discrepancies in the employment rate between people with and without SMI. People with SMI are encouraged to look for job opportunities when they are ready to go back into society. However, getting a job is not easy for them. Even if they manage to secure a position, they face numerous challenges in retaining it. Poor communication with coworkers and supervisors is a common problem in the workplace for people with SMI. While previous research has suggested that having higher social competence will result in more favorable employment outcomes (Tsang et al., 2000), improvement in social skills is essential for people with SMI to become more competitive.

Social skills training

Conceptual framework

Effective use of social skills leads to favorable responses from one's social network. People who suffer from mental illnesses and psychological disorders are often vulnerable to deficits in their social lives and psychosocial functioning. Social skills training is derived from behavior therapy principles and techniques. It aims to equip people with skills to communicate their emotions and requests effectively to other people (Kopelowicz et al., 2006). The components of social skills training are derived from the basic principles of human learning, including operant conditioning, social learning theory, social cognition, etc. The basic procedures commonly adopted in social skills training are: (1) problem identification, (2) goal setting, (3) role play, (4) positive/corrective feedback, (5) social modeling, (6) behavioral practice, (7) positive social reinforcement, (8) homework assignments, and (9) positive reinforcement and problem-solving. This training has been applied to a broad range of mental disorders and psychological problems. Specifically, it is often used for people with schizophrenia to prevent relapses and promote progress toward recovery. Social skills training has been adopted by researchers to improve the social cognition and social functioning of Chinese people with schizophrenia (Wang et al., 2013). Apart from the benefits of enhanced communication among people, social skills training can also have positive effects on the mental state and quality of life of people with schizophrenia (Almerie et al., 2015). Recent research has extended the application of social skills training to Chinese children with autism spectrum disorders with limited social interaction capability (Shum et al., 2019). The results were extremely positive, showing improvements in social competence and social functioning as well as a reduction in autistic symptoms after the intervention.

Work-related social skills training
Social interaction is a major part of people's daily living, and working is one of the main components of people's everyday social interactions. Hence, work-related social skills are essential to psychosocial functioning. People with SMI generally suffer from deficits in work-related social skills and the related consequences of employment difficulties. Given the gap in effective training and support for the employment of Chinese people with schizophrenia, work-related social skills training was developed and tested in Hong Kong (Tsang, 2001a). Later, its application was extended to people with SMI, in general (Tsang et al., 2010c). The work-related social skills training involved ten group sessions, which taught mental health service users skills necessary for job interviews, basic conversation, and social survival. The aim of this training was to improve the capability of people with SMI to handle interpersonal challenges and, hopefully, to achieve better vocational outcomes. The content of the training was developed based on a three-tier framework adapted to the Chinese sociocultural context, including basic skills, core skills, and the results subsequent to the possession of these skills (Tsang & Li, 2010). Specifically, the training involves (1) basic social skills with a focus on interpersonal communication, (2) skills in handling general and work-related situations, and (3) skills that prepare participants for social contacts (Tsang, 2001b). The effectiveness of work-related social skills training has been demonstrated through solid empirical findings. For example, previous studies have shown that the training, together with appropriate professional support, is effective in enhancing social competence and vocational outcomes (Tsang, 2001a). In addition, Tsang and Pearson (2001) provided evidence revealing that social skills training effectively enabled people with schizophrenia to receive and retain a job.

Integrated Supported Employment
Although Chinese people with SMI can achieve a higher employment rate and longer job tenure after work-related social skills training, the impact of the training-related benefits would be limited if it is applied as a stand-alone intervention. To further improve the vocational outcomes of Chinese people with SMI, an innovative model called Integrated Supported Employment (ISE) was developed (Tsang, 2008). This model combines the Individual Placement and Support (IPS) model and work-related social skills training. IPS is a well-recognized model of supported employment to help people with SMI gain and maintain employment. The employment rate after using IPS is 53%, and job tenure is 12 weeks. Since the development of the ISE model, research has been done to compare the effectiveness of the IPS and ISE programs. ISE is shown to be an

effective program for enhancing employment rates and job tenures for people with SMI. Compared to IPS, participants who went through ISE had significantly higher employment rates (79%) and longer job tenure (24 weeks) (Tsang et al., 2009). Major improvements in social skills and social competence after the ISE program were also observed, which led to successfully finding jobs (Tsang et al., 2010c). This all helped people with SMI increase their competitiveness in the employment market. Other than employment outcomes, participants' well-being and self-efficacy also improved, which ultimately led to a better quality of life for people with SMI. Most importantly, the effects of the ISE program last for years (Tsang et al., 2010c). Apart from the above empirical support based on studies in Hong Kong, ISE adapted to the mainland China context was also found to outperform IPS and treatment-as-usual in enhancing employment rates, job tenures, and psychological well-being (Zhang et al., 2017).

Further efforts have been made to add other elements to the ISE program in an attempt to increase employment rates and job tenures. For example, cognitive function training, which is a significant predictor of vocational outcomes, has been added (Au et al., 2015b). However, many outcomes did not differ significantly between the ISE program with or without cognitive function training. This might be because the ISE has already pushed the employment outcome to its upper limit. Nevertheless, the ISE program is still recognized as one of the most useful programs for people with SMI.

Concluding remarks

This chapter reviews the theoretical understanding and empirical evidence of TCM-based bodywork (*qigong*, *tai chi*, and acupressure) for stress management, the Chinese cultural roots of public stigma and self-stigma about mental illness, the culturally relevant attempts to reduce mental illness stigma among Chinese populations, and the theoretical and practical development to support social skills and employment among Chinese people with SMI. All the relevant research reviewed in the chapter can inform the promotion and maintenance of meaningful psychosocial occupation among Chinese people. According to the Model of Human Occupation (MOHO; Kielhofner, 2008), occupation is a product of the interaction between environmental factors (physical, social, and cultural) and personal factors (volition, habituation, and performance capacity). *Qigong*, *tai chi*, and acupressure are indigenous approaches with fruitful social and cultural resources in Chinese communities. The performance of these TCM-based bodywork practices aligns well with Chinese people's volition. The research on *qigong*, *tai chi*, and acupressure for stress management informs their application as additional treatment options of OT. Studies on public stigma and self-stigma about mental illness in Chinese populations reveal the phenomena related to volition, habituation, and social environment that hinder the rehabilitation of people with mental illness. Therefore, interventions aimed at reducing such stigma should include all these aspects of occupation in their treatment goals and modalities. Social skills training and supported employment are designed to enhance the volition and performance capacity of Chinese individuals with SMI in the workplace. These interventions also take into account the Chinese cultural environment, which places a high value on productivity.

More high-quality clinical studies are needed to confirm and enhance our understanding of the approaches reviewed in this chapter. It is also crucial to develop integrated programs involving the reviewed approaches to boost their treatment benefits. For example, stress management techniques can be integrated with self-stigma reduction programs to relieve psychological distress among mental health service users when facing issues concerning mental illness stigma, empowering them to cope with the difficulties associated with stigma. Another possible integration could involve ISE and interventions designed to alleviate public stigma in the workplace. A positive loop can be formed between employers/coworkers with reduced stigma and people with SMI with enhanced social skills. Occupational therapists and researchers in rehabilitation sciences are encouraged to further explore stress management, stigma, and social skills, which can lead to innovation and enhanced effectiveness in psychosocial rehabilitation.

Lastly, while TCM-based bodyworks, mental health stigma, social skills, and employment are essential topics that connect OT with Chinese culture, the review of psychosocial practice is far from exhaustive. Given the limited scope of this chapter, other topics such as groupwork and support for independent living were not covered. However, more syntheses and reviews of other areas of psychosocial OT practice in the Chinese context are needed and warranted.

References

Affleck, A., Bianchi, E., Cleckley, M., Donaldson, K., McCormack, G., & Polon, J. (1984). Stress management as a component of occupational therapy in acute care settings. *Occupational Therapy in Health Care*, 1(3), 17–41. https://doi.org/10.1080/J003v01n03_04

Agran, M., Hughes, C., Thoma, C., & Scott, L. (2016). Employment social skills: What skills are really valued? *Career Development and Transition for Exceptional Individuals*, 39(2), 111–120. https://doi.org/10.1177/2165143414546741

Almerie, M. Q., Al Marhi, M. O., Jawoosh, M., Alsabbagh, M., Matar, H. E., Maayan, N., & Bergman, H. (2015). Social skills programmes for schizophrenia. *Cochrane Database of Systematic Reviews*, (6), CD009006. https://doi.org/10.1002/14651858.CD009006.pub2

American Occupational Therapy Association. (2020). Occupational therapy practice framework: Domain and process (4th ed.). *American Journal of Occupational Therapy*, 74(Suppl. 2), 7412410010.

American Psychological Association. (n.d.). Stressor. In *APA dictionary of psychology*. Retrieved April 6, 2022, from https://dictionary.apa.org/stressor

Au, C. H., Wong, C. S. M., Law, C. W., Wong, M. C., & Chung, K. F. (2019). Self-stigma, stigma coping and functioning in remitted bipolar disorder. *General Hospital Psychiatry*, 57, 7–12. https://doi.org/10.1016/j.genhosppsych.2018.12.007

Au, D. W., Tsang, H. W., Ling, P. P., Leung, C. H., Ip, P. K., & Cheung, W. M. (2015a). Effects of acupressure on anxiety: A systematic review and meta-analysis. *Acupuncture in Medicine*, 33(5), 353–359. https://doi.org/10.1136/acupmed-2014-010720

Au, D. W., Tsang, H. W., So, W. W., Bell, M. D., Cheung, V., Yiu, M. G., Tam, K. L., & Lee, G. T. H. (2015b). Effects of integrated supported employment plus cognitive remediation training for people with schizophrenia and schizoaffective disorders. *Schizophrenia Research*, 166(1-3), 297–303. https://doi.org/10.1016/j.schres.2015.05.013

Baum, A. (1990). Stress, intrusive imagery, and chronic distress. *Health Psychology*, 9(6), 653–675. https://doi.org/10.1037//0278-6133.9.6.653

Beal, M. W. (2000). Acupuncture and Oriental body work: Traditional and modern biomedical concepts in holistic care—Conceptual frameworks and biomedical developments. *Holistic Nursing Practice*, 15(1), 78–87. https://doi.org/10.1097/00004650-200010000-00010

Bellack, A. (2004). *Social skills training for schizophrenia: A step-by-step guide* (2nd ed.). Guilford Press.

Büchter, R. B., & Messer, M. (2017). Interventions for reducing self-stigma in people with mental illnesses: A systematic review of randomized controlled trials. *German Medical Science: GMS e-Journal*, 15, Doc07. https://doi.org/10.3205/000248

Chai, X., Liu, Y., Mao, Z., & Li, S. (2021). Barriers to medication adherence for rural patients with mental disorders in eastern China: A qualitative study. *BMC Psychiatry, 21*(1), 141. https://doi.org/10.1186/s12888-021-03144-y

Chan, K., & Fung, W. (2019). The impact of experienced discrimination and self-stigma on sleep and health-related quality of life among individuals with mental disorders in Hong Kong. *Quality of Life Research, 28*(8), 2171–2182. https://doi.org/10.1007/s11136-019-02181-1

Chan, S. H. W., & Tsang, H. W. H. (2019). The beneficial effects of Qigong on elderly depression. *International Review of Neurobiology, 147*, 155–188. https://doi.org/10.1016/bs.irn.2019.06.004

Chen, E. S., Chang, W. C., Hui, C. L., Chan, S. K., Lee, E. H., & Chen, E. Y. (2016). Self-stigma and affiliate stigma in first-episode psychosis patients and their caregivers. *Social Psychiatry and Psychiatric Epidemiology, 51*(9), 1225–1231. https://doi.org/10.1007/s00127-016-1221-8

Chen, H., Fang, X., Liu, C., Hu, W., Lan, J., & Deng, L. (2014). Associations among the number of mental health problems, stigma, and seeking help from psychological services: A path analysis model among Chinese adolescents. *Children and Youth Services Review, 44*, 356–362. https://doi.org/10.1016/j.childyouth.2014.07.003

Chen, S. R., Hou, W. H., Lai, J. N., Kwong, J. S., & Lin, P. C. (2022). Effects of acupressure on anxiety: A systematic review and meta-analysis. *Journal of Integrative and Complementary Medicine, 28*(1), 25–35.

Chen, S. X., Mak, W. W., & Lam, B. C. (2020). Is it cultural context or cultural value? Unpackaging cultural influences on stigma toward mental illness and barrier to help-seeking. *Social Psychological and Personality Science, 11*(7), 1022–1031. https://doi.org/10.1177/1948550619897482

Cheung, P., Siu, A., & Brown, T. (2017). Measuring social skills of children and adolescents in a Chinese population: Preliminary evidence on the reliability and validity of the translated Chinese version of the Social Skills Improvement System-Rating Scales (SSIS-RS-C). *Research in Developmental Disabilities, 60*, 187–197. https://doi.org/10.1016/j.ridd.2016.11.019

Chien, W. T., Yeung, F. K., & Chan, A. H. (2014). Perceived stigma of patients with severe mental illness in Hong Kong: Relationships with patients' psychosocial conditions and attitudes of family caregivers and health professionals. *Administration and Policy in Mental Health and Mental Health Services Research, 41*(2), 237–251. https://doi.org/10.1007/s10488-012-0463-3

Chu, B., Marwaha, K., Sanvictores, T., & Ayers, D. (2023). Physiology, stress reaction. In *StatPearls [Internet]*. StatPearls Publishing. https://www.ncbi.nlm.nih.gov/books/NBK541120/

Church, D., Stapleton, P., Yang, A., & Gallo, F. (2018). Is tapping on acupuncture points an active ingredient in emotional freedom techniques? A systematic review and meta-analysis of comparative studies. *The Journal of Nervous and Mental Disease, 206*(10), 783–793. https://doi.org/10.1097/NMD.0000000000000878

Churchill, R., Teo, K., Kervin, L., Riadi, I., & Cosco, T. D. (2022). Exercise interventions for stress reduction in older adult populations: A systematic review of randomized controlled trials. *Health Psychology and Behavioral Medicine, 10*(1), 913–934. https://doi.org/10.1080/21642850.2022.2125874

Cohen, K. (1997). *The way of qigong: The art and science of Chinese energy healing*. Ballantine Books.

Corrigan, P. W. (2018). *The stigma effect: Unintended consequences of mental health campaigns*. Columbia University Press.

Corrigan, P. W., Bink, A. B., Schmidt, A., Jones, N., & Rüsch, N. (2016). What is the impact of self-stigma? Loss of self-respect and the "why try" effect. *Journal of Mental Health, 25*(1), 10–15. https://doi.org/10.3109/09638237.2015.1021902

Corrigan, P. W., Larson, J. E., & Rüsch, N. (2009). Self-stigma and the "why try" effect: Impact on life goals and evidence-based practices. *World Psychiatry, 8*(2), 75–81. https://doi.org/10.1002/j.2051-5545.2009.tb00218.x

Corrigan, P. W., & Rao, D. (2012). On the self-stigma of mental illness: Stages, disclosure, and strategies for change. *The Canadian Journal of Psychiatry, 57*(8), 464–469. https://doi.org/10.1177/070674371205700804

Corrigan, P. W., Tsang, H. W., Shi, K., Lam, C. S., & Larson, J. (2010). Chinese and American employers' perspectives regarding hiring people with behaviorally driven health conditions: The role of stigma. *Social Science & Medicine, 71*(12), 2162–2169. https://doi.org/10.1016/j.socscimed.2010.08.025

Corrigan, P. W., Watson, A. C., & Barr, L. (2006). The self-stigma of mental illness: Implications for self-esteem and self-efficacy. *Journal of Social and Clinical Psychology, 25*(8), 875–884. https://doi.org/10.1521/jscp.2006.25.8.875

Dong, P., & Esser, A. H. (1990). *Chi gong: The ancient Chinese way to health.* Paragon House.

Fung, K. M., Tsang, H. W., & Chan, F. (2010). Self-stigma, stages of change and psychosocial treatment adherence among Chinese people with schizophrenia: A path analysis. *Social Psychiatry and Psychiatric Epidemiology, 45*(5), 561–568. https://doi.org/10.1007/s00127-009-0098-1

Fung, K. M., Tsang, H. W., & Cheung, W. M. (2011). Randomized controlled trial of the self-stigma reduction program among individuals with schizophrenia. *Psychiatry Research, 189*(2), 208–214. https://doi.org/10.1016/j.psychres.2011.02.013

Fung, K. M., Tsang, H. W., & Corrigan, P. W. (2008). Self-stigma of people with schizophrenia as predictor of their adherence to psychosocial treatment. *Psychiatric Rehabilitation Journal, 32*(2), 95–104. https://doi.org/10.2975/32.2.2008.95.104

Fung, K. M. T., Tsang, H. W. H., Corrigan, P. W., Lam, C. S., & Cheng, W. M. (2007). Measuring self-stigma of mental illness in China and its implications for recovery. *International Journal of Social Psychiatry, 53*(5), 408–418. https://doi.org/10.1177/0020764007078342

Furnham, A., & Chan, E. (2004). Lay theories of schizophrenia: A cross-cultural comparison of British and Hong Kong Chinese attitudes, attributions and beliefs. *Social Psychiatry and Psychiatric Epidemiology, 39*(7), 543–552. https://doi.org/10.1007/s00127-004-0787-8

Gallo, F. P. (2004). *Energy psychology: Explorations at the interface of energy, cognition, behavior, and health* (2nd ed.). CRC Press.

Godoy, L. D., Rossignoli, M. T., Delfino-Pereira, P., Garcia-Cairasco, N., & de Lima Umeoka, E. H. (2018). A comprehensive overview on stress neurobiology: Basic concepts and clinical implications. *Frontiers in Behavioral Neuroscience, 12*, 127. https://doi.org/10.3389/fnbeh.2018.00127

Guan, Y., Hao, Y., Guan, Y., & Wang, H. (2020). Effects of Tai Chi on essential hypertension and related risk factors: A meta-analysis of randomized controlled trials. *Journal of Rehabilitation Medicine, 52*(5), jrm00057. https://doi.org/10.2340/16501977-2683

Guo, Y., Qu, S., & Qin, H. (2018). Study of the relationship between self-stigma and subjective quality of life for individuals with chronic schizophrenia in the community. *General Psychiatry, 31*(3), e100037. https://doi.org/10.1136/gpsych-2018-100037

Hao, J. J., & Mittelman, M. (2014). Acupuncture: Past, present, and future. *Global Advances in Health and Medicine, 3*(4), 6–8. https://doi.org/10.7453/gahmj.2014.042

Ho, R. T., Fong, T. C., Wan, A. H., Au-Yeung, F. S., Wong, C. P., Ng, W. Y., Cheung, I. K., Lo, P. H., Ng, S. M., Chan, C. L., & Chen, E. Y. (2016). A randomized controlled trial on the psychophysiological effects of physical exercise and Tai-chi in patients with chronic schizophrenia. *Schizophrenia Research, 171*(1–3), 42–49. https://doi.org/10.1016/j.schres.2016.01.038

Honda, Y., Tsuda, A., & Horiuchi, S. (2012). Effect of a four-week self-administered acupressure intervention on perceived stress over the past month. *Open Journal of Medical Psychology, 1*(3), 20–24. http://dx.doi.org/10.4236/ojmp.2012.13004

Hopton, K., & Stoneley, H. (2006). Cultural awareness in occupational therapy: The Chinese example. *British Journal of Occupational Therapy, 69*(8), 386–389. https://journals.sagepub.com/doi/epdf/10.1177/030802260606900807

Jang, Y. (1995). Chinese culture and occupational therapy. *British Journal of Occupational Therapy, 58*(3), 103–106. https://journals.sagepub.com/doi/epdf/10.1177/030802269505800303

Jorm, A. F. (2000). Mental health literacy: Public knowledge and beliefs about mental disorders. *The British Journal of Psychiatry, 177*(5), 396–401. https://doi.org/10.1192/bjp.177.5.396

Kielhofner, G. (2008). *Model of human occupation: Theory and application* (4th ed.). Lippincott Williams & Wilkins.

Kim, B., & Park, H. (2023). The effects of auricular acupressure on blood pressure, stress, and sleep in elders with essential hypertension: A randomized single-blind sham-controlled trial. *European Journal of Cardiovascular Nursing*, zvad005. https://doi.org/10.1093/eurjcn/zvad005

Kong, J., Wilson, G., Park, J., Pereira, K., Walpole, C., & Yeung, A. (2019). Treating depression with Tai Chi: State of the art and future perspectives. *Frontiers in Psychiatry, 10*, 237. https://doi.org/10.3389/fpsyt.2019.00237

Kopelowicz, A., Liberman, R., & Zarate, R. (2006). Recent advances in social skills training for schizophrenia. *Schizophrenia Bulletin, 32*(Suppl. 1), S12–S23. https://doi.org/10.1093/schbul/sbl023

Kwan, R. Y. C., Leung, M. C. P., & Lai, C. K. Y. (2017). A randomized controlled trial examining the effect of acupressure on agitation and salivary cortisol in nursing home residents with dementia. *Dementia and Geriatric Cognitive Disorders*, 44(1–2), 92–104. https://doi.org/10.1159/000478739

Kwon, C. Y., & Lee, B. (2018). Acupuncture or acupressure on *Yintang* (EX-HN 3) for anxiety: A preliminary review. *Medical Acupuncture*, 30(2), 73–79. https://www.ncbi.nlm.nih.gov/pmc/articles/PMC5908420/

Lam, C. S., Tsang, H. W., Corrigan, P. W., Lee, Y. T., Angell, B., Shi, K., Jin, S., & Larson, J. E. (2010). Chinese lay theory and mental illness stigma: Implications for research and practices. *Journal of Rehabilitation*, 76(1), 35–40. https://www.researchgate.net/publication/279544470_Chinese_lay_theory_and_mental_illness_stigma_Implications_for_research_and_practices

Lazarus, R. S., & Folkman, S. (1984). *Stress, appraisal, and coping.* Springer Publishing Company.

Li, J., Fan, Y., Zhong, H. Q., Duan, X. L., Chen, W., Evans-Lacko, S., & Thornicroft, G. (2019). Effectiveness of an anti-stigma training on improving attitudes and decreasing discrimination towards people with mental disorders among care assistant workers in Guangzhou, China. *International Journal of Mental Health Systems*, 13, 1. https://doi.org/10.1186/s13033-018-0259-2

Li, J., Huang, Y. G., Ran, M. S., Fan, Y., Chen, W., Evans-Lacko, S., & Thornicroft, G. (2018). Community-based comprehensive intervention for people with schizophrenia in Guangzhou, China: Effects on clinical symptoms, social functioning, internalized stigma and discrimination. *Asian Journal of Psychiatry*, 34, 21–30. https://doi.org/10.1016/j.ajp.2018.04.017

Li, J., Li, J., Thornicroft, G., & Huang, Y. (2014). Levels of stigma among community mental health staff in Guangzhou, China. *BMC Psychiatry*, 14, 231. https://doi.org/10.1186/s12888-014-0231-x

Li, Q., Zhao, T., Wang, X. A., Qiu, C., Zhou, B., Wang, H., & Wang, B. (2021). Study on potential of meridian acupoints of traditional Chinese medicine. *Journal of Healthcare Engineering*, 2021, 5599272. https://doi.org/10.1155/2021/5599272

Li, S., Heath, P. J., Vidales, C. A., Vogel, D. L., & Nie, Y. (2022). Measurement invariance of the Self-Stigma of Mental Illness Scale: A cross-cultural study. *International Journal of Environmental Research and Public Health*, 19(4), 2344. https://doi.org/10.3390/ijerph19042344

Liang, S. Y., & Wu, W. C. (2014). *Simplified tai chi chuan: 24 postures with applications and standard 48 postures* (2nd ed.). YMAA Publication Center, Inc.

Lin, J., Chen, T., He, J., Chung, R. C., Ma, H., & Tsang, H. W. H. (2022a). Impacts of acupressure treatment on depression: A systematic review and meta-analysis. *World Journal of Psychiatry*, 12(1), 169–186. https://doi.org/10.5498/wjp.v12.i1.169

Lin, J., Gao, Y. F., Guo, Y., Li, M., Zhu, Y., You, R., Chen, S., & Wang, S. (2022b). Effects of Qigong exercise on the physical and mental health of college students: A systematic review and meta-analysis. *BMC Complementary Medicine and Therapies*, 22(1), 287. https://doi.org/10.1186/s12906-022-03760-5

Liu, X., Clark, J., Siskind, D., Williams, G. M., Byrne, G., Yang, J. L., & Doi, S. A. (2015). A systematic review and meta-analysis of the effects of Qigong and Tai Chi for depressive symptoms. *Complementary Therapies in Medicine*, 23(4), 516–534. https://doi.org/10.1016/j.ctim.2015.05.001

Liu, X., Li, R., Cui, J., Liu, F., Smith, L., Chen, X., & Zhang, D. (2021). The effects of Tai Chi and Qigong exercise on psychological status in adolescents: A systematic review and meta-analysis. *Frontiers in Psychology*, 12, 746975. https://doi.org/10.3389/fpsyg.2021.746975

Lo, L., Suen, Y. N., Chan, S., Sum, M. Y., Cheung, C., Hui, C., Lee, E., Chang, W. C., & Chen, E. (2021). Sociodemographic correlates of public stigma about mental illness: A population study on Hong Kong's Chinese population. *BMC Psychiatry*, 21(1), 274. https://doi.org/10.1186/s12888-021-03301-3

Lu, E. Y., Lee, P., Cai, S., So, W. W. Y., Ng, B. F. L., Jensen, M. P., Cheung, W. M., & Tsang, H. W. (2020). Qigong for the treatment of depressive symptoms: Preliminary evidence of neurobiological mechanisms. *International Journal of Geriatric Psychiatry*, 35(11), 1393–1401. https://doi.org/10.1002/gps.5380

Lui, C., Wong, C., & Furnham, A. (2016). Mental health literacy in Hong Kong. *International Journal of Social Psychiatry*, 62(6), 505–511. https://doi.org/10.1177/0020764016651291

Lv, Y., Wolf, A., & Wang, X. (2013). Experienced stigma and self-stigma in Chinese patients with schizophrenia. *General Hospital Psychiatry*, *35*(1), 83–88. https://doi.org/10.1016/j.genhosppsych.2012.07.007

Ma, S., Zhu, Y., & Bresnahan, M. (2022). Chinese international students' face concerns, self-stigma, linguistic factors, and help-seeking intentions for mental health. *Health Communication*, *37*(13), 1631–1639. https://doi.org/10.1080/10410236.2021.1910167

Markus, H. R., & Kitayama, S. (1991). Culture and the self: Implications for cognition, emotion, and motivation. *Psychological Review*, *98*(2), 224–253. https://doi.org/10.1037/0033-295X.98.2.224

McFadden, K. L., Healy, K. M., Hoversten, K. P., Ito, T. A., & Hernández, T. D. (2012). Efficacy of acupressure for non-pharmacological stress reduction in college students. *Complementary Therapies in Medicine*, *20*(4), 175–182. https://doi.org/10.1016/j.ctim.2011.12.003

Mosey, A. C. (1986). *Psychosocial components of occupational therapy*. Raven Press.

National Cancer Institute. (n.d.). Chinese meridian theory. In *NCI's dictionary of cancer terms*. Retrieved March 1, 2023, from https://www.cancer.gov/publications/dictionaries/cancer-terms/def/chinese-meridian-theory

Nedeljkovic, M., Ausfeld-Hafter, B., Streitberger, K., Seiler, R., & Wirtz, P. H. (2012). Taiji practice attenuates psychobiological stress reactivity — A randomized controlled trial in healthy subjects. *Psychoneuroendocrinology*, *37*(8), 1171–1180. https://doi.org/10.1016/j.psyneuen.2011.12.007

Patriquin, M. A., & Mathew, S. J. (2017). The neurobiological mechanisms of generalized anxiety disorder and chronic stress. *Chronic Stress*, *1*, 2470547017703993. https://doi.org/10.1177/2470547017703993

Ramsey, R. (2004). Psychosocial aspects of occupational therapy (2004). *American Journal of Occupational Therapy*, *58*(6), 669–672.

Rogers, R., & Sears, S. R. (2015). Emotional Freedom Techniques for stress in students: A randomized controlled dismantling study. *Energy Psychology: Theory, Research, and Treatment*, *7*(2), 26–32.

Selye, H. (1993). History of the stress concept. In L. Goldberger, & S. Breznitz (Eds.), *Handbook of stress: Theoretical and clinical aspects* (2nd ed., pp. 7–17). Free Press.

Shum, K. K. M., Cho, W. K., Lam, L. M. O., Laugeson, E. A., Wong, W. S., & Law, L. S. (2019). Learning how to make friends for Chinese adolescents with autism spectrum disorder: A randomized controlled trial of the Hong Kong Chinese version of the PEERS® intervention. *Journal of Autism and Developmental Disorders*, *49*(2), 527–541. https://doi.org/10.1007/s10803-018-3728-1

Sirey, J. A., Bruce, M. L., Alexopoulos, G. S., Perlick, D. A., Friedman, S. J., & Meyers, B. S. (2001). Stigma as a barrier to recovery: Perceived stigma and patient-rated severity of illness as predictors of antidepressant drug adherence. *Psychiatric Services (Washington, D.C.)*, *52*(12), 1615–1620. https://doi.org/10.1176/appi.ps.52.12.1615

So, W. W. Y., Cai, S., Yau, S. Y., & Tsang, H. W. H. (2019). The neurophysiological and psychological mechanisms of qigong as a treatment for depression: A systematic review and meta-analysis. *Frontiers in Psychiatry*, *10*, 820. https://doi.org/10.3389/fpsyt.2019.00820

Song, H. J., Seo, H. J., Lee, H., Son, H., Choi, S. M., & Lee, S. (2015). Effect of self-acupressure for symptom management: A systematic review. *Complementary Therapies in Medicine*, *23*(1), 68–78. https://doi.org/10.1016/j.ctim.2014.11.002

Sun, D. Z., Li, S. D., Liu, Y., Zhang, Y., Mei, R., & Yang, M. H. (2013). Differences in the origin of philosophy between Chinese medicine and Western medicine: Exploration of the holistic advantages of Chinese medicine. *Chinese Journal of Integrative Medicine*, *19*(9), 706–711. https://doi.org/10.1007/s11655-013-1435-5

Sun, W., & Li, X. (1997). *Chi Kung: Increase your energy, improve your health*. Sterling Pub.

Tafet, G. E., & Nemeroff, C. B. (2016). The links between stress and depression: Psychoneuroendocrinological, genetic, and environmental interactions. *The Journal of Neuropsychiatry and Clinical Neurosciences*, *28*(2), 77–88. https://doi.org/10.1176/appi.neuropsych.15030053

Tam, S. F., Tsang, H. W. H., Ip, Y. C., & Chan, C. (2004). Preliminary evidence for the basis of self-concept in Chinese people with mental illness. *Quality of Life Research*, *13*(2), 497–508. https://doi.org/10.1023/B:QURE.0000018478.66085.a1

Tang, I. C., & Wu, H. C. (2012). Quality of life and self-stigma in individuals with schizophrenia. *Psychiatric Quarterly, 83*(4), 497–507. https://doi.org/10.1007/s11126-012-9218-2

Tsang, H. W., Angell, B., Corrigan, P. W., Lee, Y. T., Shi, K., Lam, C. S., Jin, S., & Fung, K. M. (2007). A cross-cultural study of employers' concerns about hiring people with psychotic disorder: Implications for recovery. *Social Psychiatry and Psychiatric Epidemiology, 42*(9), 723–733. https://doi.org/10.1007/s00127-007-0208-x

Tsang, H. W., Ching, S. C., Tang, K. H., Lam, H. T., Law, P. Y., & Wan, C. N. (2016). Therapeutic intervention for internalized stigma of severe mental illness: A systematic review and meta-analysis. *Schizophrenia Research, 173*(1–2), 45–53. https://doi.org/10.1016/j.schres.2016.02.013

Tsang, H. W. H. (2001a). Applying social skills training in the context of vocational rehabilitation for people with schizophrenia. *Journal of Nervous and Mental Disease, 189*(2), 90–98. https://doi.org/10.1097/00005053-200102000-00004

Tsang, H. W. H. (2001b). Rehab rounds: Social skills training to help mentally ill persons find and keep a job. *Psychiatric Services, 52*(7), 891–894. https://doi.org/10.1176/appi.ps.52.7.891

Tsang, H. W. H. (2008). Enhancing employment opportunities of people with mental illness through an integrated supported employment approach of individual placement and support and social skills training. *Hong Kong Medical Journal, 14*(Suppl. 3), S41–46. https://www.hkmj.org/abstracts/v14n3s3/41.htm

Tsang, H. W. H., Chan, A., Wong, A., & Liberman, R. P. (2009). Vocational outcomes of an integrated supported employment program for individuals with persistent and severe mental illness. *Journal of Behavior Therapy and Experimental Psychiatry, 40*(2), 292–305. https://doi.org/10.1016/j.jbtep.2008.12.007

Tsang, H. W. H., Chan, F., & Chan, C. C. H. (2004). Factors influencing occupational therapy students' attitudes toward persons with disabilities: A conjoint analysis. *American Journal of Occupational Therapy, 58*(4), 426–434.

Tsang, H. W. H., Fong, M. W. M., Fung, K. M. T., & Corrigan, P. W. (2010a). Reducing employers' stigma by supported employment. In C. Lloyd (Ed.), *Vocational rehabilitation and mental health* (pp. 51–64). Wiley-Blackwell. https://doi.org/10.1002/9781444319736.ch4

Tsang, H. W. H., Fung, K. M. T., & Chung, R. C. K. (2010b). Self-stigma and stages of change as predictors of treatment adherence of individuals with schizophrenia. *Psychiatry Research, 180*(1), 10–15. https://doi.org/10.1016/j.psychres.2009.09.001

Tsang, H. W. H., Fung, K. M. T., Leung, A. Y., Li, S. M. Y., & Cheung, W. M. (2010c). Three year follow-up study of an integrated supported employment for individuals with severe mental illness. *Australian and New Zealand Journal of Psychiatry, 44*(1), 49–58. https://doi.org/10.3109/00048670903393613

Tsang, H. W. H., & Li, S. M. Y. (2010). Work-related social skills and job retention. In C. Lloyd (Ed.), *Vocational rehabilitation and mental health* (pp. 157–172). Wiley-Blackwell. https://doi.org/10.1002/9781444319736.ch10

Tsang, H. W. H., Ng, B., Chiu, I. Y., & Mann, S. (2000). Predictors of post-hospital employment status for psychiatric patients in Hong Kong: From perceptions of rehabilitation professionals to empirical evidence. *International Journal of Social Psychiatry, 46*(4), 306–312. https://doi.org/10.1177/002076400004600407

Tsang, H. W. H., & Pearson, V. (2001). Work-related social skills training for people with schizophrenia in Hong Kong. *Schizophrenia Bulletin, 27*(1), 139–148. https://doi.org/10.1093/oxfordjournals.schbul.a006852

Tsang, H. W. H., Tam, P., Chan, F., & Cheung, W. M. (2003a). Stigmatizing attitudes towards individuals with mental illness in Hong Kong: Implications for their recovery. *Journal of Community Psychology, 31*(4), 383–396. https://doi.org/10.1002/jcop.10055

Tsang, H. W. H., Tam, P. K. C., Chan, F., & Cheung, W. M. (2003b). Sources of burdens on families of individuals with mental illness. *International Journal of Rehabilitation Research, 26*(2), 123–130. https://doi.org/10.1097/00004356-200306000-00007

Tsui, M. C. M., & Tsang, H. W. H. (2017). Views of people with schizophrenia and their caregivers towards the needs for psychiatric rehabilitation in urban and rural areas of mainland China. *Psychiatry Research, 258,* 72–77. https://doi.org/10.1016/j.psychres.2017.09.052

Wang, C., Bannuru, R., Ramel, J., Kupelnick, B., Scott, T., & Schmid, C. H. (2010). Tai Chi on psychological well-being: Systematic review and meta-analysis. *BMC Complementary and Alternative Medicine, 10*(1), 23. https://doi.org/10.1186/1472-6882-10-23

Wang, C. W., Chan, C. H., Ho, R. T., Chan, J. S., Ng, S. M., & Chan, C. L. (2014). Managing stress and anxiety through qigong exercise in healthy adults: A systematic review and meta-analysis of randomized controlled trials. *BMC Complementary and Alternative Medicine*, 14(1), 8. https://doi.org/10.1186/1472-6882-14-8

Wang, X., Huang, X., Jackson, T., & Chen, R. (2012). Components of implicit stigma against mental illness among Chinese students. *PLOS ONE*, 7(9), e46016. https://doi.org/10.1371/journal.pone.0046016

Wang, Y., Roberts, D. L., Xu, B., Cao, R., Yan, M., & Jiang, Q. (2013). Social cognition and interaction training for patients with stable schizophrenia in Chinese community settings. *Psychiatry Research*, 210(3), 751–755. https://doi.org/10.1016/j.psychres.2013.08.038

Warner-Schmidt, J. L., & Duman, R. S. (2006). Hippocampal neurogenesis: Opposing effects of stress and antidepressant treatment. *Hippocampus*, 16(3), 239–249. https://doi.org/10.1002/hipo.20156

Webster, C. S., Luo, A. Y., Krägeloh, C., Moir, F., & Henning, M. (2016). A systematic review of the health benefits of Tai Chi for students in higher education. *Preventive Medicine Reports*, 3, 103–112. https://doi.org/10.1016/j.pmedr.2015.12.006

Wong, D. F. K., He, X., Poon, A., & Lam, A. Y. K. (2012). Depression literacy among Chinese in Shanghai, China: A comparison with Chinese-speaking Australians in Melbourne and Chinese in Hong Kong. *Social Psychiatry and Psychiatric Epidemiology*, 47(8), 1235–1242. https://doi.org/10.1007/s00127-011-0430-4

World Health Organization. (2001). *International classification of functioning, disability and health (ICF)*. https://www.who.int/standards/classifications/international-classification-of-functioning-disability-and-health

Wu, Q., Luo, X., Chen, S., Qi, C., Yang, W., Liao, Y., Wang, X., Tang, J., Tang, Y., & Liu, T. (2020). Stigmatizing attitudes towards mental disorders among non-mental health professionals in six general hospitals in Hunan province. *Frontiers in Psychiatry*, 10, 946. https://doi.org/10.3389/fpsyt.2019.00946

Xu, Z., Huang, F., Kösters, M., & Rüsch, N. (2017a). Challenging mental health related stigma in China: Systematic review and meta-analysis. II. Interventions among people with mental illness. *Psychiatry Research*, 255, 457–464. https://doi.org/10.1016/j.psychres.2017.05.002

Xu, Z., Rüsch, N., Huang, F., & Kösters, M. (2017b). Challenging mental health related stigma in China: Systematic review and meta-analysis. I. Interventions among the general public. *Psychiatry Research*, 255, 449–456. https://doi.org/10.1016/j.psychres.2017.01.008

Yang, G., Li, W., Klupp, N., Cao, H., Liu, J., Bensoussan, A., Kiat, H., Karamacoska, D., & Chang, D. (2022). Does Tai Chi improve psychological well-being and quality of life in patients with cardiovascular disease and/or cardiovascular risk factors? A systematic review. *BMC Complementary Medicine and Therapies*, 22(1), 3. https://doi.org/10.1186/s12906-021-03482-0

Yang, L., Zhao, Y., Wang, Y., Liu, L., Zhang, X., Li, B., & Cui, R. (2015). The effects of psychological stress on depression. *Current Neuropharmacology*, 13(4), 494–504. https://www.ncbi.nlm.nih.gov/pmc/articles/PMC4790405/

Yanos, P. T., Lucksted, A., Drapalski, A. L., Roe, D., & Lysaker, P. (2015). Interventions targeting mental health self-stigma: A review and comparison. *Psychiatric Rehabilitation Journal*, 38(2), 171–178. https://doi.org/10.1037/prj0000100

Yau, M. K. S. (2007). Universality and cultural specificity in occupational therapy practice: From Hong Kong to Asia. *Hong Kong Journal of Occupational Therapy*, 17(2), 60–64. https://www.sciencedirect.com/science/article/pii/S1569186108700056

Ye, J., Cai, S., Cheung, W. M., & Tsang, H. W. H. (2019). An East meets West approach to the understanding of emotion dysregulation in depression: From perspective to scientific evidence. *Frontiers in Psychology*, 10, 574. https://doi.org/10.3389/fpsyg.2019.00574

Yee, T., Ceballos, P., & Lawless, A. (2020). Help-seeking attitudes of Chinese Americans and Chinese immigrants in the United States: The mediating role of self-stigma. *Journal of Multicultural Counseling and Development*, 48(1), 30–43. https://doi.org/10.1002/jmcd.12162

Yeung, A., Campbell, B., & Chan, J. S. (2019). The effects of Tai Chi and Qigong on anxiety and depression. In B. G. Shapero, D. Mischoulon, & C. Cusin (Eds.), *The Massachusetts general hospital guide to depression: New treatment insights and options* (pp. 211–222). Humana Press. https://doi.org/10.1007/978-3-319-97241-1

Yin, H., Wardenaar, K. J., Xu, G., Tian, H., & Schoevers, R. A. (2020). Mental health stigma and mental health knowledge in Chinese population: A cross-sectional study. *BMC Psychiatry*, *20*(1), 323. https://doi.org/10.1186/s12888-020-02705-x

Yin, Y., Zhang, W., Hu, Z., Jia, F., Li, Y., Xu, H., Zhao, S., Guo, J., Tian, D., & Qu, Z. (2014). Experiences of stigma and discrimination among caregivers of persons with schizophrenia in China: A field survey. *PLOS ONE*, *9*(9), e108527. https://doi.org/10.1371/journal.pone.0108527

Young, D. K., Ng, P. Y., Corrigan, P., Chiu, R., & Yang, S. (2020). Self-stigma reduction group for people with depression: A randomized controlled trial. *Research on Social Work Practice*, *30*(8), 846–857. https://doi.org/10.1177/1049731520941594

Young, D. K. W. (2018). Cognitive behavioral therapy group for reducing self-stigma for people with mental illness. *Research on Social Work Practice*, *28*(7), 827–837. https://doi.org/10.1177/1049731516681849

Young, D. K. W., & Ng, P. Y. N. (2016). The prevalence and predictors of self-stigma of individuals with mental health illness in two Chinese cities. *International Journal of Social Psychiatry*, *62*(2), 176–185. https://doi.org/10.1177/0020764015614596

Yu, B. C., Chio, F. H., Chan, K. K., Mak, W. W., Zhang, G., Vogel, D., & Lai, M. H. (2023). Associations between public and self-stigma of help-seeking with help-seeking attitudes and intention: A meta-analytic structural equation modeling approach. *Journal of Counseling Psychology*, *70*(1), 90–102. https://doi.org/10.1037/cou0000637

Yuen, A. S., & Mak, W. W. (2021). The effects of immersive virtual reality in reducing public stigma of mental illness in the university population of Hong Kong: Randomized controlled trial. *Journal of Medical Internet Research*, *23*(7), e23683. https://doi.org/10.2196/23683

Zeng, Y., Luo, T., Xie, H., Huang, M., & Cheng, A. S. (2014). Health benefits of qigong or tai chi for cancer patients: A systematic review and meta-analyses. *Complementary Therapies in Medicine*, *22*(1), 173–186. https://doi.org/10.1016/j.ctim.2013.11.010

Zeng, Y., Xie, X., & Cheng, A. S. (2019). Qigong or Tai Chi in cancer care: An updated systematic review and meta-analysis. *Current Oncology Reports*, *21*(6), 48. https://doi.org/10.1007/s11912-019-0786-2

Zhang, G. F., Tsui, C. M., Lu, A. J. B., Yu, L. B., Tsang, H. W. H., & Li, D. (2017). Integrated supported employment for people with schizophrenia in mainland China: A randomized controlled trial. *American Journal of Occupational Therapy*, *71*(6), 7106165020p1–7106165020p8.

Zhang, W. B., Wang, G. J., & Fuxe, K. (2015). Classic and modern meridian studies: A review of low hydraulic resistance channels along meridians and their relevance for therapeutic effects in traditional Chinese medicine. *Evidence-Based Complementary and Alternative Medicine*, *2015*, 410979. https://doi.org/10.1155/2015/410979

Zhang, Y. P., Hu, R. X., Han, M., Lai, B. Y., Liang, S. B., Chen, B. J., Robinson, N., Chen, K., & Liu, J. P. (2020). Evidence base of clinical studies on Qi Gong: A bibliometric analysis. *Complementary Therapies in Medicine*, *50*, 102392. https://doi.org/10.1016/j.ctim.2020.102392

Zhang, Z., Sun, K., Jatchavala, C., Koh, J., Chia, Y., Bose, J., Li, Z., Tan, W., Wang, S., Chu, W., Wang, J., Tran, B., & Ho, R. (2019). Overview of stigma against psychiatric illnesses and advancements of anti-stigma activities in six Asian societies. *International Journal of Environmental Research and Public Health*, *17*(1), 280. https://doi.org/10.3390/ijerph17010280

Zou, L., Sasaki, J. E., Wang, H., Xiao, Z., Fang, Q., & Zhang, M. (2017). A systematic review and meta-analysis of Baduanjin Qigong for health benefits: Randomized controlled trials. *Evidence-Based Complementary and Alternative Medicine*, *2017*, 4548706. https://doi.org/10.1155/2017/4548706

CHAPTER 6

Return to the home and community

Stella Wai Chee Cheng, Bobby Hin Po Ng, and Eddie Yip Kuen Hai

Introduction

This chapter includes the following four main sections:

1   The role of occupational therapists in the return to the home and community
2   Common assessments
   ■   Assessment for basic activities of daily living
   ■   Assessment for instrumental activities of daily living
   ■   Functional Independence Measure
   ■   Home safety assessment
3   Discharge planning and preparation
   ■   Guide for occupational therapists in discharge planning and preparation
4   Home visit and environmental modification
   ■   Use of standardized assessments
   ■   Use of non-standardized assessments
   ■   Assessment of accessibility
   ■   Safety considerations
   ■   Case study on home assessment and modification

The role of occupational therapists in the return to the home and community

A safe return to the home and community is one of the key goals of occupational therapy (OT) for clients following their hospital admission. In Hong Kong, there are over 36,000 hospital beds and over 83% of them are managed by the Hospital Authority (HA), which is the public hospital service provider (Department of Health, 2022). The elderly population of those aged 65 or above accounted for 50% of the inpatient

DOI: 10.4324/9781032721170-9

discharges from the HA in 2019 (Hospital Authority, 2021). To reduce the burden on the public healthcare service, it is important to ensure the speedy and safe discharge of clients.

When clients' medical conditions are stabilized, occupational therapists will assess whether they can perform their required basic activities of daily living (BADL), such as self-hygiene, going to the toilet, and bathing, as well as instrumental activities of daily living (IADL), such as cooking, financial management, and household cleaning, both at home and in the community after being discharged from the hospital. In case they do not meet the required level of performance after training, assistive devices to support clients in BADL and IADL can be arranged, and modification of the living environment can be recommended.

There were 13.1% and 25.2% of the elderly population living alone or with a spouse, respectively, and 8.1% were living in non-domestic households or institutions in Hong Kong according to the *2016 Population By-census Thematic Report: Older Persons* (Census and Statistics Department, 2018). It is therefore crucial for occupational therapists to interview the clients and their family members to gain an understanding of the social support available and their discharge destination preference.

Common assessments

To determine whether clients reach the acceptable level of performance to return to the home or community, BADL, IADL, and environmental risk assessments have to be arranged. In the following section, the most commonly used assessment tools, including the Modified Barthel Index, the Hong Kong Chinese Version of the Lawton Instrumental Activities of Daily Living Scale, and the Chinese Home Falls and Accidents Screening Tool, will be introduced.

Assessment for basic activities of daily living

The most common BADL assessment tool used in Hong Kong is the Modified Barthel Index (MBI) or the Chinese Version of the Modified Barthel Index (MBI-C). The Barthel Index was introduced by Mahoney F. L. and Barthel D. W. in 1965. It was modified into the MBI for better sensitivity and reliability by Shah et al. (1989). The MBI consists of ten items, each with five ratings. The MBI-C is based on the MBI but with a slight modification to consider Hong Kong Chinese culture, such as items on feeding and stair climbing. The MBI-C is also considered a reliable assessment of BADL, with construct validity and inter-rater reliability for stroke clients (Leung et al., 2007).

Details of the MBI commonly used in Hong Kong hospitals are tabulated in Table 6.1. Occupational therapists can refer to the item description in the assessment and identify aspects of BADL that require special attention and training before discharge. The total score indicates the performance level of a client, with 100 being independent and 20 or below being totally dependent. The total score can also be used as an indicator for the discharge destination. A lower performance level usually indicates a higher need for institutional care. However, if the client's family is capable of providing the level of care required, the client can still be discharged for home care.

Table 6.1 Item description based on the MBI

Item	Score	Description
Feeding	0	Dependent in all aspects and needs to be fed.
	2	Can manipulate an eating device usually a spoon but someone must provide active assistance during the meal.
	5	Able to feed self with supervision. Assistance is required with associated tasks such as putting milk/sugar into tea, putting salt/pepper into food, spreading butter, turning a plate, or other "set-up" activities.
	8	Independent in feeding with prepared tray except maybe cutting meat, opening milk cartons or jar lids, etc. Presence of another person is not required.
	10	The patient can feed self from a tray or table when someone puts the food within reach. The patient may put on an assistive device if needed (e.g., for cutting meat).
Personal hygiene	0	The patient is unable to attend to personal hygiene and dependent in all aspects.
	1	Assistance is required in all steps of personal hygiene.
	3	Some assistance is required in one or more steps of personal hygiene.
	4	The patient is able to conduct his/her own personal hygiene but requires minimal assistance before and/or after the operation.
	5	The patient can wash his/her hands and face, comb hair, clean teeth, and shave. A male patient may use any kind of razor but must insert the blade, or plug in the razor without help, as well as retrieve it from the drawer or cabinet. A female patient may apply make-up, if used, but needs not braid or style her hair.
Dressing	0	The patient is dependent in all aspects of dressing and unable to participate in the activity.
	2	The patient is able to participate to some degree but dependent in all aspects of dressing.
	5	Assistance is needed in putting on and/or removing any clothing.
	8	Only minimal assistance is required in fastening clothing such as buttons, zips, bra, and shoes.
	10	The patient is able to put on, remove, and fasten clothing, tie shoelaces, or put on, fasten, and remove corsets, braces as required.
Chair/bed transfer	0	Unable to participate in transfer. Two attendants are required to transfer the patient with or without a mechanical device.
	3	Able to participate but maximum assistance of one other person is required in all aspects of the transfer.
	8	The transfer requires the assistance of one other person. Assistance may be required in any aspects of the transfer.
	12	The presence of another person is required either as a confidence measure, or to provide supervision for safety.
	15	The patient can safely approach the bed in a wheelchair, lock the brakes, lift the foot rests, move safely in bed, lie down, come to a sitting position on either side of the bed, change position of the wheelchair, and transfer back into it safely. The patient must be independent in all phases of the activity.

Table 6.1 Item description based on the MBI (*continued*)

Item	Score	Description
Bowel	0	The patient is bowel incontinent.
	2	The patient needs help to assume an appropriate position, and needs help with bowel movement facilitatory techniques.
	5	The patient can assume an appropriate position, but cannot use facilitatory techniques or clean self without assistance, and has frequent accidents. Assistance is required with incontinence aids such as pads etc.
	8	The patient may require supervision with the use of suppositories or take an enema when necessary.
	10	The patient can control bowel and has no accidents, can use suppositories or take an enema when necessary.
Bladder	0	The patient is dependent in bladder management, is incontinent, or has an indwelling catheter.
	2	The patient is incontinent but can be assisted with the application of an internal or external device.
	5	The patient is generally dry by day, but not at night, and needs some assistance with devices.
	8	The patient is generally dry by day and night, but may have an occasional accident, or needs minimal assistance with internal or external devices.
	10	The patient is able to control bladder day and night, and/or is independent with internal or external devices.
On & off toilet	0	Fully dependent in toileting.
	2	Assistance is required in all aspects of toileting.
	5	Assistance may be required in management of clothing, transferring, or washing hands.
	8	Supervision may be required for safety with normal toilet. A commode may be used at night but assistance is required for emptying and cleaning it.
	10	The patient is able to get on and off the toilet, fasten and unfasten clothes, prevent soiling of clothes, and use toilet paper without help. If necessary, the patient may use a bedpan, commode, or urinal at night but must be able to use them independently.
Bathing self	0	Total dependent in bathing self.
	1	Assistance is required in all aspects of bathing.
	3	Assistance is required in either transfer to shower/bath or in washing and drying, including inability to complete the task because of conditions of the disease etc.
	4	Supervision is required for safety, such as in adjusting water temperature or in transfer.
	5	The patient may use a bathtub, a shower, or take a complete sponge bath but must be able to perform all the steps alone.
Stairs	0	The patient is unable to climb stairs.
	2	Assistance is required in all aspects of stair climbing, including assistance with walking aids.
	5	The patient is able to ascend/descend but is unable to carry walking aids, and needs supervision or assistance.

Table 6.1 Item description based on the MBI (*continued*)

Item	Score	Description
	8	Generally, no assistance is required. Occasional supervision is required for safety due to morning stiffness, shortness of breath etc.
	10	The patient is able to go up and down a flight of stairs safely without help or supervision. The patient is able to use handrails, canes or crutches when needed and is able to carry the devices required as he/she ascends or descends.
Ambulation	0	Dependent in ambulation.
	3	Constant presence of one or more assistants is required during ambulation.
	8	Assistance is required in reaching walking aids and/or their manipulation. One person is required to help.
	12	The patient is independent in ambulation but unable to walk 50 yards without help. Or supervision is needed for confidence or safety in hazardous situations.
	15	The patient, if indicated, must be able to wear braces, lock and unlock them, assume a standing position, sit down, and place the necessary aids in position for use. The patient must be able to walk, with the use of walking aids if indicated, for 50 yards without help or supervision.
Wheelchair (only use this item if patient is rated 0 for ambulation and can use a wheelchair)	0	Dependent in wheelchair maneuvering.
	1	The patient can propel self for a short distance on a flat surface but assistance is required for all other wheelchair maneuvers.
	3	Presence of one person is necessary and constant assistance is required to maneuver the wheelchair to a table, bed etc.
	4	The patient can propel self for a reasonable distance over regularly encountered terrain. Minimal assistance may still be required in "tight corners".
	5	The patient can propel wheelchair independently including going around corners, turning around, maneuvering to a table, bed, toilet etc. The patient must be able to push the wheelchair for 50 yards.

Grading according to total score:

0–20	21–60	61–90	91–99	100
Totally dependent	Severely dependent	Moderately dependent	Slightly dependent	Independent

Assessment for instrumental activities of daily living

For IADL, the most commonly adopted assessment in Hong Kong is the Hong Kong Chinese Version of the Lawton Instrumental Activities of Daily Living Scale (HKCV-Lawton IADL), which is based on the Lawton Instrumental Activities of Daily Living Scale (Lawton IADL) introduced by Lawton and Brody in 1969. This is a widely used and easy-to-administer self-report or surrogate-report assessment instrument for more complex daily functional tasks. The Lawton IADL was later modified to include nine items with a three-point ordinal scale and was included in the Multilevel Assessment Instrument (Lawton et al., 1982). The nine items are: use of a telephone, use of public transport, shopping, medication management, money management, meal preparation, housework, laundry, and handyman work. The HKCV-Lawton IADL further modified the Lawton IADL to a four-point scale that is considered to have better test–retest reliability and internal consistency (Tong & Man, 2002), with 0 indicating totally dependent, 1 indicating help required, 2 indicating perform with difficulties, and 3 indicating totally independent (Table 6.2). The HKCV-Lawton IADL helps therapists, clients, and their caregivers identify areas in daily tasks with

Table 6.2 The HKCV-Lawton IADL

項目 *Item*	評分 *Score* 0/1/2/3
(1) 你能唔能夠自己用電話呢? (包括找電話號碼、打及接聽電話。) Can you use your telephone? (Including finding the numbers, making and receiving calls.)	
(2) 你能唔能夠自己搭車呢? (包括自己上到正確的車、俾車錢、買車票、上或落車。) Can you use public transport by yourself? (Including finding the correct transport, paying, getting on and off the vehicle.)	
(3) 你能唔能夠自己買嘢呢? (包括自己揀貨品、俾錢及攞番屋企。) Can you buy your daily necessities? (Including selecting items, paying and getting the items back home.)	
(4) 你能唔能夠自己煮食呢? (包括諗食甚麼、準備材料、煮熟食物及放入碗碟內。) Can you cook a meal? (Including planning the menu, preparing the ingredients, cooking and putting the food in a bowl or a dish.)	
(5) 你能唔能夠自己做家務呢? (包括簡單家務如抹檯、執床、洗碗及更重家務如抹地和窗。) Can you perform household chores? (Including simple household work such as wiping the table, making the bed, washing dishes, and heavier work such as mopping the floor and cleaning windows.)	
(6) 你能唔能夠自己應付簡單的家居維修呢? (例如換燈膽、上緊螺絲等。) Can you handle simple household maintenance work? (Including changing lightbulbs, tightening loose screws.)	
(7) 你能唔能夠自己洗衫呢? (包括清洗及曬自己的衫、床單或被。) Can you do laundry? (Including washing and hanging clothes and bed linen.)	
(8) 你能唔能夠自己服用藥物呢? (包括依照指示在指定時間內服用正確的分量。) Can you handle your own medications? (Including following the correct schedule and dosage.)	
(9) 你能唔能夠自己處理自己的財務呢? (包括錢銀找續、交租、交水電費及到銀行提款。) Can you handle your finance? (Including money transactions, paying the rent, settling water and electricity bills, and getting money from the bank.)	

Table 6.2 The HKCV-Lawton IADL (*continued*)

評分標準 Scoring criteria:

0	完全不能自己做	Totally dependent
1	需要一些幫忙	Need help
2	可以自己做，但做的時候有困難	Can perform but encounter difficulties
3	不需要任何幫忙	Totally independent

which clients need support in order to live safely in the community. Items that are not applicable can be omitted.

Functional Independence Measure

The Functional Independence Measure (FIM™) (Granger & Hamilton, 1992) adopts a seven-point ordinal scale with equal increments to assess occupational performance for 13 motor items and five cognition items. The motor items are grouped into four sub-domains: self-care (grooming, feeding, bathing, dressing – upper body, dressing – lower body, and going to the toilet), sphincter management (bowel and bladder management), transfer (bed, chair, wheelchair, toilet, bath/shower), and locomotion (walking/wheelchair and stairs). The cognition items are grouped into communication (comprehension and expression) and social cognition (social interaction, problem-solving, and memory). The definition of the seven-point ordinal scale is based on the percentage of the client's participation in a certain ADL, as shown below:

Independence	*Modified dependence*	*Complete dependence*
7: Complete independence (timely, safely)	5: Supervision (Participation = 100%)	2: Maximal assistance (Participation = 25%+)
6: Modified independence (device)	4: Minimal assistance (Participation = 75%+)	1: Total assistance (Participation = less than 25%)
	3: Moderate assistance (Participation = 50%+)	

The FIM™ is used in several hospitals in Hong Kong to monitor the rehabilitation progress of clients. Clinicians need to be trained to administer the FIM™, and a subscription fee is required to use it. It is used by multidisciplinary teams in rehabilitation settings as outcome measures. Occupational therapists are usually responsible for the measurement of the self-care aspect. As subscription fee is required, it is not commonly used in hospitals and rehabilitation settings in Hong Kong.

Home safety assessment

Home safety assessments are routinely carried out, particularly for elderly clients with fall histories who have been admitted to hospitals or accident and emergency departments. The most commonly used assessment is the Chinese Home Falls and Accidents Screening Tool (Chinese HOME-FAST). This is based on the Home Falls and Accidents Screening Tool (HOME-FAST) developed in Australia in 2000 (Mackenzie et al., 2000). The Chinese HOME-FAST consists of 20 self-reported questions in yes-or-no format

(Table 6.3). If more than seven positive responses are recorded, further home assessment through a home visit is indicated (Lai et al., 2020). In some situations, therapists gather information on home safety by interviewing the clients or their caregivers.

In summary, the BADL and IADL assessments provide important information on the functional status of the client, which is essential in discharge planning. Considering that environmental risks are equally important, if the client requires support in BADL or IADL, home support services such as bathing or meals on wheels can be arranged. Home visits will be considered if environmental risks are identified. In situations where

Table 6.3 The Chinese HOME-FAST

請細閱以下每條題目，並請從"是"/"否"當中選出合適你的答案。 *Please read the statements and tick Yes/No.*	是 *Yes*	否 *No*
(1) 家居內的走廊和通道"是"/"否"沒有雜物阻塞? (包括沒有傢俬、雜物和電線，會阻礙室內房門的開關。) Walkways free of obstacles? (Any furniture, clutter and electric wires blocking the way including the doorway?)		
(2) 家居內的地面狀態"是"/"否"良好? (地板是否沒有破損，也沒有滑溜的感覺?) Floor coverings in good condition? (Any broken floor tiles and slippery floor?)		
(3) 上床和下床時"是"/"否"安全? (床是否有適當的高度，及不需要借助其他東西起床?) Can get in and out of bed easily and safely? (Appropriate bed height; do not need to rely on other support to get out of bed?)		
(4) 家居內的座椅"是"/"否"安全? (座椅的高度是否合適? 坐墊的保養是否合適?) Are the chairs safe to sit on? (Appropriate chair height; seat cushions appropriately maintained?)		
(5) 家居內的燈光"是"/"否"充足? (是否使用75W 或者以上的燈光光線，而且家中也沒有眩光或反光?) Is lighting sufficient? (Using light bulbs of 75W or above; no glare or reflective light at home?)		
(6) 晚間進出家居時的燈光"是"/"否"充足? (是否有75W 或者以上的燈光光線?) Is lighting at night sufficient? (Using light bulbs of 75W or above?)		
(7) 在家居如廁時，站立和坐下廁所 (或蹲下踎廁) 的時候，"是"/"否"安全? (座廁是否有合適高度，不需要借助其他東西從座廁站起?) Can get on and off the toilet (or squat) easily and safely? (Appropriate toilet seat height; no need to rely on other support to get up?)		
(8) 在家居洗澡時，進出洗澡區"是"/"否"安全? (是否可以跨過花灑缸或浴缸的邊緣，並安全的使用沐浴設施?) Can get in and out of the bathing facility safely? (Can step over and get in the bathtub or shower tray and use the facility safely?)		
(9) 進入廁所和浴室時"是"/"否"安全? (包括沒有雜物和地布，也不會阻礙廁所門的開關。) Can get in the toilet and bathroom safely? (Including no obstacles and floor cloth and no obstruction to the door.)		

Table 6.3 The Chinese HOME-FAST (*continued*)

請細閱以下每條題目，並請從 "是"／"否" 當中選出合適你的答案。 *Please read the statements and tick Yes/No.*	是 *Yes*	否 *No*

(10) 浴室和廁所位置 "是"／"否" 有安裝扶手? (扶手是否牢固地安裝在牆上，而不是使用毛巾架?)

Are handrails installed in the bathroom and toilet area? (Are the handrails securely installed on the walls and towel racks are not used as support?)

(11) 浴室和廁所位置 "是"／"否" 有使用防滑墊? (是否有塑膠材料的防滑墊，或者在地面貼上防滑沙紙?)

Are non-slip mats available in the bathroom and toilet area? (Plastic non-slip mats or non-slip adhesive taps?)

(12) 廁所的位置 "是"／"否" 靠近在睡房旁邊? (廁所和睡房相距，是否少於4米 [約10尺] 的距離?)

Is the toilet in proximity to the bedroom? (Is the distance between the toilet and bedroom less than 4 meters or 10 feet?)

(13) 需要使用廚房的物品時，這些物品 "是"／"否" 容易拿到? (是否不需要過分伸張身體，或者彎曲腰背?)

Can easily reach items in the kitchen that are used regularly? (Without overstretching the body or bending the back?)

(14) 將食物從廚房拿到飯枱時 "是"／"否" 容易? (是否沒有傢俬和雜物，會阻礙從廚房到飯枱的路線?)

Can carry meals easily and safely from the kitchen to the dining area? (No obstruction of the way by furniture or clutter?)

(15) 家居內的梯級 "是"／"否" 有安裝扶手? (這條題目只是提供給在家居室內有梯級的人士填寫。)

Is the staircase inside the house with handrails? (Only applicable to those with a staircase inside the house.)

(16) 居住單位或房子樓層的梯級 "是"／"否" 有安裝扶手? (居住同一層的樓梯是否有安裝扶手?)

Is the staircase of the building with handrails? (Is the staircase of the same floor with handrails?)

(17) 梯級的邊緣 "是"／"否" 清晰和容易看到? (梯級的邊緣位置，是否沒有其他的花紋會阻礙視線?)

Are the edges of the steps easily identified? (Any other signs blocking the edges of the stairs?)

(18) 家居門口 "是"／"否" 安全和容易進出? (家居的門框是否穩固? 門鎖的位置是否適中?)

Can use the entrance doors safely and easily? (Is the door frame secure? Are the door locks in appropriate locations?)

(19) 在家中 "是"／"否" 有穿著合適的拖鞋或家居鞋? (是否穿著合適尺碼和沒有破損的鞋履?)

Is the person currently wearing well-fitting slippers or shoes? (In an appropriate size and not torn?)

(20) 在家中 "是"／"否" 有需要照顧寵物的飲食和清潔? (這條題目只是提供給有需要照顧寵物的人士填寫。) ("否" 代表正面的回覆。)

Are there pets at home that require care, feeding and cleaning? (Only applicable to those with pets.) ("No" as a positive response.)

there are safety issues, such as a lack of supervision for high fall-risk clients or the elderly with severe cognitive impairment, arrangement of daycare facilities or even institutional care may be required.

Discharge planning and preparation

Discharge planning and preparation is a key process in hospital settings, with the former being one of the roles of occupational therapists working in hospitals. There is preliminary evidence supporting the value of OT in discharge planning, including reducing resources, improving satisfaction, and avoiding unplanned re-admissions. In recent years, there has been a growing number of publications highlighting and supporting the role of occupational therapists in facilitating hospital discharge, particularly among elderly clients (Crennan & MacRae, 2010; Moats & Doble, 2006; Wales et al., 2012; 2018). There is also preliminary evidence supporting discharge planning among the elderly and the contribution of occupational therapists in helping to prevent unplanned hospital re-admissions (Rogers et al., 2017).

In the medical literature, discharge planning sometimes refers to the "development of an individualized care plan prior to leaving the hospital for home or any agreed environment in order to arrange what the client needs for a smooth transition from one level of care to another". "Any agreed environment" implies that clients may not necessarily be discharged to home, but to an old age home or a residential care institution. Discharge planning is an essential process to ensure a smooth transition from one level of care to another. It is important to understand that discharge from the hospital does not necessarily mean that clients have reached full recovery. It only implies that hospital care is not required as the medical condition is stable. The healthcare team typically aims to facilitate a client's discharge from the hospital as early as possible to minimize the hazards and risks associated with hospitalization, particularly for frail elderly clients (Creditor, 1993; Labella et al., 2011). On the other hand, promote further recovery, there is the need to ensure the continuity of care, including medical, nursing, and rehabilitation care, after clients are discharged from the hospital.

Both clients and their caregivers often experience significant stress when clients are discharged home, especially if they have acquired new disabilities due to major illnesses or injuries. These clients typically require assistance in personal care activities, which can add to the stress for their families. The situation would be more complicated for clients who are considered as mentally incapacitated persons (MIP). The healthcare team needs to identify any potential abuse of MIP. The abuse can come in various forms, including physical, psychological, financial, and sexual, as well as neglect or abandonment. Whenever there is an indication of abuse, a guardian, usually a social worker, will be appointed to take care of all the issues of this MIP.

Overall, in discharge planning, occupational therapists are required to strike a balance between the benefits of being discharged back home and the stress caused to the family members or caregivers.

Guide for occupational therapists in discharge planning and preparation

Intervention by occupational therapists in discharge planning can be divided into two phases: planning and preparation.

Discharge planning refers to the process of compromising on a plan. It involves communication or counseling processes to help clients and their families decide on crucial issues including:

(1) Where: the destination or residence upon discharge; is the client going back home or resettling in an institution?
(2) Who: the caregiver of the client when he/she is back home; would this be the old partner or a hired helper?
(3) What: the caring duties that the family is required to take up, the types of assistive devices such as a hospital bed and wheelchair, and the types of community care service that would be required upon discharge.

Discharge preparation refers to the process and work related to the implementation of the compromised discharge plan. To ensure continuity of care, it is essential to communicate extensively with stakeholders and to provide training and coaching for caregivers.

To help therapists understand the process and provide a reference guide for practice, discharge planning and preparation are divided into five steps. Steps 1 to 3 focus on planning, which involves counseling and engaging with clients and their families in making decisions. Steps 4 and 5 concern discharge preparation and implementation of the discharge plan.

Step 1: Explore the wishes, worries, stresses, and values of both clients and their caregivers

This exploration step should begin at the very start of the discharge planning process as it is fundamental and critically important. The information gathered during this step will help therapists in making recommendations in Step 3. This exploration process typically involves counseling and engaging with clients and their families. By demonstrating understanding and expressing a commitment to support clients and their families through challenges, occupational therapists can build trust and establish a stronger therapeutic relationship.

Step 2: Determine the right moment to initiate discussion of a discharge plan

The ideal scenario would involve the medical officer or clients and their families initiating discussions about discharge or proposing a clear discharge plan, indicating their readiness to take action. However, this is not commonly observed. Therefore, therapists need to identify the right moment to start discussing a discharge plan. If the discussion occurs too early, clients and their caregivers may not be prepared and could feel distressed. On the other hand, if it happens too late, occupational therapists may lack sufficient time to complete the necessary preparations, potentially compromising the continuity of care. Identifying the right time can be straightforward if therapists have validated the following information:

(1) Medical condition and progress: whether optimal treatment has been provided to clients and they are responding to treatment.
(2) Rehabilitation potential and progress: the trend and extent of the short-term and long-term functional recovery of the clients. This would help therapists make

valid recommendations about the plan for further therapy, including settings, intensity, etc.

(3) Long-term care needs: the various caring activities that caregivers are required to provide when clients are discharged back home. The following list highlights the common needs of frail elderly clients.

- ADL-transfer, including toilet and bathtub transfer, and functional mobility
- Feeding, nutrition, and hydration (considering artificial hydration and nutrition versus careful hand feeding)
- Bladder and bowel management, including incontinence management
- Pressure sore prevention and management
- Some medical procedures for continuation of care in home settings:
  - Insulin injections for diabetes mellitus
  - Inhalers for respiratory conditions
  - Home oxygen therapy for clients requiring oxygen supplementation
  - Non-invasive positive pressure ventilation, such as using bilevel positive airway pressure (BiPAP)
  - Renal replacement therapy, such as continuous ambulatory peritoneal dialysis (CAPD)

The above information can be obtained through the Comprehensive Geriatric Assessment (CGA). CGA refers to a "multidimensional diagnostic process focused on determining an older person's medical, psychological, and functional capability in order to develop a coordinated and integrated plan for treatment as well as long-term follow-up". CGA was developed based on the assumption that "older people often have more complex multi-system problems, and are at increased risk for morbidity and mortality, and need comprehensive interventions that take into account the bio-psychosocial components of health" (Stuck et al., 1993). In daily practice, besides observation, interviewing, and physical examination, occupational therapists also use various standardized assessment tools to facilitate CGA. Table 6.4 shows the milestones in the development of some commonly used tools for CGA. Once the therapist has obtained the information discussed in Steps 1 and 2, they can proceed to Step 3.

Step 3: Discuss with clients and caregivers to develop a tentative discharge plan
A guiding communication or counseling style is recommended for the discussion. Guiding means therapists refrain from giving directions or expert advice based on their professional assessment directly. Instead, they try to help clients and caregivers see the benefits and challenges of the discharge plan and make their own decisions. They also respect clients' autonomy to choose the option that best meets their needs, provided that they are well informed. Motivational Interviewing (MI) is an example of a guiding communication or counseling style. There are preliminary reports on the potential effect of MI on improving client satisfaction and long-term compliance (Taylor et al.,

Table 6.4 Milestones in the development of standardized tools for CGA

Year	Standardized tool	Assessment area
1963	Katz Activities of Daily Living (ADL)	ADL
1965	Barthel Index (BI)	ADL
1969	Lawton Instrumental Activities of Daily Living (IADL)	ADL
1975	Mini-mental State Examination (MMSE)	Cognition
1983	Geriatric Depression Scale (GDS)	Mood
1984	Functional Independence Measure (FIM™)	ADL, mobility, and cognition
1986	Get Up and Go (GUG)	Mobility
1986	Tinetti Performance-oriented Mobility Assessment (POMA)	Mobility and balance
1990	Confusion Assessment Method (CAM)	Cognition
1994	Mini Nutritional Assessment (MNA)	Others
1995	Hierarchical Assessment of Balance and Mobility (HABAM)	Mobility and balance
1998	Executive Clock Drawing Task (CLOX)	Cognition
2000	Androgen Deficiency in Aging Males (ADAM)	Others
2005	Clinical Frailty Scale (CFS)	Others

2021; Vellone et al., 2020). The ultimate goal is to help clients and caregivers decide on the discharge destination, who will be the primary caregiver, the types of assistive devices, the types of community care service, etc. Occupational therapists should be familiar with all the possible options so that they can give professional advice and provide relevant information when requested by clients and their caregivers.

Step 4: Follow through with the plan and schedule an expected date of discharge
Once a tentative plan has been made, the therapist can bring it back to the team for further discussion and amendment. The team then follows through with the plan. Occupational therapists are usually responsible for arranging trials of various assistive devices, applying for social funding to support these devices, conducting caregiver training, prescribing home modifications, initiating referrals for continuity of care by community care services, and initiating referrals for further rehabilitation. A sample application letter for home modification of a public housing unit in Hong Kong is provided in Figure 6.1.

Step 5: Trouble-shooting on or near the date of discharge
This is a crucial step because it ensures every part of the plan is implemented as scheduled. If any problem is left unidentified, clients may be at risk. For example, if clients are discharged back home without proper assistive devices and services to support them, health and safety issues may arise.

In summary, discharge planning and preparation can be carried out in five steps, as indicated in Figure 6.2. Both clients and their caregivers should be involved. During the process, occupational therapists take on a guiding role and respect clients' and their caregivers' decisions.

醫院管理局
HOSPITAL
AUTHORITY

九龍醫院
KOWLOON HOSPITAL

Our Reference: XXXXXXXXXXXX

Your Reference:

領先物業服務有限公司
XXXXXXXXXXXXXXX
Fax. XXXXXXXX
Tel. XXXXXXXX

Date   22 December 2015

Request for Home Modification for
Tenant: XXXXXXX (HKID. XXXXXXX)
Unit: XXXXXXXXXXXXXXXXXXXXXXXXXXXX

     I write, on behalf of MS. XXXXXXXXXXXXXXXX, to request for the following modifications in the captioned unit:

| Items: | Install of totally 3 grabrails; 2 within shower area and another 1 by the entrance of the shower area
Within the shower area
Grabrail 1 (*Diagram 1 & 2*):
    <u>Dimension</u>: Length 24", Diameter 1.25"
    <u>Orientation</u>: Vertical
    <u>Location</u>: 28" away from the side wall of the shower area, and, its low-end 24" from the base of the shower base.
Grabrail 2 (*Diagram 1 & 2*):
    <u>Dimension</u>: Length 18", Diameter 1.25"
    <u>Orientation</u>: Horizontal
    <u>Location</u>: its tail-end 4" away from the back wall of the toilet, and, 24" from the base of the shower base.
By the Entrance of the shower area
Grabrail 3 (*Diagram 1 & 3*):
    <u>Dimension</u>: Length 24", Diameter 1.25"
    <u>Orientation</u>: Vertical
    <u>Location</u>: 4" away of the front entrance of the shower area and its low-end 24" from the floor |
| Justification: | To allow accessibility and ensure safety in bathing of the tenant; who relies on quadripod and firm support in mobility due to a prior brain injury leading to weakness of the left side limbs. |

    Related diagrams (**Diagram 1 , 2 & 3**), illustrating the requested modifications, are attached for your reference. In case of any query and needs for clarification, please feel free to contact the undersigned, at:

Correspondence: Occupational Therapy Department, Kowloon Hospital (Rehabilitation Building)
                      147A Argyle Street, Kowloon
Fax.   2624 7142
Tel.   3129 7122

XXXXXXXXXXXXXXXX
Occupational Therapist
Kowloon Hospital

(a)

Figure 6.1 A sample application letter for home modification of a local public housing unit (a), with three diagrams illustrating the requested modifications (b–d)

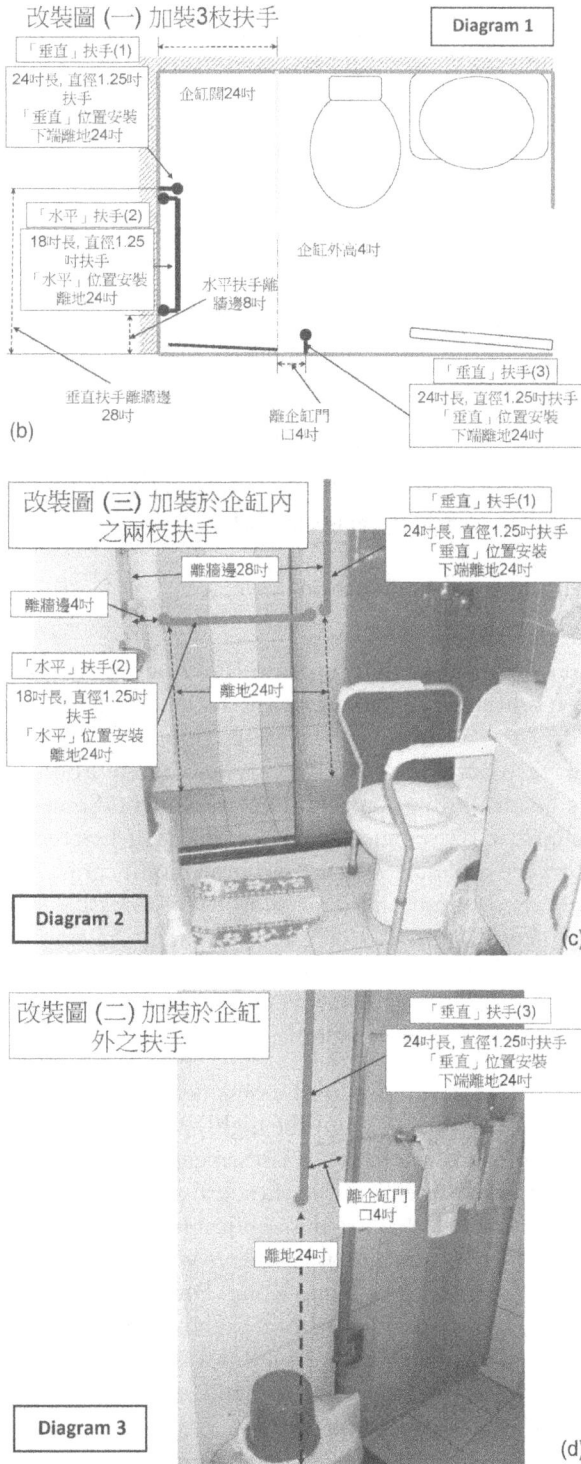

改裝圖 (一) 加裝3枝扶手

Diagram 1

「垂直」扶手(1)

24吋長, 直徑1.25吋
扶手
「垂直」位置安裝
下端離地24吋

企缸闊24吋

「水平」扶手(2)

18吋長, 直徑1.25
吋扶手
「水平」位置安裝
離地24吋

企缸外高4吋

水平扶手離
牆邊8吋

垂直扶手離牆邊
28吋

離企缸門
口4吋

「垂直」扶手(3)

24吋長, 直徑1.25吋扶手
「垂直」位置安裝
下端離地24吋

(b)

改裝圖 (三) 加裝於企缸內
之兩枝扶手

「垂直」扶手(1)

24吋長, 直徑1.25吋扶手
「垂直」位置安裝
下端離地24吋

離牆邊28吋

離牆邊4吋

「水平」扶手(2)

18吋長, 直徑1.25吋
扶手
「水平」位置安裝
離地24吋

離地24吋

Diagram 2

(c)

改裝圖 (二) 加裝於企缸
外之扶手

「垂直」扶手(3)

24吋長, 直徑1.25吋扶手
「垂直」位置安裝
下端離地24吋

離企缸門
口4吋

離地24吋

Diagram 3

(d)

Figure 6.1 A sample application letter for home modification of a local public housing unit (a), with three diagrams illustrating the requested modifications (b–d) (*continued*)

Step 1: Explore the wishes, worries, stresses, and values of both clients and their caregivers

⬇

Step 2: Determine the right moment to initiate discussion of a discharge plan

⬇

Step 3: Discuss with clients and caregivers to develop a tentative discharge plan

⬇

Step 4: Follow through with the plan and schedule an expected date of discharge

⬇

Step 5: Trouble-shooting on or near the date of discharge

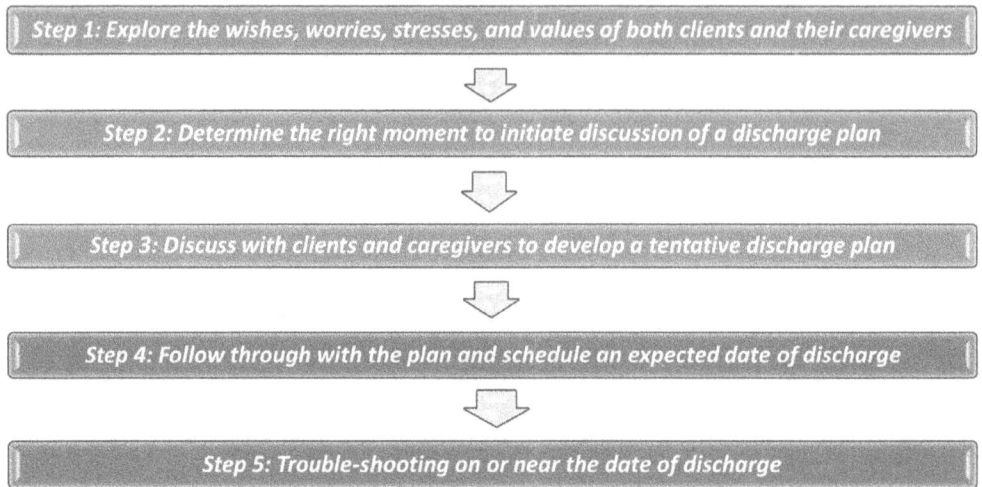

Figure 6.2 A guide for occupational therapists in discharge planning and preparation

Home visit and environmental modification

Use of standardized assessments

Based on the Person-Environment-Occupation (PEO) model developed by Law et al. (1996), apart from modifying the person factor, such as body functions, occupational therapists can modify the environment factor to improve the fitness of the occupational performance transaction. Before modifying the environment for clients, the OT process always begins with an appropriate assessment. Some occupational therapists may use standardized assessments, while some will use their clinical judgment on-site to provide advice and suggestions on home modification. In Hong Kong, the two most commonly used standardized environmental assessments are the Westmead Home Safety Assessment (Clemson, 1997) and the Safety Assessment of Function and the Environment for Rehabilitation–Health Outcome Measurement and Evaluation (SAFER-HOME) (Chiu & Oliver, 2006). There are two limitations when applying these standardized assessments in environmental assessment:

(1) The basic construct of a standardized assessment is always designed to include every possible aspect. However, given the highly diverse nature of every household condition, the comprehensiveness of the assessment is always too lengthy. Therapists might have to skip several items in the standardized environmental assessment or put an "N/A" next to items that are not applicable.

(2) These standardized environmental assessments were designed in foreign countries that are markedly different from Hong Kong. For instance, Hong Kong is densely populated, and the living space of each household unit is significantly limited. A major problem faced by clients with disabilities is accessibility to their residential areas. Therefore, therapists may need to make extra remarks in addition to the standardized items in the assessment form.

Despite their limitations, these standardized assessments can serve as good references or checklists for occupational therapists in performing home assessments, as they cover every possible problem that clients may face when they interact with the environment.

Use of non-standardized assessments

Most occupational therapists in Hong Kong prefer to use a non-standardized home assessment based on observation and clinical judgment. Although it may not be as comprehensive as the standardized ones, it is more flexible and can be custom-made to suit clients with various clinical conditions. For example, for spinal cord injury clients who are wheelchair-bound, the focus of the home assessment may be accessibility to the building and to various areas inside the flat. For clients with dementia, the focus would be on the risk of performing daily activities and the environmental support for the loss of memory. For clients with COPD requiring oxygen therapy, the focus would be on the feasibility of using the oxygen devices at home. Based on the above examples, it is clear that home assessment is never a "one size fits all" solution. Due to the uniqueness of each scenario, there is no rigid way to perform a home assessment. Occupational therapists should always bear in mind the PEO interaction to identify components in the environment that would be a challenge for the client in terms of their person and occupation factors.

Assessment of accessibility

Accessibility is always the first thing to consider for clients with various clinical conditions. In Hong Kong, the Buildings Department published the *Design Manual: Barrier Free Access 2008 (2021 Edition)* for designers and architects to use as a reference when building barrier-free environments (Buildings Department, 2021). The manual applies to "all common areas of buildings of more than four storeys" for domestic buildings and serves as the gold standard when designing public barrier-free environments. However, it is not advisable to use the numeric data in the manual as guidelines for assessing clients' individual home environments because household space is often quite limited. In many circumstances, occupational therapists need to critically and creatively formulate solutions to address the clients' needs within the environmental limitations. Therefore, when assessing the accessibility of the home environment, the first thing to do is to assess clients' personal factors, such as anthropometric data, strength, balance, walking ability, and types of walking aids. This information can help therapists judge the minimum space required by the clients. Second, therapists should also have a clear understanding of clients' occupational performance, as well as the need to perform various occupations during a normal day. Occupational therapists can only judge whether the environment is suitable for clients after analyzing their person and occupation factors. For example, the focus of the assessment would be different between a man who is dependent on BADL and a housewife. For the man with dependent BADL, the focus would be on the adequacy of space for his caregivers to take care of him, including the use of assistive devices. For the housewife, the focus would be on the accessibility of the kitchen and household utensils.

Safety considerations

In addition to accessibility, how safe a person is when performing an occupation within the environment is also critical. The best way to assess safety during the performance of an occupation is to ask the client to perform the necessary occupation in the actual environment, such as performing toilet and bathtub transfer in his/her own home. When the client is performing the toilet or bathtub transfer, the therapist can assess whether the client's person factor (e.g., his/her ability) matches the environment factor (e.g., the toilet or bathtub height). If the PEO transaction is unmatched, occupational therapists can decide whether to alter the person factor, the environment factor, the occupation factor, or to alter a combination of them. In situations where occupational therapists cannot perform an assessment in the actual home environment, such as during a pandemic, they might ask the clients or their families to take photos and then offer advice according to the photos provided. However, this method should only be considered a temporary measure under special situations as the therapists cannot see the PEO transaction accurately. When the situation allows, a follow-up home visit by hospital-based or community-based occupational therapists should be arranged.

Case study on home assessment and modification
The case below serves to illustrate the clinical reasoning process in home assessment and modification.

Mr. Li is a stroke client with right-sided weakness. He was observed to be unsafe in performing bathtub transfer. The possible reasons may be:

(1) Mr. Li does not have adequate strength over his affected side (P);
(2) Mr. Li cannot perform the transfer using his previous method (O); or
(3) The height of the bathtub is too high for Mr. Li (E).

To remedy the situation, an occupational therapist can provide training to Mr. Li to improve the strength of his affected limbs (P). The therapist may need to assess Mr. Li's rehabilitation potential first and see if the chance of improvement is high. It might take a long time to improve Mr. Li's strength. Apart from enhancing the P factor, the therapist can also consider modifying the way Mr. Li gets into the bathtub, i.e., modifying the O factor. As already mentioned, Mr. Li cannot use his previous means of getting into the bathtub because of his right-sided weakness. Repetitive training of bathtub transfer can be provided to Mr. Li but the effectiveness of the training depends on his rehabilitation potential. Alternatively, to address the O factor, Mr. Li could adopt adaptive methods such as sitting on the water closet instead of getting into the bathtub to take a shower. Making environmental modifications to address the E factor can also be considered. Occupational therapists are frequently expected to provide recommendations for environmental modification. As the home environment varies among families, the E factor should be considered individually. Two options for environmental modification can be suggested to Mr. Li:

(1) Remove the bathtub and replace it with a shower cubicle so that the client does not need to climb into the bathtub; or
(2) Use a bath board so that the client can sit on it for transferring into the bathtub.

There are several conditions for consideration when choosing between these two modifications. Many people believe that removing the bathtub would be easier. However, due to building designs varying, it may not be so easy to remove the bathtub in most flats in

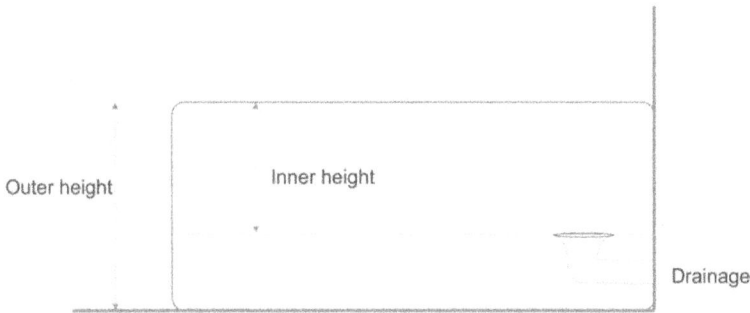

Figure 6.3 A side view of a common bathtub design showing a large discrepancy between the inner height and the outer height

Hong Kong. To check the feasibility of removing the bathtub, we might need to examine the original building plan. That said, it is often difficult to obtain the original building plan, even if it still exists. An alternative method is to examine the discrepancy between the inner height and the outer height of the bathtub. A large discrepancy implies that there may be drainage pipes built under the bathtub, as illustrated in Figure 6.3, which is common in public housing estates across Hong Kong. Upon removing the bathtub, it might be found that the floor is not completely level. Mr. Li would therefore still need to climb a step to enter the shower area, as illustrated in Figure 6.4, increasing the risk of falls.

In some private housing units, bathtubs are installed in a sunken position, meaning the drainage is located below the floor of the client's flat, as illustrated in Figure 6.5. The therapist may find that the outer height and the inner height of the bathtub are nearly identical. Removing the bathtub will level the floor of the shower area, significantly reducing the risk of falls and making bathing easier, as illustrated in Figure 6.6. To ensure maximum safety, it may also be beneficial to consider installing handrails and providing a shower chair so that the client can take a shower while seated.

The therapist may have other concerns that prevent him from recommending the removal of the bathtub, such as the preference of Mr. Li and his family, or the time required for the modification. The family may be reluctant to remove the bathtub because they are renting the flat. In this situation, the right to make alterations belongs to the flat owner. If they make changes, they will need to restore the flat to its original

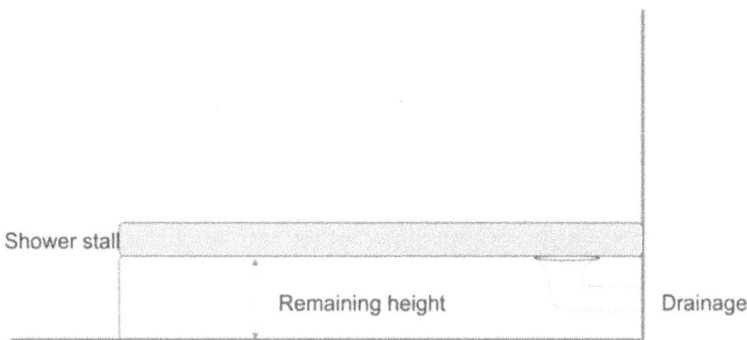

Figure 6.4 A side view of the shower area after removing the bathtub, leaving a remaining height

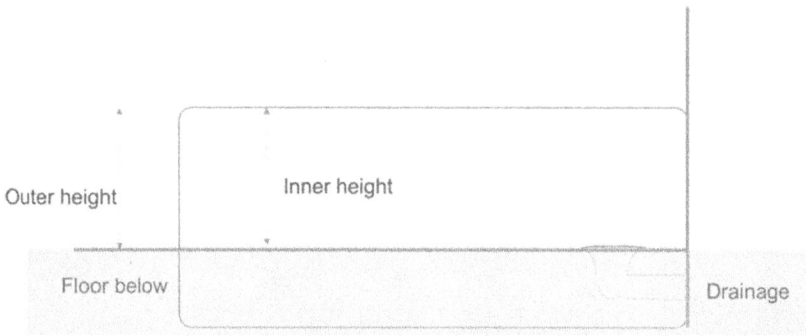

Figure 6.5 Another design showing the drainage built beneath the floor of the client's flat, typically concealed by a false ceiling in the flat below

condition at their own expense when they move out, which may deter them from spending extra money on reinstalling the bathtub. Therefore, the therapist should be sensitive to Mr. Li's feelings as he may regard any changes made for his benefit as a burden on his family. The therapist should try to find a balance between necessary modifications and adaptations, keeping changes to a minimum to avoid causing inconvenience to the family members who share the flat with Mr. Li.

If Mr. Li is discharged at short notice, construction work may not be completed in time. In this case, the therapist may need to recommend a different type of modification that is easier and quicker to implement for a safe discharge. If the bathtub must remain for any of the reasons mentioned above, adaptive devices can be considered. The most common adaptive device is a bath board, which comes in various designs but should be securely fixed to the bathtub with at least two rubber legs. The width of the bath board should match the width of the bathtub, otherwise it may pose a fall risk during transfers. Additionally, the height of the bathtub should be carefully assessed. It is not recommended to use bath boards on bathtubs with an outer height of less than 14 inches or 355 mm. For lower bathtubs, a bath bench that can be adjusted to a more suitable height of around 18 inches or 450 mm is recommended instead. The bath bench should be positioned across the low bathtub, with one side placed inside the bathtub and the other outside, allowing the client to sit on the edge of the bath bench first before gradually moving into the bathtub for showering.

Figure 6.6 Removal of the bathtub and replacement with a shower stall would eliminate nearly all of the height that the client needs to overcome

As mentioned above, regardless of whether the bathtub is removed or not, appropriate handrails should be installed to ensure safe transfers for the client. Therapists should also consider other practical issues such as water splashing, which could create safety concerns if only a bath board is recommended without addressing the shower curtain. If Mr. Li's rehabilitation potential is good or is expected to improve soon, environmental modifications should be carefully considered as suggestions made at this point may not suit his future needs.

In summary, home assessment involves not only assessing the physical environment but also understanding the PEO transaction within the home context. Besides the client's needs, therapists should also consider the needs of family members who share the same living space.

Summary

Helping clients to return to the home or community is a vital role of occupational therapists within the multidisciplinary care team. This chapter has discussed commonly used assessments in Hong Kong hospitals that prepare clients for discharge. It also provides therapists with guiding principles for planning safe discharges and creating supportive home environments for clients with residual disabilities after their hospital stay. While assessment tools and considerations for environmental modifications may vary between countries, the essential components for safe discharge and community reintegration remain consistent. These components include accurate and efficient assessments of clients' functional capacities, careful consideration of the home environment and available social support, and the education and empowerment of family members to assist in the clients' transition back to their communities.

References

Buildings Department, Hong Kong SAR Government. (2021). *Design manual: Barrier free access 2008* (2021 edition). https://www.bd.gov.hk/doc/en/resources/codes-and-references/code-and-design-manuals/BFA2008_e.pdf

Census and Statistics Department, Hong Kong SAR Government. (2018). *2016 Population by-census thematic report: Older persons.* https://www.statistics.gov.hk/pub/B11201052016XXXXB0100.pdf

Chiu, T., & Oliver, R. (2006). Factor analysis and construct validity of the SAFER-HOME. *OTJR: Occupation, Participation and Health, 26*(4), 132–142. https://doi.org/10.1177/153944920602600403

Clemson, L. (1997). *Home fall hazards: A guide to identifying fall hazards in the homes of elderly people and an accompaniment to the assessment tool, the Westmead Home Safety Assessment (WeHSA).* Co-ordinates Publications.

Creditor, M. C. (1993). Hazards of hospitalization of the elderly. *Annals of Internal Medicine, 118*(3), 219–223.

Crennan, M., & MacRae, A. (2010). Occupational therapy discharge assessment of elderly patients from acute care hospitals. *Physical & Occupational Therapy in Geriatrics, 28*(1), 33–43. https://doi.org/10.3109/02703180903381060

Department of Health, Hong Kong SAR Government. (2022). *Health facts of Hong Kong 2022 edition.* https://www.dh.gov.hk/english/statistics/statistics_hs/files/2022.pdf

Granger, C. V., & Hamilton, B. B. (1992). UDS report. The Uniform Data System for Medical Rehabilitation Report of First Admissions for 1990. *American Journal of Physical Medicine & Rehabilitation, 71*(2), 108–113.

Hospital Authority, Hong Kong SAR Government. (2021). *Hospital Authority strategic plan 2022-2027*. https://www.ha.org.hk/haho/ho/ap/HA_StrategicPlan2022-2027_Eng_211216.pdf

Labella, A. M., Merel, S. E., & Phelan, E. A. (2011). Ten ways to improve the care of elderly patients in the hospital. *Journal of Hospital Medicine, 6*(6), 351–357. https://doi.org/10.1002/jhm.900

Lai, F. H. Y., Yan, E. W. H., Mackenzie, L., Fong, K. N. K., Kranz, G. S., Ho, E. C. W., Fan, S. H. U., & Lee, A. T. K. (2020). Reliability, validity, and clinical utility of a self-reported screening tool in the prediction of fall incidence in older adults. *Disability and Rehabilitation, 42*(21), 3098–3105. https://doi.org/10.1080/09638288.2019.1582721

Law, M., Cooper, B., Strong, S., Stewart, D., Rigby, P., & Letts, L. (1996). The Person-Environment-Occupation model: A transactive approach to occupational performance. *Canadian Journal of Occupational Therapy, 63*(1), 9–23. https://doi.org/10.1177/000841749606300103

Lawton, M. P., & Brody, E. M. (1969). Assessment of older people: Self-maintaining and instrumental activities of daily living. *The Gerontologist, 9*(3, Part 1), 179–186. https://doi.org/10.1093/geront/9.3_Part_1.179

Lawton, M. P., Moss, M., Fulcomer, M., & Kleban, M. H. (1982). A research and service oriented multilevel assessment instrument. *Journal of Gerontology, 37*(1), 91–99. https://doi.org/10.1093/geronj/37.1.91

Leung, S. O. C., Chan, C. C. H., & Shah, S. (2007). Development of a Chinese version of the Modified Barthel Index — Validity and reliability. *Clinical Rehabilitation, 21*(10), 912–922. https://doi.org/10.1177/0269215507077286

Mackenzie, L., Byles, J., & Higginbotham, N. (2000). Designing the Home Falls and Accidents Screening Tool (HOME FAST): Selecting the items. *British Journal of Occupational Therapy, 63*(6), 260–269. https://doi.org/10.1177/030802260006300604

Moats, G., & Doble, S. (2006). Discharge planning with older adults: Toward a negotiated model of decision making. *Canadian Journal of Occupational Therapy, 73*(5), 303–311. https://doi.org/10.1177/000841740607300507

Rogers, A. T., Bai, G., Lavin, R. A., & Anderson, G. F. (2017). Higher hospital spending on occupational therapy is associated with lower readmission rates. *Medical Care Research and Review, 74*(6), 668–686. https://doi.org/10.1177/1077558716666981

Shah, S., Vanclay, F., & Cooper, B. (1989). Improving the sensitivity of the Barthel Index for stroke rehabilitation. *Journal of Clinical Epidemiology, 42*(8), 703–709.

Stuck, A. E., Siu, A. L., Wieland, G. D., Rubenstein, L. Z., & Adams, J. (1993). Comprehensive geriatric assessment: A meta-analysis of controlled trials. *The Lancet, 342*(8878), 1032–1036. https://doi.org/10.1016/0140-6736(93)92884-V

Taylor, N. F., O'Halloran, P. D., Watts, J. J., Morris, R., Peiris, C. L., Porter, J., Prendergast, L. A., Harding, K. E., Snowdon, D. A., Ekegren, C. L., Hau, R., Mudiyanselage, S. B., Rimayanti, M. U., Noeske, K. E., Snowdon, M., Kim, D., & Shields, N. (2021). Motivational interviewing with community-dwelling older adults after hip fracture (MIHip): Protocol for a randomised controlled trial. *BMJ Open, 11*(6), e047970. https://doi.org/10.1136/bmjopen-2020-047970

Tong, A. Y. C., & Man, D. W. K. (2002). The validation of the Hong Kong Chinese Version of the Lawton Instrumental Activities of Daily Living Scale for institutionalized elderly persons. *OTJR: Occupation, Participation and Health, 22*(4), 132–142. https://doi.org/10.1177/153944920202200402

Vellone, E., Rebora, P., Ausili, D., Zeffiro, V., Pucciarelli, G., Caggianelli, G., Masci, S., Alvaro, R., & Riegel, B. (2020). Motivational interviewing to improve self-care in heart failure patients (MOTIVATE-HF): A randomized controlled trial. *ESC Heart Failure, 7*(3), 1309–1318. https://doi.org/10.1002/ehf2.12733

Wales, K., Clemson, L., Lannin, N. A., Cameron, I. D., Salked, G., Gitlin, L., Rubenstein, L., Barras, S., Mackenzie, L., & Davies, C. (2012). Occupational therapy discharge planning for older adults: A protocol for a randomised trial and economic evaluation. *BMC Geriatrics, 12*(1), 34. https://doi.org/10.1186/1471-2318-12-34

Wales, K., Salkeld, G., Clemson, L., Lannin, N. A., Gitlin, L., Rubenstein, L., Howard, K., Howell, M., & Cameron, I. D. (2018). A trial based economic evaluation of occupational therapy discharge planning for older adults: The HOME randomized trial. *Clinical Rehabilitation, 32*(7), 919–929. https://doi.org/10.1177/0269215518764249

CHAPTER 7

Return to work

Andy Shu Kei Cheng and Yanwen Xu

Introduction

Work is a productive activity valued by individuals and society. The ability to participate in productive activity contributes significantly to both the physical and psychological well-being of a person (Figueredo et al., 2020). It has benefits such as creative skills development, financial gain, and social status. People also bring their values to employment. When a person is injured at work, there are changes in all aspects of that individual's functioning, whether the injury is short-term or long-term, permanent or temporary, serious or minor. The changes for the worker are complex and may be physical, psychological, social, or financial. These changes all interrelate and affect one another. For example, following an injury, there will be appointments with a doctor, occupational therapist, and physiotherapist, which may necessitate the reorganization of the family's routine. Furthermore, the pattern of family interactions may change as family members take on new tasks, roles, and responsibilities. All these changes can lead to stress. The potential negative consequences from being out of work extend well beyond the loss of financial rewards to include the loss of self-esteem and self-worth (Jeong et al., 2019; Peteet, 2000).

The employer and the management of the workplace may also be affected by the injury. There are both direct and indirect costs of injury, including the medical expenses for the rehabilitation of the injured worker, loss of production due to the loss of the injured worker's skills, salary paid to the non-productive worker, and legal costs for litigation. Staff morale and the reputation of the company may also be affected. Successful work resumption is important, not only because it provides financial benefit to the injured worker but also because it brings other benefits, including health and quality of life gains, re-establishment of one's sense of self in society, and the ability to perform other life roles within the family and community (Gewurtz et al., 2018). However, the return to work (RTW) of an injured worker, especially those with chronic symptoms, can be conceptualized as a complex human behavioral change, involving physical

DOI: 10.4324/9781032721170-10

recovery, motivation, behavior, and interaction with a number of factors in the workplace (Aasdahl et al., 2022). For every rehabilitation professional, particularly occupational therapists, one of the overriding duties is to optimize the productive capacity of an individual and prevent the development of work disability so that the individual can have a safe and timely RTW.

Rehabilitation programs for injured workers

There are a range of terms related to various rehabilitation programs for injured workers, namely vocational rehabilitation, occupational rehabilitation, and work rehabilitation. These terms are frequently used during the rehabilitation process of injured workers. The choice of term very much depends on the preference of the particular organization, government, or funding agency, and the terms are often used interchangeably in many countries. However, in practice, there are subtle differences between them.

Vocational rehabilitation

The goal of vocational rehabilitation is employment with another employer, either with the same, modified, or different work tasks (Scully et al., 1999). In 1998, the International Labour Organization (ILO) defined vocational rehabilitation by stating its objective as referring to any programs that enable a person with a disability to secure and retain suitable employment (International Labour Organization, 1998). Vocational rehabilitation can, therefore, be regarded as a formal training program designed to help individuals of working age with physical or mental disabilities to compete successfully against others in order to earn a livelihood. In the United States, vocational rehabilitation is a federal/state-funded program providing services to help individuals with disabilities enter or return to employment. According to the Americans with Disabilities Act, vocational rehabilitation programs take an active leadership role in advocating for the rights of individuals with disabilities, removing the physical and attitudinal barriers that often confront them, and publicizing their abilities and accomplishments to society.

Occupational rehabilitation

Occupational rehabilitation is distinguished from vocational rehabilitation in that the main goal of the intervention is to return injured workers to their pre-injury employer (Harrison & Allen, 2003). It is broadly defined as a managed process involving early intervention with appropriate and timely services based on assessed needs and is aimed at maintaining injured or ill employees in, or returning them to, suitable employment (National Occupational Health and Safety Commission, 1995). The main goal of occupational rehabilitation is to enable workers to keep their jobs or to return to gainful employment after an accident, injury, or the onset of an unfavorable health condition in order to prevent work disability. In other words, the situational definition of work disability is a person's inability to remain at work or RTW during the course of or after an injury/illness. The ILO provides objectives for occupational rehabilitation as a process that enables a person with a disability to secure and retain suitable employment and embodies the idea of integration or reintegration of the person into society. Occupational rehabilitation may include specialized vocational guidance and counseling, vocational training and placement, and employment (International Labour Organization, 1983). It is a process consisting of medical, psychological, social, and occupational activities among sick or injured people with work histories to re-establish their work capacity to return to the workforce. It also plays a key role in various settings such as mental health (Crowther et al., 2001), and may even be a critical determinant in engaging individuals to work but who have not worked prior to the health event (e.g., due to childhood-onset conditions, intellectual disability, etc.) (Anderson et al., 2009).

Work rehabilitation

Work rehabilitation, sometimes referred to as work hardening, is provided to injured workers after medical rehabilitation in order to prepare them to RTW. It is a basic component of the occupational rehabilitation process (see Figure 7.1). Work-hardening programs are rooted in the Moral Treatment movement of the late 1800s, when people who were "mentally and muscularly flabby" engaged in a "period of training or hardening up" in order to restore occupational capacity (Hanson & Walker, 1992). The aim of these programs was to rehabilitate injured workers, returning them to productive work as soon as possible. In 1977, Dr. Leonard Matheson was the first to describe a work-hardening program that he had established at Rancho Los Amigos Hospital in Downey (Helm-Williams, 1993). Later, in 1985, Matheson et al. defined work hardening as work-oriented treatment programs that have an outcome that is measured in terms of an improvement in the client's productivity (Matheson et al., 1985). In 1986, the American Occupational Therapy Association (AOTA) Commission on Practice published work-hardening guidelines. These guidelines defined a work-hardening program as:

> an individual, work-oriented activity process that involves a client in simulated or actual work tasks. These tasks are structured and graded progressively to increase psychological, physical and emotional tolerance and improve endurance and work feasibility.
>
> *(American Occupational Therapy Association, 1986, p. 841)*

In March 1988, the National Advisory Committee of the United States, which is a multidisciplinary body consisting of occupational therapists, physical therapists, rehabilitation counselors, administrators, rehabilitation nurses, psychologists, and attorneys, together with the Commission on Accreditation of Rehabilitation Facilities (CARF), expanded the definition of the concept of work hardening as follows:

> Work hardening is a highly structured, goal oriented, individualised treatment programme designed to maximise the individual's ability to return to work. Work hardening programmes, which are interdisciplinary in nature, use real or simulated work activities in conjunction with conditioning tasks that are graded to progressively improve the biomechanical, neuromuscular, cardiovascular/metabolic and psychosocial functions of the individual. Work hardening provides a transition between acute care and return to work while addressing the issues of productivity, safety, physical tolerances, and work behaviors.
>
> *(Commission on Accreditation of Rehabilitation Facilities, 1988, p. 1)*

This definition makes it explicit that an individualized work-oriented activity by means of simulated or actual work tasks is the main treatment modality used to help an individual RTW. These simulated work tasks can range from general to specific tasks, and only part of the body is involved in the general simulation tasks. For example, a general work simulation of a lifting task can be structured by putting a load on a clinical table and asking the injured worker to lift and lower the weight to and from waist height only. Initially, this may primarily involve the arms and only a portion of the actual lifting the worker must do on the job. In a specific work simulation, the simulated work environment may be totally different. A corner of the therapy room may be arranged as a warehouse with various sizes of boxes or goods placed on shelves of varying heights. The worker may be asked to retrieve different items from the shelves. By doing so, the worker will be required to use the entire body, including the back, legs, and arms, to lift and lower various boxes or goods with or without using a ladder. These simulations also train cognitive functions.

Specific work simulations are more advantageous than general work simulations in preparing the injured worker to RTW. However, it is impossible to accommodate all the possible work tasks or to simulate all working environments in the clinical setting. Consequently, worksite or workplace work-hardening programs are now identified as the therapeutic environment of choice as actual work duties and the real work environment can be used as the rehabilitation medium. The inherent benefits of workplace rehabilitation include the injured workers' ongoing interaction with the workplace, their coworkers, and supervisors so that the psychological bond between workers and the work environment is not weakened. There is evidence to suggest that in order to facilitate the RTW process, clinical interventions need to have a tie-in to the workplace (Franche et al., 2005). Durand and Loisel (2001) indicated the importance of placing the worksite in the center of the work-hardening program since workplace factors are critical for successful work rehabilitation. However, the therapist should carefully monitor the progress of the worker to prevent deterioration in their condition during this process. The majority of the current work-hardening programs are underpinned by the Stage Model of Industrial Rehabilitation (Matheson, 1986). This model was developed by Leonard Matheson as a way to describe the occupational rehabilitation process as a gradual transition from "patient" to "worker". There are eight stages in the occupational rehabilitation process, beginning at the point at which pathology is identified and extending to the point at which earning capacity is determined (Table 7.1).

At Stage One, the pathology with which an injured worker presents is assessed. Pathology is defined as an injury or disease process. At Stage Two, the injured worker's impairment is measured in terms of his/her anatomy, physiology, and psychology. Impairment is defined as the measurable consequence of pathology taken as a disruption of physical or mental integrity. Stage Three concerns the assessment of the functional limitations presented by the patient. The injured worker's reports of symptoms and limitations are corroborated through observation of function. Functional limitation is defined as the inability to perform functional activities and is measured in terms of general tasks that are not specifically tied to any one role but are found in many of the injured worker's roles. For instance, the phrase "unable to lift more than 20 pounds from floor to shoulder level" is a description of a functional limitation. The consequences of this finding in terms of role effects are considered at the next stage in

Table 7.1 The Stage Model of Industrial Rehabilitation (Matheson, 1986)

Stage	Area assessed	Measured by or in terms of ...
One	Pathology	Studies of tissue and bone.
Two	Impairment	Anatomy, physiology, and psyche.
Three	Functional limitation	Symptoms and limitations.
Four	Occupational disability	Social consequences of functional limitations.
Five	Vocational feasibility	Acceptability of the patient as an employee in the most general sense.
Six	Employability	Ability to become employed.
Seven	Vocational handicap	Ability to perform a particular job.
Eight	Earning capacity	Earned income measured over expected worklife.

the process. At Stage Four, the disability that the patient presents with is evaluated. Disability is defined as the social consequence of the injured worker's functional limitations. Disability is a question of the manner in which these functional limitations affect the patient's customary roles, such as a work role or family role. Disability is based on the evaluation of impairment provided at a prior stage.

Stage Five is concerned with the assessment of the injured worker's feasibility for competitive employment, which is defined in general terms as the acceptability of the patient (as an employee) to an employer. Special attention is paid to the work behavior of the employee-to-be. Stage Five is a transitional stage where the injured worker is no longer considered a "patient" but is now a "worker". This is the first stage in which the injured worker is formally assessed in terms that are used by potential employers. The injured worker's work behavior is considered in general terms with issues of productivity, safety, and interpersonal behavior of primary importance. Stage Six involves the injured worker's employability, i.e., his ability to become employed within a particular labor market. Stage Six is distinct from Stage Five (feasibility for competitive employment) in that feasibility is concerned with the general acceptability of the person as an employee in any occupation, while employability is concerned with the ability of a person to become employed within a particular labor market. It may be feasible for a person to seek competitive employment but be unemployable because no occupations exist in the particular labor market for which he/she qualifies. For example, an older worker who is able to seek employment often cannot find employment because of an age bias in the labor market.

Stage Seven concerns the vocational handicap, or the ability to become employed in a particular occupation. The nature and severity of the handicap are wholly determined by the interface between the worker and the job. The issue here is, "How well does the injured worker match his/her particular job?" The last stage, Stage Eight, involves earning capacity, which is measured in terms of work-generated income over the worker's lifetime. The Stage Model is useful to delineate some of the more important differences between occupational rehabilitation, which is based on a vocational model, and a traditional "medical model" approach.

If we consider that the two most general categories of tasks involved in rehabilitation are "evaluation" and "development", the medical model's focus is on the first three stages, while the vocational model's focus is on Stage Six and Stage Seven. In other words, work-hardening programs are provided to injured workers after medical rehabilitation in order to prepare them to RTW. It is a basic component of the occupational rehabilitation process.

The present form of work-hardening programs is deeply influenced by this model, which identifies and addresses the various stages of progression in the rehabilitation process. An injured worker can be referred to work hardening at any point from Stage Two (impairment) to Stage Seven (vocational handicap). From whichever point the injured worker enters the program, the goal of work hardening is to progress him/her through the remainder of the stages to emerge as a worker. As a result, an injured worker's productivity can improve during and after work hardening through the following techniques:

(1) *Decreasing secondary impairment effects*: Impairment is often magnified through disuse. Work hardening improves strength, flexibility, and endurance.
(2) *Decreasing functional limitations*: The injured worker's style of work and the quality of his/her work behavior often exacerbate functional impairment due to the injury. Work hardening helps the injured worker learn effective adaptive behaviors.
(3) *Decreasing disability*: Disability is the impact of functional impairment on the injured worker's societal roles, among which work roles are prominent. Work hardening helps the injured worker re-establish many of these roles. Improvement in these other areas generalizes to work roles and results in a concomitant decrease in work-related disability.
(4) *Improvement of vocational feasibility*: Most injured workers with work injuries have not worked for several months. Thus, work hardening identifies and addresses potential problems with productivity, increases safety in the workplace, and strengthens interpersonal relations.
(5) *Improvement of employability*: Most injured workers cannot RTW because of suboptimal work ability, including work strength, work skills, and work tolerances (e.g., the ability to lift, carry, and stand) compared with those of other workers in the general labor market. Work hardening identifies and develops these work tolerances.
(6) *Decreasing vocational handicap*: The match between the injured worker and the job can be improved by increasing the worker's level of function and modifying the job's critical work demands. Work hardening involves collaboration between both the injured worker and the employer to address these issues effectively.

Based on this model, there are two types of work-hardening programs: Feasibility Development Work Hardening and Employability Development Work Hardening (Ogden-Niemeyer & Jacobs, 1989). The overall objectives and program content of these programs vary. They can also be tailored based on the injured workers' readiness for work, as assessed by the Stage of Change Model, to determine the most suitable work-hardening program.

Feasibility Development Work Hardening focuses on workers at Stage Five (feasibility), where injured workers lack a defined worker role and may be grappling with their own ability to RTW, heavily influenced by a strong sick or patient role. The primary objective of this work-hardening program is to help injured workers develop sufficient work behaviors to be considered acceptable employees in a general sense. The major problem areas that underlie observed non-feasible behaviors include severe deconditioning or low functional level, poor activity control of symptoms, lack of worker role identification, and decrease in self-esteem or depression. Conversely, Employability Development Work Hardening addresses injured workers at Stage Six (employability), where injured workers already have had a worker role and are prepared to work again. The primary objective of this work-hardening program is to help injured workers reduce their impairments and improve specific areas of functioning where they have demonstrated poor performance, including developing physical capacity, work efficiency, symptom control, and selected work skills; improving the match between the individual and a selected occupational group or job through the development of the individual's capabilities or job modification; and helping them RTW.

As the field of work rehabilitation has evolved, a new model of work-hardening programs has emerged. This model is based on the therapeutic use of modified work programs and incorporates the concept of workplace rehabilitation for the management of occupational rotator cuff injuries. The aim is to promote effective physical and functional restoration, ultimately facilitating a successful RTW outcome. In the context of work rehabilitation for injured workers with physical disabilities, rehabilitation professionals strive to prepare these workers for RTW to the best of their ability. However, many injured workers may expect to achieve 100% recovery before resuming their jobs, which may not be a realistic expectation. A randomized controlled trial was conducted to investigate the effect of a workplace-based rehabilitation program on the RTW outcome of injured workers, which program is based on the therapeutic use of actual work facilities, the work environment, and the functions of a job coach (Cheng & Hung, 2007). A total of 103 workers with shoulder injuries were recruited and randomly assigned into hospital-based or workplace-based work-hardening groups. The hospital-based group was given traditional generic work-hardening training, while the workplace-based group received workplace-based work-hardening training. After four weeks, a higher RTW rate was obtained in the workplace-based group compared to the hospital-based group (71.4% versus 37%, $p < 0.01$). A statistically significant difference ($p < 0.05$) was also noted in the lowering of self-reported shoulder problems and functional work capabilities in the workplace-based group versus the hospital-based group. The result of this study showed that the workplace-based rehabilitation program appeared to be more effective in facilitating the RTW process of the injured workers as assessed immediately following the intervention. This approach specifically addresses many of the psychosocial workplace factors commonly associated with separation from the work routine. It helps minimize the influence of peer groups and employers on the injured workers' rehabilitation process. To explain the significant treatment effect of the workplace-based work-hardening program, it is possible that self-efficacy or the individual's confidence in engaging in RTW and in the activities that will maintain RTW was the process underlying the change in both groups. Therefore, a greater sense of self-efficacy could have occurred in the workplace-based work-hardening group. As mentioned before, the attitude of the injured worker in terms of his/her possible RTW is a crucial determinant of the likelihood of RTW. RTW self-efficacy and attitude regarding recovery may have had a significant impact on the RTW rate. During on-site workplace training, the injured worker could test his/her work ability in a real work situation instead of an artificial clinical environment before making the decision to RTW.

Furthermore, the presence of a job coach in the workplace-based work-hardening group played a significant role in facilitating the RTW decision of the injured worker.

The job coach acted like a second supervisor, trainer, educator, or support person to the injured worker. The job coach provided advice about proper biomechanics, safe work practices, and the appropriate pacing of work activities in the workplace. Through on-site supervision and assessment of the worker's performance, the job coach could provide more relevant and objective information to both the injured worker and his/her supervisors. In addition, the job coach could advocate for the injured worker to promote understanding and tolerance of his/her situation, offer additional information to the employer, and keep the employer informed about the activities undertaken to restore the worker's level of functioning. More importantly, concerns about RTW issues such as work arrangements, colleagues' perceptions, and relationships with supervisors could also be addressed during on-site training and with the presence of the job coach. These supportive conditions did influence the injured worker's decisions and thus facilitated the experiential process of change, leading to the behavioral process of change in making an attempt to RTW.

Workplace-based work-hardening programs are a further development of work rehabilitation programs. The results of the abovementioned randomized controlled trial confirmed that workplace-based rehabilitation intervention is more effective than conventional clinic-based rehabilitation programs in terms of the prevention of further work disability, an improvement in functional capabilities, and a decrease in perceived pain and disability. More importantly, many of the psychosocial problems associated with separation from the work routine, peer group, or employer are minimized by the presence of the job coach. Therapeutic use of actual work facilities and the work environment can facilitate the successful RTW process of the injured worker.

Last but not least, it is necessary to highlight that the CARF, an independent, nonprofit accreditor of health and human services, has used the term "occupational rehabilitation" instead of "work hardening" since 1995 (King, 1998), and occupational rehabilitation has been divided into a general occupational rehabilitation program versus a comprehensive occupational rehabilitation program. The former is usually offered at the onset of an injury or illness but may also be provided at any time throughout the recovery phase. It focuses on functional restoration and RTW. The goals of the program include but are not limited to improvement of cardiopulmonary and neuromusculoskeletal functions (strength, endurance, movement, flexibility, stability, and motor control functions), education of the persons served, and symptom relief. Services offered by the program may include the time-limited use of passive modalities with progression to active treatment or simulated/real work (CARF International, 2006). The latter, however, is an interdisciplinary, outcome-focused, and individualized program provided by occupational rehabilitation specialists. The goals of the program are to deal with the medical, psychological, behavioral, physical, functional, and vocational components of employability and RTW. It is often conducted under a simulated/real work situation to address the complexities of the persons served and their work environments (CARF International, 2006).

The occupational rehabilitation process

Chan (2001) provided a schematic description of the occupational rehabilitation process (Figure 7.1). The process has several components, including vocational guidance (e.g., counseling), work retraining, education, ergonomics, and psychosocial programs

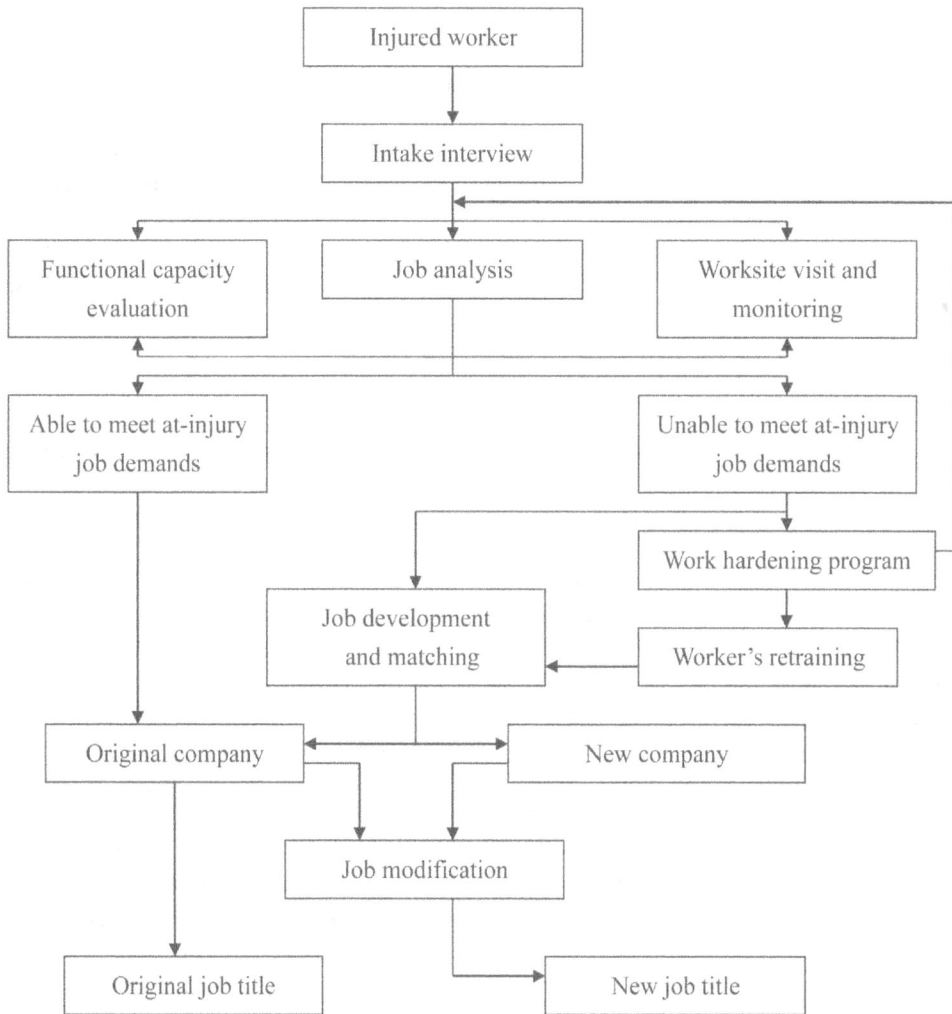

Figure 7.1 The occupational rehabilitation process (adapted from Chan, 2001)

(Marnetoft et al., 2001). Important factors that need to be considered within occupational rehabilitation may include personal and psychosocial factors, medical factors, the employer and the workplace, and socioeconomic factors (Khorshidi et al., 2019; Selander et al., 2002). The application of occupational rehabilitation can be useful for various health conditions such as those that are physical or psychological in nature (Beveridge & Fabian, 2007). Occupational rehabilitation is a complex collection of interventions that require more than one discipline to ensure success in returning or engaging a worker toward gainful employment. It is often a multi-tiered process that consists of multiple players and relates the functioning of the individual worker with his/her work role in the broadest sense. A successful occupational rehabilitation program relies on the interrelationship between several elements, such as workplace commitment, accommodations made by the employer, RTW coordinators and planners, supervisors, early intervention, and effective communication between the employer and healthcare provider (Franche et al., 2004). Studies have shown that there are numerous benefits of occupational rehabilitation. For example, it has been found to reduce lost workdays and work-related disability, facilitating an earlier RTW (Karrholm et al., 2008; Norrefalk et al., 2008). Early occupational rehabilitation is linked to sustained employment (DeSouza et al., 2007) and has been proven to decrease workers' sickness absence over time (Bultmann et al., 2009; Jensen et al., 2009; Suoyrjo et al., 2009). In terms of economics, occupational rehabilitation has been found to have favorable cost-benefit ratios (Turner-Stokes, 2008), potentially leading to cost savings for employers.

According to Figure 7.1, job analysis and functional capacity evaluation (FCE) are identified as two critical steps in starting the process.

Job analysis

Job analysis or work analysis is a method for collecting work information, identifying the activities that comprise work tasks, and describing the knowledge, skills, and abilities required of workers for successful work performance. Occupational therapists use job analysis as a basis for evaluating injured workers, planning rehabilitative programs, structuring pre-employment screening protocols, developing transitional work plans, and conducting environmental modification and risk management programs (Lysaght, 1997). Chan (2005) explained that FCE was for the injured worker, and job analysis was for the work tasks that were performed by the worker prior to the injury. The concept of work analysis is not exclusive to the rehabilitation field; work information is the basic data used by industry, governmental and private agencies, and employee organizations for many human resource programs (U.S. Department of Labor, 1991). For example, human resources specialists use work analysis for selection purposes to establish training requirements, develop performance appraisals, and identify benchmark employment when establishing pay grades in work evaluation systems. Vocational counselors use work analysis for career counseling in schools, and for advising disabled or unemployed workers on potential new occupations. Curriculum developers in academic and industry settings use work analysis to match training objectives to specific groups of students.

Work information can be collected in four ways. First, it can be collected from the injured worker. The most direct way is to obtain work information during the initial intake interview. However, the therapist may find it difficult to understand the various technical terms for a particular job or the nickname of a specific tool. Second, work information can be collected from the employer. However, work information is often written by human resources managers in such a way that it primarily provides descriptions of the duties or responsibilities of a given post. It seldom provides any quantitative information about the work demands, such as the weight of a load or the frequency or duration of a repetitive task. Third, work information can be collected from the Dictionary of Occupational Titles (DOT), which was developed in the 1930s. It was intended to help deal with the economic crisis of the Great Depression by helping the new public employment system link skill supply and skill demand (U.S. Department of Labor, 1993) and provide a comprehensive system for describing all occupations. The Dictionary continues to be updated, and between the mid-1960s and the mid-1970s, over 75,000 on-site work analyses were conducted by analysts in United States

Employment Service centers across America. DOT is now in its fourth edition, comprising approximately 12,800 job descriptions. According to the United States Employment Service, work information in the DOT includes:

(1) the worker's relationship to data, people, and things;
(2) the methodologies and techniques employed;
(3) the machines, tools, equipment, and work aids used;
(4) the materials, products, subject matter, or services which result; and
(5) the work attributes that contribute to successful work performance.

The techniques for obtaining and presenting this information are known as work analysis (U.S. Department of Labor, 1991).

However, there are shortcomings in using this information. The accuracy with which the DOT can reflect work requirements in the local Hong Kong context is open to question. Lo and Lam (2000) conducted a study to examine the content validity of the DOT as applied to employment as a painter in Hong Kong. After both an expert panel review and a field study, they concluded that there was a significant discrepancy in the work information between Hong Kong and the United States. Lee and Chan (2003) undertook a further study using the DOT to compare the physical demands of formwork carpentry in Hong Kong with those in the United States. The work information of formwork carpentry was collected through the Dictionary of Occupational Titles Physical Demand Questionnaire (DOT-PDQ) and on-site visits. An agreement of 84.6% with the original DOT was obtained, although it should be noted that their study was limited as it compared only the physical demand components of the job. Last but not least, work information can be collected from an on-site work analysis. Work information collected in this way is considered to be the most objective and valid. The therapist can bring equipment such as force gauges, weight scales, stopwatches, tape measures, cameras, and video recorders to the workplace to quantify the task demands and make a functional work analysis. However, this method is usually the last resort and only used for problematic cases as it is costly and labor-intensive.

Functional capacity evaluation

The purpose of work analysis is to form the target areas for the rehabilitation of injured workers. The data obtained serves as the basis from which the RTW decision can be made. To provide an objective and pertinent decision, FCE is needed. It provides an objective measurement system to match physical abilities with essential and critical work demands (Cheng & Cheng, 2010). Performance-based FCE is commonly used to determine the physical work abilities of individuals who have sustained musculoskeletal injury (Gross, 2004) and has become part of common clinical practice in several areas of occupational and rehabilitation medicine for individuals who have sustained musculoskeletal diseases (Echeita et al., 2018).

FCE was developed in the late 1970s when the American Workers' Compensation Administration became alarmed at the increasing delays in workers' returning to work after injury and the subsequent increased cost. A major factor for these delays was the difficulty physicians had in deciding when an injured worker could RTW or in determining the level of work that the worker could sustain upon his/her return

(Schonstein & Kenny, 2001). To address this problem, therapists compiled existing and self-developed tests into a battery of tests and named them FCEs (Reneman & Dijkstra, 2003). The primary purpose of FCEs is to establish a functional profile of the injured worker through the administration of standardized assessment protocols in order to determine the current safe vocational levels or demonstrated work ability of the injured worker. This maximum safe level of work performance is determined from both psychophysical and kinesio-physical perspectives. From the psychophysical point of view, it is believed that the worker is able to judge his or her own safety maximum. From the kinesio-physical point of view, the professional administering the test can base his/her judgment on observation and experience to determine the worker's maximum level of performance (Schonstein & Kenny, 2001).

The goal of testing must be established prior to the testing. If no specific job is identified to which the worker will return, a general FCE should be conducted, which quantifies worker traits and acts as a baseline capacity evaluation. The common physical demands that are tested may include sitting, standing, walking, balancing, climbing, kneeling, stooping, crouching, reaching, lifting, carrying, pushing, pulling, motor coordination, fine dexterity, grasping, and pitching (Hart et al., 1993). However, if the specific job to which the worker is returning is known and a functional work description or analysis has identified the critical work demands, a more specific FCE could be considered, such as a work capacity evaluation (WCE). In WCE, work simulations are conducted over a significant time period within a simulated work environment. The assessments usually cover physical, mental, psychological, and emotional aspects. Other work attributes such as work habits, full-day workplace tolerance, and daily attendance may also be included.

Nowadays, there is a wide variety of FCE equipment available on the market. Tramposh (1991) distinguished between a "work-sample" approach and a "work-system" approach to this equipment. Examples of the "work-sample" approach include the WEST, VALPAR, and Singer work samples. Examples of the "work-system" approach include the Key Functional Assessments, Isernhagen Work Systems Evaluation, BTE Work Simulator, LIDO Work Simulator, ARCON, Blankenship FCE, and B-200 (Innes & Straker, 1999). In Hong Kong, the FCE equipment used will depend on the problems faced by injured workers, the availability of the assessment tools, the knowledge of the rehabilitation specialists, and the established norms or references used with the instrument. Sometimes, the rehabilitation specialists who perform FCEs have to develop their own approach using whatever equipment is available in the clinical setting, as well as their own experience, to develop simulated "work-stations" to assist the assessment. In Hong Kong, the common FCE protocols include the Baltimore Therapeutic Equipment (BTE) (Primus RS or EVAL), ARCON, and VALPAR, among others.

The BTE Primus RS is advanced equipment integrating assessment, rehabilitation, and training and is widely used in hospitals and rehabilitation centers (Suda et al., 2017; Torpel et al., 2017). It consists of three major components: (1) a variable resistance device or exercise head that can be raised or lowered on two shafts; (2) various attachments that can be mounted on the exercise head in multiple positions to simulate several combinations of movements; and (3) a console with a microprocessor and a control panel that allows selection of the desired resistance and measures performance by quantifying the force exerted, work done, and power output while the task is being performed (Figure 7.2).

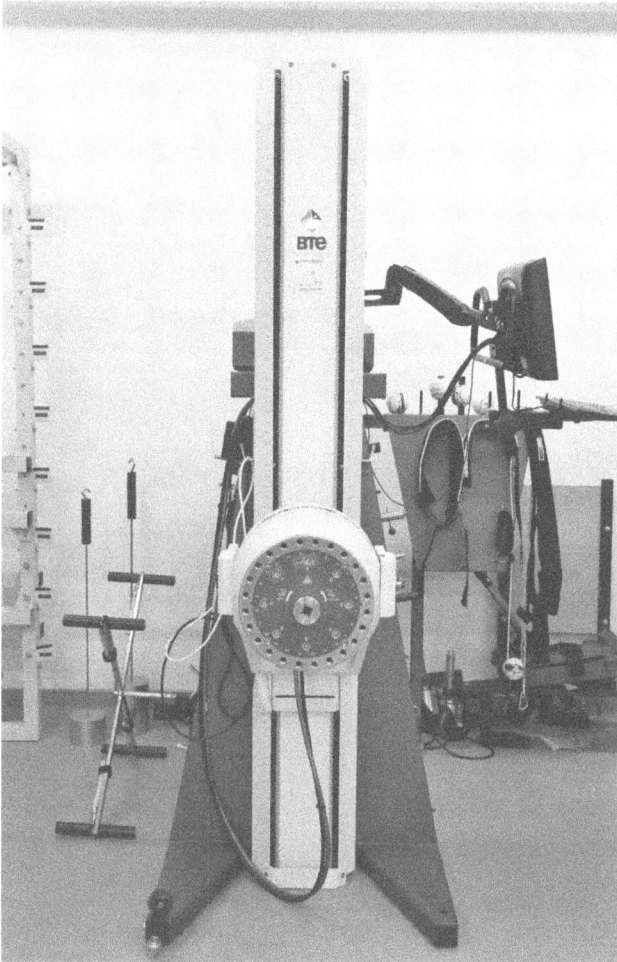

Figure 7.2 The BTE Primus RS

ARCON is a computerized instrument for FCE. It is commonly used by occupational therapists and physiotherapists in Hong Kong. The free-standing testing platform is designed to evaluate both static and dynamic whole-body strength. Static strength testing is a safe and accurate method to determine maximum voluntary effort (Harber & SooHoo, 1984) (Figure 7.3). The range of motion system measures the active range of motion of a specific joint through an electronic goniometer (Figure 7.4). Standardized protocols and instructions that come with the system can help the evaluator follow an established testing pattern, thereby enhancing both inter- and intra-tester reliability. ARCON hardware interfaces directly with software to produce reports and can be used to compare normative data from the American Medical Association's (AMA) guide to the evaluation of permanent impairment or the database acceptable to the National Institute of Occupational Safety and Health (NIOSH). The computer will automatically and instantaneously calculate validity measures such as standard deviation and the coefficient of variation (CV). These calculations are based on the objective

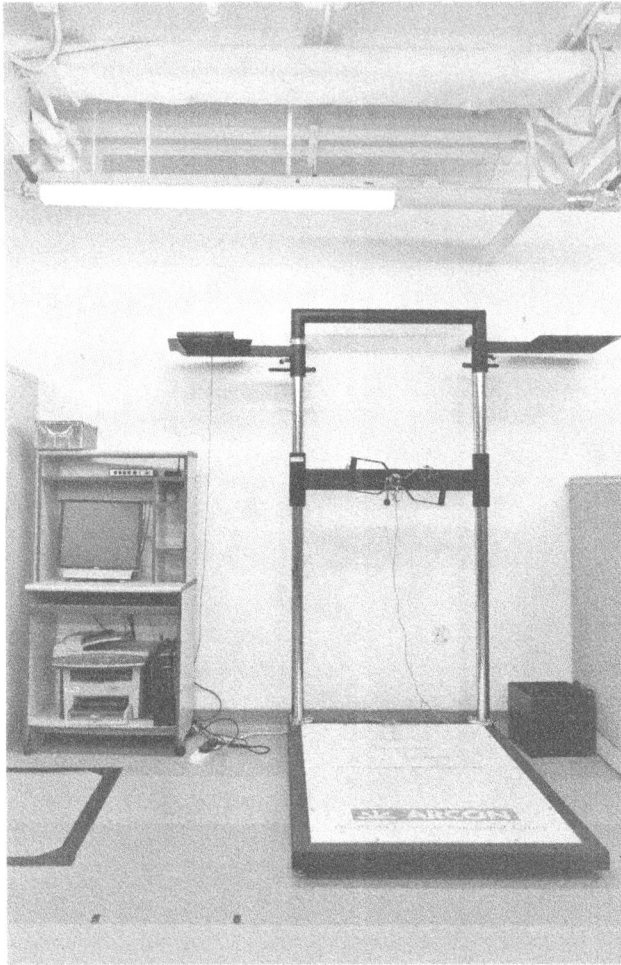

Figure 7.3 The ARCON system

analysis of discrete data points. These validity checks are used to identify whether the effort made by the client is consistent, valid, and reproducible.

The VALPAR Component Work Samples (VCWS) are criterion-referenced instruments (Figure 7.5). The focus of criterion-referenced instruments is not to compare individuals but to determine whether individuals can perform certain tasks of interest, defined in terms of a domain of known criteria (Christopherson & Hayes, 1992). The work samples were designed to simulate various work factors based on the most widely used system of work classification and analysis, as defined in the U.S. Department of Labor Dictionary of Occupational Titles (DOT). These work samples contain tasks conducive to a form of work rate analysis known as Methods-Time Measurement (MTM) developed by industrial engineers. It is used as a source of standard time for simulation around the world (Machado et al., 2019) and results in a time standard for the completion of the work sample according to the standard instructions. This time standard can be viewed as the rate of work percent score.

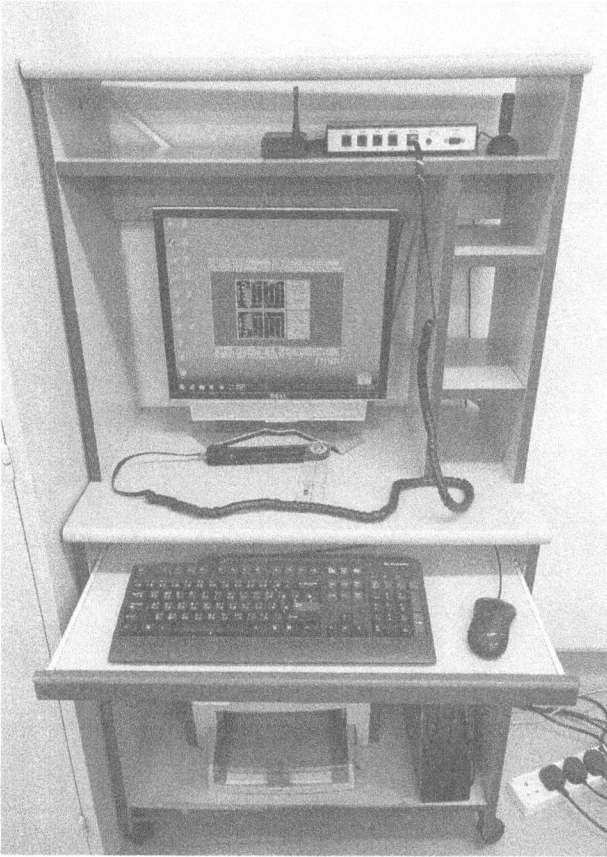

Figure 7.4 The ARCON range of motion test and its peripheral electronic goniometer

The reliability of the FCE results is frequently questioned by rehabilitation professionals for two reasons. First, there is the problem of validating that the effort made by the person being evaluated is true and is their maximal effort. Second, there is the problem of ensuring the test's reliability through test-retest reliability and/or inter-rater reliability. King and Berryhill (1991) stated that the components of functional evaluations must address the question of the person's effort. These components should be chosen based on statistical support of their ability to delineate clearly between the individual who has put maximum voluntary effort into the evaluation and one who has not. The CV is a statistical method used to evaluate effort consistency. It consists of the standard deviation of three average exertion measurements for a given task divided by the mean of these measurements and expressed as a percentage. A greater CV indicates greater variability and lower consistency. A threshold or cut-off value is usually established for the CV, above which the effort is considered inconsistent enough to be regarded as sub-maximal effort (Shechtman et al., 2006). Based on the NIOSH guideline for validity, test results that exhibit a CV greater than or equal to 15% cannot be considered valid, consistent, and reproducible.

Test-retest and inter-rater reliability of determining levels of safe, maximal ability are considered the most important forms of FCE test consistency (Velozo, 1993).

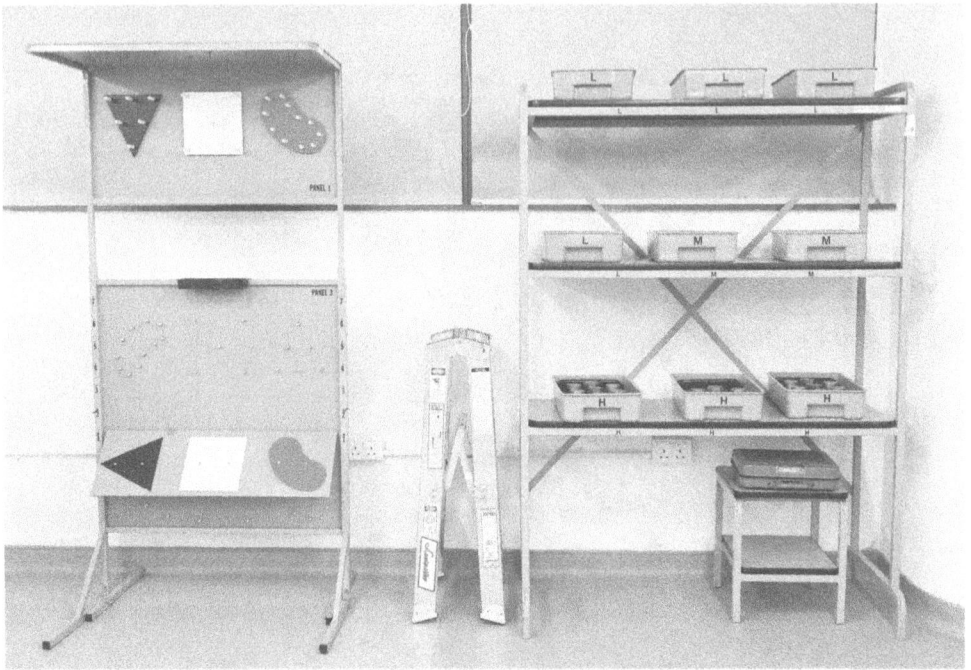

Figure 7.5 Examples of the VALPAR Component Work Samples (VCWS 9 [left] and VCWS 19 [right])

Brouwer et al. (2003) studied the reliability of therapists in assessing safe work levels using complete FCE protocols for people with low back and other musculoskeletal disorders. They reported that there was acceptable agreement on the vast majority of tasks in the protocol studies. Gross and Battie (2002) investigated the test–retest reliability of the judgments of safe, maximal effort on FCE lifting tests performed by people with low back pain. They also reported that acceptable agreement was achieved for clinical use. Gross (2004) concluded that the reliability of safe, maximum performance determinations seems acceptable when an operational definition is provided to raters. With advances in modern technology, much of the FCE equipment has become computerized, featuring built-in software for standardized operational definitions of each test and databases for various norms and industrial standards. This allows for automatic data analysis. In addition, using the FCE equipment often requires the operator to undergo formal training before an evaluation can be conducted. This further improves the reliability of the FCE.

Regarding the validity of FCEs, all forms of validity are appropriate and should be considered or constructed if a specific FCE protocol is developed. Innes and Straker (1999) noted that face and content validity are required to demonstrate the relevance of the assessment to the client, therapist, employer, insurer, and others involved in assisting injured workers safely RTW. Criterion-related validity is crucial for demonstrating that the results of the FCE can predict successful RTW. Construct validity, on the other hand, detects changes in injured workers following treatment and evaluates whether the instrument accurately measures the intended constructs.

Self-perceived functional capabilities

Functional capacity can be measured by self-report and is based on performance. Individuals' beliefs about the severity of their health conditions, or their abilities and limitations, play a significant role in the level of presenting disability (van der Meer et al., 2014). Research has shown that individuals' perceptions of the severity of their health conditions (van der Giezen et al., 2000) or the extent of their physical limitations (Feuerstein et al., 2003) are significant predictors of RTW outcomes. Treatment-related reductions in perceived disability have been associated with a higher probability of RTW (McGonagle et al., 2015). Viola et al. (2000) investigated 1,063 clients with shoulder injuries. They found that occupational shoulder injuries covered by workers' compensation had significantly lower self-addressed shoulder function and health status than shoulder conditions not related to on-the-job injuries. Cook et al. (2002) highlighted that several scales were developed to measure shoulder outcomes, including the Shoulder Pain and Disability Index (SPADI), the University of California at Los Angeles (UCLA) Shoulder Score, the Constant-Murley Scale (CMS), and the American Shoulder and Elbow Society (ASES) Shoulder Index. Among them, the SPADI was most commonly used in examining outcomes in clients with shoulder pathologies. The Spinal Function Sort (SFS) pictorial questionnaire is commonly used in Hong Kong to measure the self-perceived functional capabilities of clients with low back pain. It contains pictures representing both work-related tasks and activities of daily living (Oesch et al., 2010). The person is asked to look at each picture and rate his/her abilities related to a task or activity. The SFS is predictive of future work status (Lassfolk et al., 2021).

Return to work and disability management

The last part of the occupational rehabilitation process (Figure 7.1) is work re-entry or RTW. Ideally, after work-hardening programs, the gap between the work demands and work ability of injured workers will be significantly reduced. However, some remain incapacitated or have ongoing functional limitations. In other words, they may have varying degrees of work disability. RTW following a work disability is an important yet complicated issue. Its success can be affected by the motivation, interests, and concerns of various RTW stakeholders (Cheng et al., 2011), who are defined as any person, organization, or agency that stands to gain or lose based on the results of the RTW process (Young et al., 2005).

Work disability management is a term that originated in the 1980s as a response by self-insured employers in the United States to the rising costs of disability and injury (Habeck & Hunt, 1999). Franche and Krause (2002) described work disability management as a proactive, employer-based approach developed to:

(1) prevent the occurrence of accidents and disability;
(2) provide early intervention services for health and disability risk factors; and
(3) foster coordinated rehabilitative and administrative strategies to promote cost-effective restoration and RTW.

Referring to the International Classification of Functioning, Disability and Health (ICF), disability is characterized as the outcome or result of a complex relationship

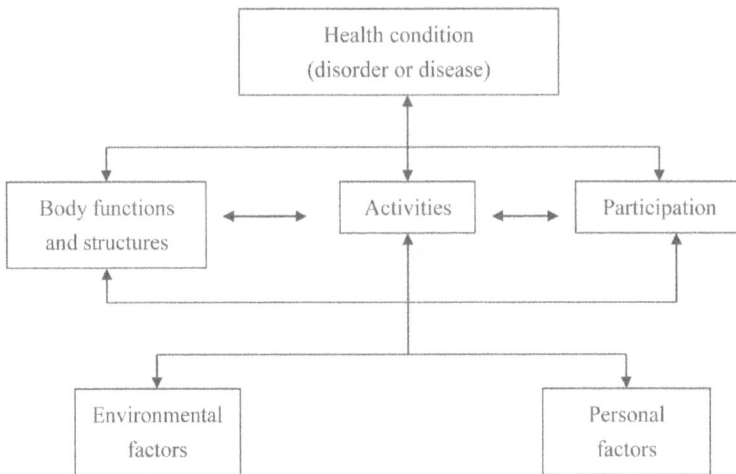

Figure 7.6 The World Health Organization's International Classification of Functioning, Disability and Health (World Health Organization, 2001)

between an individual's health condition and personal and external factors (World Health Organization, 2001). Work disability, therefore, could be considered as a dynamic interaction between bodily functions and structures and the ability to perform activities and participate in society (Figure 7.6). This model provides a measurement domain for judging work disability following musculoskeletal injury, including evaluations at the level of occupational activity and participation in the actual work environment.

The model also indicates that function is influenced not only by injury to bodily structures, but also by environmental factors. Because of this relationship, various environments may have a significantly different impact on the same individual with a given health condition. An environment with barriers, or without facilitators, will restrict the individual's performance. On the other hand, environments that facilitate RTW may increase the individual's performance. Therefore, a health condition or work disability would no longer be a disability if barriers could be removed and facilitators provided in the workplace. Within this context, disability management can simply be described as any measures that facilitate environmental adaptations and accommodations that resolve work disability and promote worker reintegration and retention.

Work disability management is an employer-directed process that uses organizational systems to promote prevention and rehabilitation, focusing on interventions at the worksite. As mentioned previously, rehabilitation at the workplace facilitates better adaptation of the injured worker when he/she returns to work as the occupational bond has been maintained. However, organizational factors could also influence the external loading on the injured worker in terms of the organization of tasks, work pace, characteristics of interpersonal interactions, and the utilization of ergonomic principles. Workplace culture could be a barrier to RTW. Amick et al. (2000) found that a people-oriented culture, safety climate, disability management policies and practices, and ergonomic practices created an "organizational ecology" that was predictive of the incidence of work disability and the duration and cost of work disability. Supervisors can play an important role during the RTW of injured workers to aid injured workers in accessing healthcare services and providing reasonable job accommodation (Nastasia et al., 2021). Shaw et al. (2003) noted the significance of the supervisors' role from the employees' perspective. They concluded that the effort of on-site health services or others to facilitate RTW could not be substituted for the involvement of frontline supervisors in the planning process.

Rehabilitation plans should include all the interventions that have to be made for the sick-listed client (worker) to RTW (Larsson & Gard, 2003). Many of these interventions use modified work programs as a key element in the rehabilitation process (van Duijn et al., 2004). Various terms are used for these modified work programs, although most of the programs are similar in nature. The most frequently used terms include "light duty", "limited duty work", and "transitional work".

Light duty is any temporary or permanent activity that is less demanding than that of regular or full duty, which enables a disabled worker to perform a role according to a set of conditions prescribed by a healthcare provider. Light duty positions are paid work and are performed in a competitive work environment. They range from adaptations of the worker's pre-injury duties to working in an entirely different role at the same company or a different company, either pre-existing or specially created for the disabled worker (Krause et al., 1998). Limited duty work, however, is any role that is appropriate to an injured worker's skills, interests, and capabilities. New work may be designed for workers who cannot return to their original duties. These new roles may be either temporary (for a specified time such as a few weeks or months) or permanent (when the worker will not be able to return to the original role) (Randolph & Dalton, 1989). Transitional work is any combination of tasks, functions, or jobs that a worker who has functional restrictions can perform safely, for pay, and without the risk of injury to themselves or other workers. Transitional work options include designated roles or work tasks that are modified, over time, to accommodate the injured worker during the physical recovery process (Shrey & Hursh, 1999).

Other terms that may be used to describe a modified work program include "lighter duty", "modified duty", "restricted duty", "alternate duty", and "alternative duty". Whatever the modified work program is called, the core idea is that the work undertaken by the worker with temporary or permanent disability is modified in order to accommodate the current medical condition to facilitate a safe and early RTW. This process should include a transitional work plan or worker's work task assignment together with graded work exposure in which the hours, duties, or performance expectations of a role are gradually increased until the worker is ready for regular or full duty. If the worker cannot return to his/her original work, permanent placement in another role can be offered.

Provision of modified work programs is a critical administrative measure or organizational policy in workplace disability management. Krause et al. (1998) reported on a systematic review and critical appraisal of the scientific literature on modified work programs published since 1975. The main finding of this review was that modified work programs are effective in helping workers with temporary or permanent disabilities to RTW. The workers with access to modified work return to their work roles roughly twice as often as those without access to any form of modified duties. The number of work days lost per disabling injury is also cut in half when companies implement modified work programs. The importance of modified work programs is that through graded work exposure, the injured workers can test their abilities and regain their confidence. The programs provide a transitional process that allows injured workers to be rehabilitated and to prepare for eventual return to full-duty work. Durand and Loisel (2001) conducted a study on "Therapeutic Return to Work (TRW) programmes" for chronic low back pain clients. Their programs linked graded work exposure with functional restoration therapy as the treatment media. A higher statistical significance was found in returning and maintaining regular work for those clients receiving TRW than for those receiving functional restoration therapy only.

Conclusions

Returning to work after a compensable occupational injury is a complex and multifactorial process. In some extreme cases, people are forced to leave their jobs permanently. Individuals who are unable to return to their workplace impose a burden on their families and society. In addition to the monetary costs associated with loss of work due to work disability, there may also be certain negative psychological consequences for the injured workers, which, in turn, not only decrease their self-esteem and motivation but also cause anxiety in their families. Therefore, addressing work-related issues among injured workers is relevant because work is a key component of their recovery. Work contributes to greater well-being and enhances one's sense of normalcy and daily structure, control, identity, and meaning.

References

Aasdahl, L., Fimland, M. S., & Røe, C. (2022). The readiness for return to work scale; Does it help in evaluation of return to work? *Journal of Occupational Rehabilitation*, 32(3), 426–437. https://doi.org/10.1007/s10926-021-10009-4

American Occupational Therapy Association. (1986). Work hardening guidelines. *The American Journal of Occupational Therapy*, 40, 841–843.

Amick, B. C., Habeck, R. V., Hunt, A., Fossel, A. H., Chapin, A., Keller, R. B., & Katz, J. N. (2000). Measuring the impact of organizational behaviors on work disability prevention and management. *Journal of Occupational Rehabilitation*, 10(1), 21–38. https://doi.org/10.1023/A:1009437728024

Anderson, V., Brown, S., Newitt, H., & Hoile, H. (2009). Educational, vocational, psychosocial, and quality-of-life outcomes for adult survivors of childhood traumatic brain injury. *Journal of Head Trauma Rehabilitation*, 24(5), 303–312. https://doi.org/10.1097/HTR.0b013e3181ada830

Beveridge, S., & Fabian, E. (2007). Vocational rehabilitation outcomes: Relationship between individualized plan for employment goals and employment outcomes. *Rehabilitation Counseling Bulletin*, 50(4), 238–246. https://doi.org/10.1177/00343552070500040501

Brouwer, S., Reneman, M. F., Dijkstra, P. U., Groothoff, J. W., Schellekens, J. M. H., & Goeken, L. N. H. (2003). Test-retest reliability of the Isernhagen Work Systems Functional Capacity Evaluation in patients with chronic low back pain. *Journal of Occupational Rehabilitation*, 13(4), 207–218. https://doi.org/10.1023/a:1026264519996

Bultmann, U., Sherson, D., Olsen, J., Hansen, C. L., Lund, T., & Kilsgaard, J. (2009). Coordinated and tailored work rehabilitation: A randomized controlled trial with economic evaluation undertaken with workers on sick leave due to musculoskeletal disorders. *Journal of Occupational Rehabilitation*, 19(1), 81–93. https://doi.org/10.1007/s10926-009-9162-7

CARF International. (2006). *Medical rehabilitation standards manual. July 2006-June 2007.* CARF.

Chan, C. C. H. (2001). Introduction to process of occupational rehabilitation. In C. C. H. Chan, K. Y. L. Hui, E. K. S. Lo, S. Y. Lo, & T. W. W. Kwok (Eds.), *Cumulative trauma at work* (pp. 41–54). Hong Kong Workers' Health Centre.

Chan, C. C. H. (2005, April). *A review and implications of occupational rehabilitation systems* [Paper presentation]. National Symposium on Work Injury Rehabilitation, Guangzhou, China.

Cheng, A. S. K., & Cheng, S. W. C. (2010). The predictive validity of job-specific functional capacity evaluation on the employment status of patients with nonspecific low back pain. *Journal of Occupational and Environmental Medicine, 52*(7), 719–724. https://doi.org/10.1097/JOM.0b013e3181e48d47

Cheng, A. S. K., & Hung, L. K. (2007). Randomized controlled trial of workplace-based rehabilitation for work-related rotator cuff disorder. *Journal of Occupational Rehabilitation, 17*(3), 487–503. https://doi.org/10.1007/s10926-007-9085-0

Cheng, A. S. K., Loisel, P., & Feuerstein, M. (2011). Return-to-work activities in a Chinese cultural context. *Journal of Occupational Rehabilitation, 21*, S44–S54. https://doi.org/10.1007/s10926-010-9272-2

Christopherson, B. B., & Hayes, P. D. (1992). *Valpar component work samples: Uses in allied health*. Valpar International Corporation.

Commission on Accreditation of Rehabilitation Facilities. (1988). *National Advisory Committee recommendations for work hardening programs*. Commission on Accreditation of Rehabilitation Facilities.

Cook, K. F., Roddey, T. S., Olson, S. L., Gartsman, G. M., Valenzuela, F. F. T., & Hanten, W. P. (2002). Reliability by surgical status of self-reported outcomes in patients who have shoulder pathologies. *Journal of Orthopaedic & Sports Physical Therapy, 32*(7), 336–346. https://www.jospt.org/doi/10.2519/jospt.2002.32.7.336

Crowther, R., Marshall, M., Bond, G. R., & Huxley, P. (2001). Vocational rehabilitation for people with severe mental illness. *Cochrane Database of Systematic Reviews, 2001*(2), CD003080. https://doi.org/10.1002/14651858.CD003080

DeSouza, M., Sycamore, M., Little, S., & Kirker, S. G. B. (2007). The Papworth early rehabilitation programme: Vocational outcomes. *Disability and Rehabilitation, 29*(8), 671–677. https://doi.org/10.1080/09638280600926538

Durand, M. J., & Loisel, P. (2001). Therapeutic return to work: Rehabilitation in the workplace. *Work, 17*(1), 57–63.

Echeita, J. A., Bethge, M., van Holland, B. J., Gross, D. P., Kool, J., Oesch, P., Trippolini, M. A., Chapman, E., Cheng, A. S. K., Sellars, R., Spavins, M., Streibelt, M., van der Wurff, P., & Reneman, M. F. (2018). Functional capacity evaluation in different societal contexts: Results of a multicountry study. *Journal of Occupational Rehabilitation, 29*(1), 222–236. https://doi.org/10.1007/s10926-018-9782-x

Feuerstein, M., Shaw, W. S., Lincoln, A. E., Miller, V. L., & Wood, P. M. (2003). Clinical and workplace factors associated with a return to modified duty in work-related upper extremity disorders. *Pain, 102*(1), 51–61. https://doi.org/10.1016/s0304-3959(02)00339-1

Figueredo, J.-M., García-Ael, C., Gragnano, A., & Topa, G. (2020). Well-being at work after return to work (RTW): A systematic review. *International Journal of Environmental Research and Public Health, 17*(20), 7490. https://doi.org/10.3390/ijerph17207490

Franche, R. L., Cullen, K., Clarke, J., Irvin, E., Sinclair, S., & Frank, J., The Institute for Work & Health (IWH) Workplace-Based RTW Intervention Literature Review Research Team. (2005). Workplace-based return-to-work interventions: A systematic review of the quantitative literature. *Journal of Occupational Rehabilitation, 15*(4), 607–631. https://doi.org/10.1007/s10926-005-8038-8

Franche, R. L., Cullen, K., Clarke, J., MacEachen, E., Frank, J., Sinclair, S., & Reardon, R. (2004). *Workplace-based return-to-work interventions: A systematic review of the quantitative and qualitative literature. Summary* (pp. 5–9). Institute for Work & Health. https://www.iwh.on.ca/sites/iwh/files/iwh/reports/iwh_summary_rtw_interventions_2004.pdf

Franche, R. L., & Krause, N. (2002). Readiness for return to work following injury or illness: Conceptualizing the interpersonal impact of health care, workplace, and insurance factors. *Journal of Occupational Rehabilitation, 12*(4), 233–256. https://doi.org/10.1023/a:1020270407044

Gewurtz, R. E., Premji, S., & Holness, D. L. (2018). The experiences of workers who do not successfully return to work following a work-related injury. *Work*, *61*(4), 537–549. https://doi.org/10.3233/WOR-182824

Gross, D. P. (2004). Measurement properties of performance-based assessment of functional capacity. *Journal of Occupational Rehabilitation*, *14*(3), 165–174. https://doi.org/10.1023/b:joor.0000022759.30446.4f

Gross, D. P., & Battie, M. C. (2002). Reliability of safe maximum lifting determinations of a functional capacity evaluation. *Physical Therapy*, *82*(4), 364–371. https://doi.org/10.1093/ptj/82.4.364

Habeck, R. V., & Hunt, H. A. (1999). Disability management perspectives: Developing accommodating work environments through disability management. *American Rehabilitation*, *25*(1), 18–25. https://core.ac.uk/download/pdf/217635742.pdf

Hanson, C. S., & Walker, K. F. (1992). The history of work in physical dysfunction. *The American Journal of Occupational Therapy*, *46*(1), 56–62.

Harber, P., & SooHoo, K. (1984). Static ergonomic strength testing in evaluating occupational back pain. *Journal of Occupational Medicine*, *26*(12), 877–884. https://doi.org/10.1097/00043764-198412000-00005

Harrison, K., & Allen, S. (2003). Features of occupational rehabilitation systems in Australia: A map through the maze. *Work*, *21*(2), 141–152.

Hart, D. L., Isernhagen, S. J., & Matheson, L. N. (1993). Guidelines for functional capacity evaluation of people with medical conditions. *Journal of Orthopaedic & Sports Physical Therapy*, *18*(6), 682–686. https://www.jospt.org/doi/10.2519/jospt.1993.18.6.682

Helm-Williams, P. (1993). Industrial rehabilitation: Developing guidelines. *PT-Magazine of Physical Therapy*, *1*(3), 65–68.

Innes, E., & Straker, L. (1999). Validity of work-related assessments. *Work*, *13*(2), 125–152. https://content.iospress.com/articles/work/wor00050

International Labour Organization. (1983). *Convention 159: Convention concerning vocational rehabilitation and employment (disabled persons)*. Adopted by the International Labour Conference at its 69th session, Geneva, 20 June 1983.

International Labour Organization. (1998). *Vocational rehabilitation and employment of disabled persons*. International Labour Conference, 86th session, Geneva, June 1998.

Jensen, I. B., Busch, H., Bodin, L., Hagberg, J., Nygren, A., & Bergstrom, G. (2009). Cost effectiveness of two rehabilitation programmes for neck and back pain patients: A seven year follow-up. *Pain*, *142*(3), 202–208. https://doi.org/10.1016/j.pain.2008.12.015

Jeong, I., Yoon, J.-H., Roh, J., Rhie, J., & Won, J.-U. (2019). Association between the return-to-work hierarchy and self-rated health, self-esteem, and self-efficacy. *International Archives of Occupational and Environmental Health*, *92*(5), 709–716. https://doi.org/10.1007/s00420-019-01406-7

Karrholm, J., Ekholm, K., Ekholm, J., Bergroth, A., & Ekholm, K. S. (2008). Systematic co-operation between employer, occupational health service and social insurance office: A 6-year follow-up of vocational rehabilitation for people on sick-leave, including economic benefits. *Journal of Rehabilitation Medicine*, *40*(8), 628–636. https://doi.org/10.2340/16501977-0233

Khorshidi, H. A., Marembo, M., & Aickelin, U. (2019). Predictors of return to work for occupational rehabilitation users in work-related injury insurance claims: Insights from mental health. *Journal of Occupational Rehabilitation*, *29*(4), 740–753. https://doi.org/10.1007/s10926-019-09835-4

King, J. W., & Berryhill, B. H. (1991). Assessing maximum effort in upper-extremity functional testing. *Work*, *1*(3), 65–76.

King, P. M. (1998). Work hardening and work conditioning. In P. M. King (Ed.), *Sourcebook of occupational rehabilitation* (pp. 257–273). Plenum Press.

Krause, N., Dasinger, L. K., & Neuhauser, F. (1998). Modified work and return to work: A review of the literature. *Journal of Occupational Rehabilitation*, *8*(2), 113–139. https://doi.org/10.1023/A:1023015622987

Larsson, A., & Gard, G. (2003). How can the rehabilitation planning process at the workplace be improved? A qualitative study from employers' perspective. *Journal of Occupational Rehabilitation*, *13*(3), 169–181. https://doi.org/10.1023/A:1024953218252

Lassfolk, M., Escorpizo, R., Korniloff, K., & Reneman, M. (2021). Linking the Spinal Function Sort and Functional Capacity Evaluation tests to the International Classification of Functioning, Disability and Health Core Set of Vocational Rehabilitation. *Journal of Occupational Rehabilitation, 31*(1), 166–174. https://doi.org/10.1007/s10926-020-09905-y

Lee, G. K. L., & Chan, C. C. H. (2003). Use of Dictionary of Occupational Titles (DOT) on formwork carpentry — A comparison between the United States and Hong Kong. *Work, 20*(2), 103–110.

Lo, E. K. S., & Lam, P. C. W. (2000). Validity of the Dictionary of Occupational Titles as applied to construction site workers in Hong Kong. *Work, 14*(3), 191–201.

Lysaght, R. (1997). Job analysis in occupational therapy: Stepping into the complex world of business and industry. *American Journal of Occupational Therapy, 51*(7), 569–575.

Machado, R. H. C., Helleno, A. L., de Oliveira, M. C., dos Santos, M. S. C., & da Costa Dias, R. M. (2019). Analysis of the influence of standard time variability on the reliability of the simulation of assembly operations in manufacturing systems. *Human Factors, 61*(4), 627–641. https://doi.org/10.1177/0018720819829596

Marnetoft, S. U., Selander, J., Bergroth, A., & Ekholm, J. (2001). Factors associated with successful vocational rehabilitation in a Swedish rural area. *Journal of Rehabilitation Medicine, 33*(2), 71–78. https://doi.org/10.1080/165019701750098902

Matheson, L. N. (1986). *Work capacity evaluation: Systematic approach to industrial rehabilitation. Developed to accompany the Work Capacity Evaluation Workshop.* Employment and Rehabilitation Institute of California.

Matheson, L. N., Ogden, L. D., Violette, K., & Schultz, K. (1985). Work hardening: Occupational therapy in industrial rehabilitation. *American Journal of Occupational Therapy, 39*(5), 314–321.

McGonagle, A. K., Fisher, G. G., Barnes-Farrell, J. L., & Grosch, J. W. (2015). Individual and work factors related to perceived work ability and labor force outcomes. *Journal of Applied Psychology, 100*(2), 376–398. https://doi.org/10.1037/a0037974

Nastasia, I., Coutu, M.-F., Rives, R., Dubé, J., Gaspard, S., & Quilicot, A. (2021). Role and responsibilities of supervisors in the sustainable return to work of workers following a work-related musculoskeletal disorder. *Journal of Occupational Rehabilitation, 31*(1), 107–118. https://doi.org/10.1007/s10926-020-09896-w

National Occupational Health and Safety Commission. (1995). *Uniform guidelines for accreditation of rehabilitation providers.* Australian Government Publishing Service.

Norrefalk, J. R., Ekholm, K., Linder, J., Borg, K., & Ekholm, J. (2008). Evaluation of a multi-professional rehabilitation programme for persistent musculoskeletal-related pain: Economic benefits of return to work. *Journal of Rehabilitation Medicine, 40*(1), 15–22. https://doi.org/10.2340/16501977-0131

Oesch, P. R., Hilfiker, R., Kool, J. P., Bachmann, S., & Hagen, K. B. (2010). Perceived functional ability assessed with the spinal function sort: Is it valid for European rehabilitation settings in patients with non-specific non-acute low back pain? *European Spine Journal, 19*(9), 1527–1533. https://doi.org/10.1007/s00586-010-1429-3

Ogden-Niemeyer, L., & Jacobs, K. (1989). *Work hardening: State of the art.* Slack Inc.

Peteet, J. R. (2000). Cancer and the meaning of work. *General Hospital Psychiatry, 22*(3), 200–205. https://doi.org/10.1016/S0163-8343(00)00076-1

Randolph, S. A., & Dalton, P. C. (1989). Limited duty work: An innovative approach to early return to work. *American Association of Occupational Health Nurses Journal, 37*(11), 446–453. https://doi.org/10.1177/216507998903701101

Reneman, M. F., & Dijkstra, P. U. (2003). Introduction to the special issue on functional capacity evaluations: From expert based to evidence based. *Journal of Occupational Rehabilitation, 13*(4), 203–206. https://doi.org/10.1023/A:1026266303157

Schonstein, E., & Kenny, D. T. (2001). The value of functional and work place assessments in achieving a timely return to work for workers with back pain. *Work, 16*(1), 31–38.

Scully, S. M., Habeck, R. V., & Leahy, M. J. (1999). Knowledge and skill areas associated with disability management practice for rehabilitation counselors. *Rehabilitation Counseling Bulletin, 43*(1), 20–29. https://doi.org/10.1177/003435529904300105

Selander, J., Marnetoft, S.-U., Bergroth, A., & Ekholm, J. (2002). Return to work following vocational rehabilitation for neck, back and shoulder problems: Risk factors reviewed. *Disability and Rehabilitation, 24*(14), 704–712. https://doi.org/10.1080/09638280210124284

Shaw, W. S., Robertson, M. M., Pransky, G., & McLellan, R. K. (2003). Employee perspectives on the role of supervisors to prevent workplace disability after injuries. *Journal of Occupational Rehabilitation, 13*(3), 129–142. https://doi.org/10.1023/A:1024997000505

Shechtman, O., Anton, S. D., Kanasky, W. F. Jr, & Robinson, M. E. (2006). The use of the coefficient of variation in detecting sincerity of effort: A meta-analysis. *Work, 26*(4), 335–341.

Shrey, D. E., & Hursh, N. C. (1999). Workplace disability management: International trends and perspectives. *Journal of Occupational Rehabilitation, 9*(1), 45–59. https://doi.org/10.1023/A:1021393432243

Suda, A. J., Prajitno, J., Grutzner, P. A., & Tinelli, M. (2017). Good isometric and isokinetic power restoration after distal biceps tendon repair with anchors. *Archives of Orthopaedic and Trauma Surgery, 137*, 939–944. https://doi.org/10.1007/s00402-017-2724-9

Suoyrjo, H., Oksanen, T., Hinkka, K., Kivimaki, M., Klaukka, T., Pentti, J., & Vahtera, J. (2009). The effectiveness of vocationally oriented multidisciplinary intervention on sickness absence and early retirement among employees at risk: An observational study. *Occupational and Environmental Medicine, 66*(4), 235–242. https://doi.org/10.1136/oem.2007.038067

Torpel, A., Becker, T., Thiers, A., Hamacher, D., & Schega, L. (2017). Intersession reliability of isokinetic strength testing in knee and elbow extension and flexion using the BTE PrimusRS. *Journal of Sport Rehabilitation, 26*(4), 1–14.

Tramposh, A. K. (1991). The functional capacity evaluation: Measuring maximal work abilities. *Spine, 5*(3), 437–448.

Turner-Stokes, L. (2008). Evidence for the effectiveness of multi-disciplinary rehabilitation following acquired brain injury: A synthesis of two systematic approaches. *Journal of Rehabilitation Medicine, 40*(9), 691–701. https://doi.org/10.2340/16501977-0265

U.S. Department of Labor. (1991). *The revised handbook for analyzing jobs.* U.S. Department of Labor.

U.S. Department of Labor. (1993). *The new DOT: A database of occupational titles for the twenty-first century.* U.S. Department of Labor.

van der Giezen, A. M., Bouter, L. M., & Nijhuis, F. J. N. (2000). Prediction of return-to-work of low back pain patients sicklisted for 3-4 months. *Pain, 87*(3), 285–294. https://doi.org/10.1016/S0304-3959(00)00292-X

van der Meer, S., Reneman, M. F., Verhoeven, J., & van der Palen, J. (2014). Relationship between self-reported disability and functional capacity in patients with whiplash associated disorder. *Journal of Occupational Rehabilitation, 24*(3), 419–424. https://doi.org/10.1007/s10926-013-9473-6

van Duijn, M., Miedema, H., Elders, L., & Burdorf, A. (2004). Barriers for early return-to-work of workers with musculoskeletal disorders according to occupational health physicians and human resource managers. *Journal of Occupational Rehabilitation, 14*(1), 31–41. https://doi.org/10.1023/B:JOOR.0000015009.00933.16

Velozo, C. A. (1993). Work evaluations: Critique of the state of the art of functional assessment of work. *American Journal of Occupational Therapy, 47*(3), 203–209.

Viola, R. W., Boatright, K. C., Smith, K. L., Sidles, J. A., & Matsen, F. A. (2000). Do shoulder patients insured by workers' compensation present with worse self-assessed function and health status? *Journal of Shoulder and Elbow Surgery, 9*(5), 368–372. https://doi.org/10.1067/mse.2000.107391

World Health Organization. (2001). *International classification of functioning, disability and health.* World Health Organization. https://www.who.int/standards/classifications/international-classification-of-functioning-disability-and-health

Young, A. E., Wasiak, R., Roessler, R. T., McPherson, K. M., Anema, J. R., & van Poppel, M. N. M. (2005). Return-to-work outcomes following work disability: Stakeholder motivations, interests and concerns. *Journal of Occupational Rehabilitation, 15*(4), 543–556. https://doi.org/10.1007/s10926-005-8033-0

Case illustration

Musculoskeletal injuries related to work rehabilitation

Andy Shu Kei Cheng and Melva Yin Mei Yip

Case background

Case diagnosis and history of present illness

Mr. Cheng is a 29-year-old who used to work as a structural steelworker (扎鐵工人) on a construction site. He suffered an injury on duty three months ago when he fell from a height of two meters and landed on his outstretched right hand. A radiological examination in the Accident and Emergency Department of a public hospital revealed a displaced scaphoid fracture in the wrist. He was then transferred to the Department of Orthopedics and Traumatology. Percutaneous screw fixation was performed by an orthopedic surgeon to manage his unstable scaphoid fracture. This technique was reported to be a safe and effective method when a manual reduction is possible. It is also a less invasive option compared to the standard open technique (Matson et al., 2017). Unlike conservative treatment, this technique promotes better fracture healing and allows for an earlier return to work (RTW) by significantly reducing the need for wrist and thumb immobilization. It also minimizes the risk of devascularization of fracture fragments and preserves the integrity of surrounding ligaments and capsules (Puopolo & Rettig, 2003–2004).

Mr. Cheng received physiotherapy after the operation. The range of motion and strength of his right wrist showed significant improvement. However, he complained of muscle weakness in his right upper limb when performing certain daily tasks, a dull ache in the fracture site, and stabbing pain from the right wrist to the neck and upper back. The pain made it difficult for him to sleep at night. He was greatly concerned about his condition and told his doctor that he was unable to RTW as a structural steelworker as the work demands were very high. However, a radiological examination of the fracture site showed that Mr. Cheng's scaphoid fracture was well-healed. There was neither avascular necrosis nor malunion. Therefore, his doctor referred him to occupational therapy (OT) for work assessment and rehabilitation.

DOI: 10.4324/9781032721170-12

Table 8.1 Hand assessment during the intake interview

	Right side (dominant)	Left side (non-dominant)
Wrist extension/flexion	80°/85°	80°/90°
Wrist radial deviation/ulnar deviation	5°/20°	10°/25°
Thumb abduction	40°	40°
Thumb opposition	To proximal interphalangeal (PIP) joint of little finger	To base of little finger
First web space (cm)	16	17
Tip pinch (kg)	2	7
Power grip (kg)	10	34

Presentation of client

When Mr. Cheng's case occupational therapist met him during the initial assessment session, the range of motion in his right hand was comparable with his left hand. However, there was a significant decrease in right-hand power grip and pinch (Table 8.1). Usually, the grip power of the dominant hand is eight to nine percent higher than that of the non-dominant hand (Incel et al., 2002). He also complained of residual pain. Despite this being a common symptom after a scaphoid fracture, which could be a result of intraoperative articular damage after surgery (Barton, 2004), the pain location was somewhat diffuse. It spread from the whole right upper limb to the neck and upper back. The intensity of the pain was up to eight out of ten according to the visual analog scale. These residual symptoms affected his daily living performance. For instance, his right hand was relatively weak when wringing a towel, preventing him from drying it thoroughly. This caused him to lose confidence in returning to work as a structural steelworker because the job requires vigorous use of the hands. Being young, he was also concerned about his future.

Relevant history

Medical history

Mr. Cheng had been an active smoker since he was a teenager and used to smoke three to four cigarettes per day. Otherwise, he had good prior health. After fracturing his wrist, he was advised to quit or reduce smoking, and now only smokes one to two cigarettes per day.

Work history

Mr. Cheng is a Form Six graduate with fairly good academic results in the Hong Kong Diploma of Secondary Education Examination (HKDSE). He had been a casual worker with an unstable employment record for the first few years after graduation from secondary school. Two years ago, he was introduced by a friend to work as a structural steelworker in a construction company. He found that the nature of the job was stimulating and the salary rewarding. As such, he stayed at the same company and received annual salary increases.

Social history

Mr. Cheng is single and lives with his family in a private flat. His parents work full-time, and his older brother is married and has moved out. Mr. Cheng is currently on sick leave but has denied experiencing any immediate financial difficulties.

Psychological status

Mr. Cheng has expressed concerns about his future and was ambivalent about his RTW. On the one hand, he felt that working on a construction site as a structural steelworker matched his interests and outgoing personality, and the salary was rewarding. On the other hand, he was concerned about his residual symptoms and muscle weakness.

Assessment

Assessments relevant to the diagnosis

After three months of rehabilitation, Mr. Cheng's doctor assessed his right hand and noted that the fracture site was consolidated and stable enough for further work rehabilitation. A detailed initial assessment was then performed by an occupational therapist in the work rehabilitation team. A hand assessment was conducted first as it provided essential information about his physical recovery in general (Table 8.1). It also served as a foundation for formulating a further work rehabilitation plan.

Assessments that lead to intervention decisions

Work readiness

The Lam Assessment of Employment Readiness (LASER) was used to assess Mr. Cheng's readiness to work. LASER contains 14 items that describe behaviors in the pre-contemplation (six statements), contemplation (four statements), and action stages (four statements). Mr. Cheng was asked to rate each item on a five-point Likert scale with 1 indicating "strongly disagree" to 5 indicating "strongly agree". The scores were then tabulated and assigned various subscores representing the corresponding stages, creating a continuous measure (Chan et al., 2006). The highest subscore represented Mr. Cheng's tendency toward the corresponding stage. The assessment results showed that Mr. Cheng was at the contemplation stage. He was considering the pros and cons of working but had not yet participated in any related action to RTW. This finding was in line with his current psychological status of being ambivalent about RTW.

Job analysis

With reference to both international and local databases of job definitions, which include the Occupational Information Network developed by the US Department of Labor (O*NET OnLine, https://www.onetonline.org/) and the Construction Workers Registration Ordinance in Hong Kong (Department of Justice, 2021), the major job tasks which would likely be affected by Mr. Cheng's right-hand injury are identified below:

(1) Cutting and bending the required rebars with a steel bar bending machine after measurement.

(2) Lifting rebars manually to a designated construction site or machine.
(3) Aligning rebars in position by wrapping wires on them with a wire twister.
(4) Fastening steel members to the hoist cable using a rope or chain.
(5) Placing and binding steel structures, such as floor panels, walls, columns, arrays, and stairs.

The working environment of a structural steelworker is mostly outdoors, where the demand and level of exhaustion are greatly affected by the weather. Mr. Cheng had to withstand prolonged work at high temperatures in the summer months. The noise produced by the construction machine was also an environmental factor. His daily working hours fluctuated from 8 to 20 hours since overtime work was sometimes required. Mr. Cheng needed to have good physical strength and endurance in order to carry rebars that weighed 10–40 kg by himself, or ~120 kg with co-workers, depending on the size and length of the rebars. Apart from the physical demands, a certain degree of cognitive ability is also required to be a structural steelworker. Mr. Cheng was required to understand the instructions and blueprints given to him by his supervisor to accurately cut the necessary steel and align the rebars accordingly. Basic calculations were needed when measuring the length of the rebars and the distance between them. Based on the diagnosis and Mr. Cheng's concern about his newly healed right scaphoid fracture, the job analysis mainly focused on his physical work demands. Although his injury did not directly affect other performance components, such as cognitive and social aspects, the case occupational therapist needed to be sensitive to any secondary effects on his psychosocial well-being, including mental stress due to prolonged sick leave. Table 8.2 summarizes the job analysis of a structural steelworker.

Critical job demands

There were two principles that the case occupational therapist had to consider when determining the critical job demands that would likely be affected by the injury when

Table 8.2 Job analysis of a structural steelworker

Job title:
Structural steelworker

Occupational group:
Construction

Working schedule:
Five working days per week
Eight standard working hours per day from 9 am to 6 pm

Main working locations:
Outdoor construction sites

Licensing:
Test Certificate for Bar Bender and Fixer issued by Construction Industry Council

Physical demand category level:
Very heavy

Table 8.2 Job analysis of a structural steelworker (*continued*)

Demands	N	O	F	C	Description
(1) Standing				+	■ Major position of work for fixing and wiring rebars.
(2) Walking		+			■ Walking to various working areas on the construction site.
(3) Walking up and down stairs		+			■ Walking to working areas at various heights.
(4) Sitting		+			■ Sitting on steel bars to tie rebars.
(5) Climbing		+			■ Climbing onto steel beams and girders to perform high-level bolting and riveting. ■ Climbing up and down a steel cage.
(6) Balancing			+		■ Maintaining balance when carrying steel or working on an uneven surface or narrow base.
(7) Squatting		+			■ Fixing and wiring rebars below waist level.
(8) Kneeling		+			
(9) Crouching		+			
(10) Crawling	+				■ Not required.
(11) Reaching			+		■ Reaching for equipment. ■ Fixing and wiring rebars at various levels and directions.
(12) Handling			+		■ Manipulation of handheld tools, including
(13) Fingering			+		an angle grinder, power shear, flame cutting equipment, manual rebar cutter and bender, pliers, and rebar tie wire twister. ■ Screw turning of metal parts (bolts or welded pieces). ■ Fastening structural steel members with wires.
(14) Lifting			+		■ Lifting steel bars ~10–30 kg in weight (frequently). ■ Lifting steel bars ~40 kg in weight (occasionally). ■ Level of lifting: from floor to shoulder level.
(15) Carrying		+			■ Carrying rebars ~120 kg at shoulder or waist level with co-workers.
(16) Pushing			+		■ Pushing and pulling metal rebars when handling
(17) Pulling			+		them with a bending machine or pliers. ■ Positioning of rebar wires.

Abbreviations: N = Never; O = Occasional (0–33% of work); F = Frequent (34–66% of work); C = Constant (67–100% of work).

Mr. Cheng was going to RTW as a structural steelworker. The first principle was the necessity of the job post, which included (1) work tasks that could not be shared with co-workers or delegated to others and (2) tasks with minimal flexibility in adjustment, such as reducing working speed or adjusting loading. The second principle was the degree of physical loading and level of strenuousness on Mr. Cheng's injured wrist, particularly in relation to (1) his limited functional performance after the injury, which concerned mainly his right hand, wrist, and forearm strength and (2) the risk of reinjury in the case

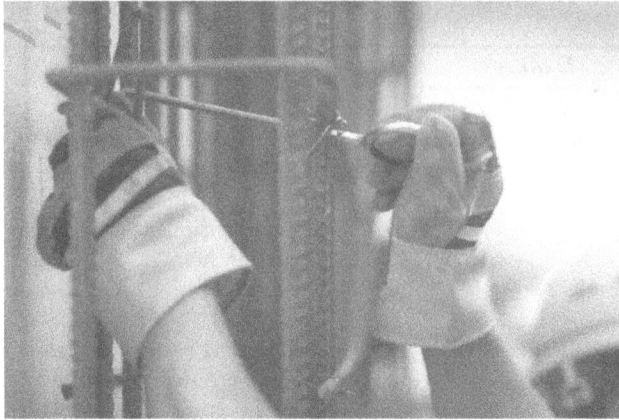

Figure 8.1 Fastening structural steel members with wires using a twister

of overloading, such as repetitive, resistive, or forceful right thumb, wrist, or forearm movements. As a result, the following critical job demands were identified.

Handling and fingering

The first critical job demand was handling and fingering, which requires good finger dexterity, wrist movements, and pinch and grip strength. Mr. Cheng was required to turn screws by rotating bolts or welded pieces and to fasten structural steel members with wires using a twister (Figure 8.1). He was also required to grip various manual tools and steel bars constantly and steadily with strong and repetitive thumb and wrist movements. Mr. Cheng might not be able to fulfill the job demand of repeated gripping against resistance for a long period of working time. Additionally, his newly healed right hand would be at risk of overloading due to repetitive and resistive thumb, wrist, and forearm movements when manipulating handheld tools.

Pushing and pulling

The second critical job demand was related to rebars. Specifically, each rebar used on the construction site needed to be cut or bent into particular shapes by a steel bar bending machine (Figure 8.2) according to the architectural drawings. Further fine-tuning using

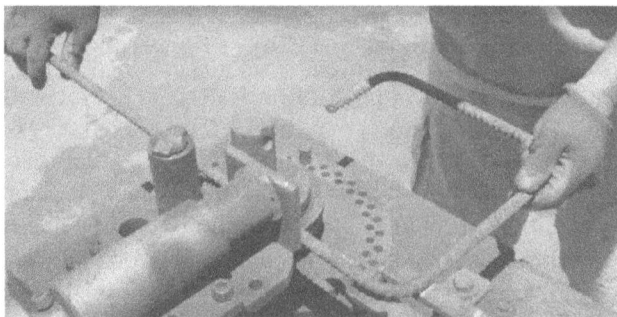

Figure 8.2 Bending rebars using a steel bar bending machine

a hickey bar or even bare hands might also be needed. Mr. Cheng had to bend wires and steel bars frequently with either tools or his bare hands. In view of his diminished grip power and wrist strength, his performance in those tasks would be hindered as the actions demand flexible and forceful wrist and thumb motions in holding, pushing, and pulling the steel bars or tools to a particular position or in a particular direction.

Lifting and carrying

The third critical job demand was bilateral lifting and carrying rebars of various weights. Mr. Cheng needed to lift and carry steel columns and beams of various weights around the construction area. If a rebar had to be lifted from floor level, he had to hold it with both hands in a squatting position, and then lift it up to waist level and finally over the shoulder. For a thicker or longer rebar that could not be lifted by a single person, it would be lifted by two or more workers together. Mr. Cheng's reduced grip endurance and strength would affect his ability to lift heavy objects and sustain the posture of carrying them from one place to another. Therefore, it was challenging and risky for him to lift and carry heavy objects such as rebars.

Work capacity evaluation

After obtaining Mr. Cheng's job information and critical job demands, a work capacity evaluation (WCE), i.e., a more specific form of functional capacity evaluation, was conducted. According to the hand assessment and job analysis results of Mr. Cheng, the following work-related tasks were suggested to be included in the WCE to check for any discrepancy between his work capacity and the minimal job requirements.

(1) Handling and fingering (including tool gripping)
(2) Pushing and pulling
(3) Lifting and carrying

As the aim of the WCE was to test Mr. Cheng's functional capacity at the maximal level, safety measures needed to be taken, which included pre-WCE assessments and the preparation of Mr. Cheng for the WCE. For example, measurement of his blood pressure and heart rate needed to be performed as a preliminary screening for cardiac conditions. Second, Mr. Cheng had to complete the Physical Activity Readiness Questionnaire (PAR-Q) before the WCE assessment (Appendix 8.1). This is a self-reporting screening tool used to uncover exercise-related risks and safety concerns according to a client's health history, active symptoms, and risk factors.

An assessment of pain was also conducted because it could indicate potential issues that might hinder his performance in the WCE. The location, type, and intensity of the pain were recorded by the Ransford Pain Drawing (Appendix 8.2). Lastly, warm-up exercises such as stretching of wrists, fingers, and arms before the test were performed. In response to the problems identified in the previous section, a progressive loading format was adopted, along with a mixed approach that combined psychophysical and kinesiophysical methods. In the mixed approach, the case occupational therapist encouraged Mr. Cheng to exert maximal effort to help determine his physical limits by expressing his rate of perceived exertion (RPE). Safety should always be the highest priority.

Evaluation of handling and fingering (including pinching and gripping)

As Mr. Cheng had to handle various handheld tools such as a manual rebar cutter and bender, pliers, and a rebar tie wire twister, he needed to have strong proximal stability, gripping strength, and endurance, all of which are vital in tool handling. The BTE Primus RS attachment #162 was used. Calibration should be done before using the BTE to ensure measurement validity. The work head of the BTE Primus RS was first positioned at Mr. Cheng's waist level, and then the attachment was oriented in a 45° angulated downward position. Mr. Cheng was required to stand sideways to the work head and grasp the handles with his elbows in flexion and wrists in slight ulnar deviation to simulate the action (Figure 8.3).

After giving a demonstration with a verbal description of the required actions to Mr. Cheng, his peak isometric strength (PIS) was measured with the good hand first and then the injured one. He had to grip as hard as he could and hold on for five seconds. A ten-second rest was allowed after each trial. The average PIS in three trials was calculated for each hand. Afterward, testing of dynamic endurance was performed for both hands by setting the resistance at 30% of the isometric average of each hand and the pace at 45 repetitions per minute. A computer screen was shown to Mr. Cheng, and he was required to grip through the full range of motion and grip at the pace shown on the screen until three consecutive bars fell below the expected value; then he was asked to stop. To prevent exhaustion, only one trial was performed for each hand.

The BTE Primus RS attachment #400 lathe crank was used to simulate complicated movements (including wrist circumduction and finger dexterity) during rebar wire tying with a twister. Mr. Cheng was required to clench his fist and hold the small handle of the lathe crank between the second and third fingers of his right hand. He then had to rotate the lathe crank using repeated wrist circumduction. The power of this action was assessed using a concentric–eccentric mode to simulate the twisting motions performed when securing rebar junctions with a tie wire twister. He was asked to rotate the lathe crank as quickly as possible (three times within ten seconds, with a ten-second break in between trials) because speedy motions were normal for a structural steelworker.

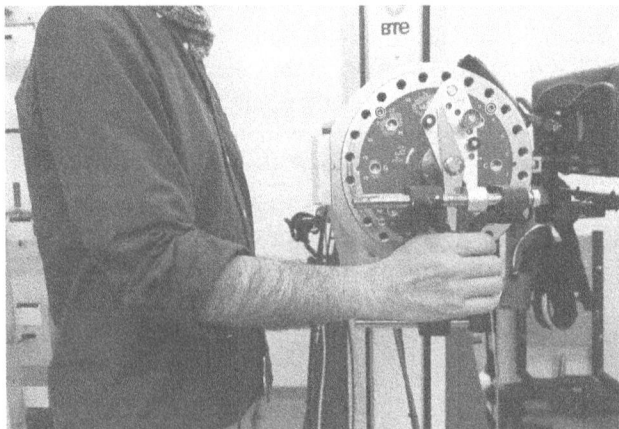

Figure 8.3 Assessment of gripping strength

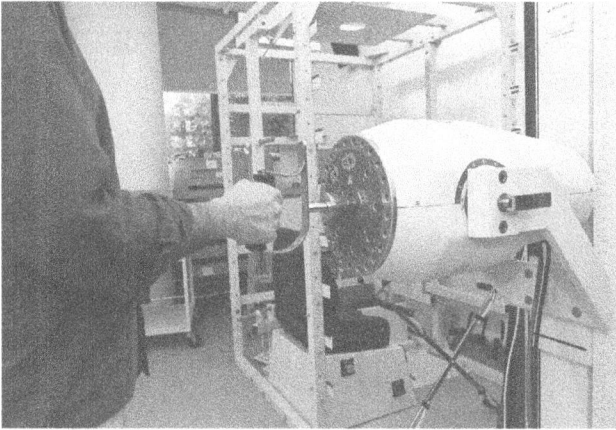

Figure 8.4 Twisting wire action assessment

Furthermore, the wiring action was further assessed by the BTE Primus RS attachment #601 to simulate the critical job demand of tying rebars, which requires frequent and prolonged supination and pronation. The attachment was positioned vertically and at Mr. Cheng's waist level (Figure 8.4). The case occupational therapist had to make sure Mr. Cheng's forearm was in flexion and aligned with the axis of rotation of the attachment shaft. A verbal instruction and demonstration of movement were given to Mr. Cheng, and the PIS was first measured with the good hand (left hand) followed by the injured hand (right hand). The average PIS was then calculated. After that, a dynamic endurance test was conducted by setting the resistance at 30% of the isometric strength average with three sets of 50 repetitions. This endurance test was only conducted on the right hand since the wire twister was only manipulated by the right hand at work. In addition, a dynamic strength test was unnecessary since the wire twister is relatively light (less than 2.5 kg) and its manipulation, though repetitive and long-lasting, does not require the powerful contraction of muscle fibers.

The VALPAR Component Work Sample #4 (VCWS-4) was also used to assess the range of motion and work tolerance of the upper extremities, including shoulders, arms, elbows, wrists, hands, and fingers. This work sample represented light work and assessed fingering, reaching, and depth perception, which simulated Mr. Cheng's real-world job tasks, including screw turning with bolts or welded pieces and fastening structural steel members with wires. The VCWS-4 includes a 12-inch work box cube with an open back and a five-inch opening in the front, with various thread and machine bolt sizes (Figure 8.5). Mr. Cheng was asked to pick up one nut at a time, reach through the opening of the work box, and screw the nut down snugly against the box. Since occlusion of vision was not applicable for Mr. Cheng's real-world job tasks, he was allowed to reach through the square opening of the work box instead of the circular opening. After screwing in nuts of various sizes onto various planes, he was asked to remove the nuts using one hand at a time and place them back into the storage compartment. There were eight assemblies (four for each hand) and one disassembly for both hands. The time needed for the assembly was recorded.

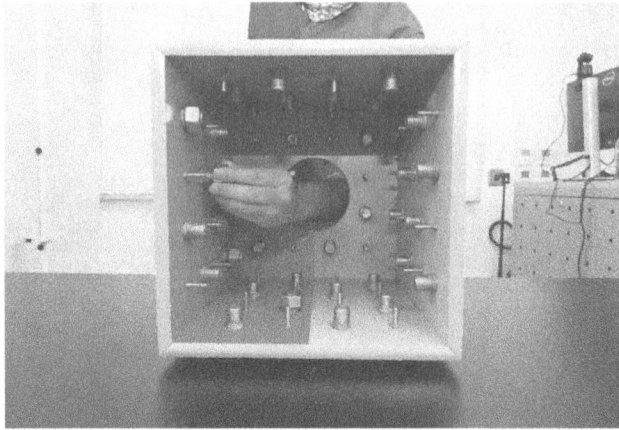

Figure 8.5 Assessment of the range of motion and work tolerance of the upper extremity

Evaluation of pushing and pulling

Being a structural steelworker, Mr. Cheng was required to bend rebars using a bending machine, pliers, or his bare hands. To simulate these work tasks, the BTE Primus RS attachment #701 and attachment #802 (Figure 8.6) were used. The plate of movement should be the same as in real-world work tasks. The typical setup for bending rebars on a construction site was having the exercise head of a socket wrench set at Mr. Cheng's waist level. He then faced the BTE slightly offset to the left or right depending on which side was being tested. During the test, his shoulder was positioned in a slight abduction

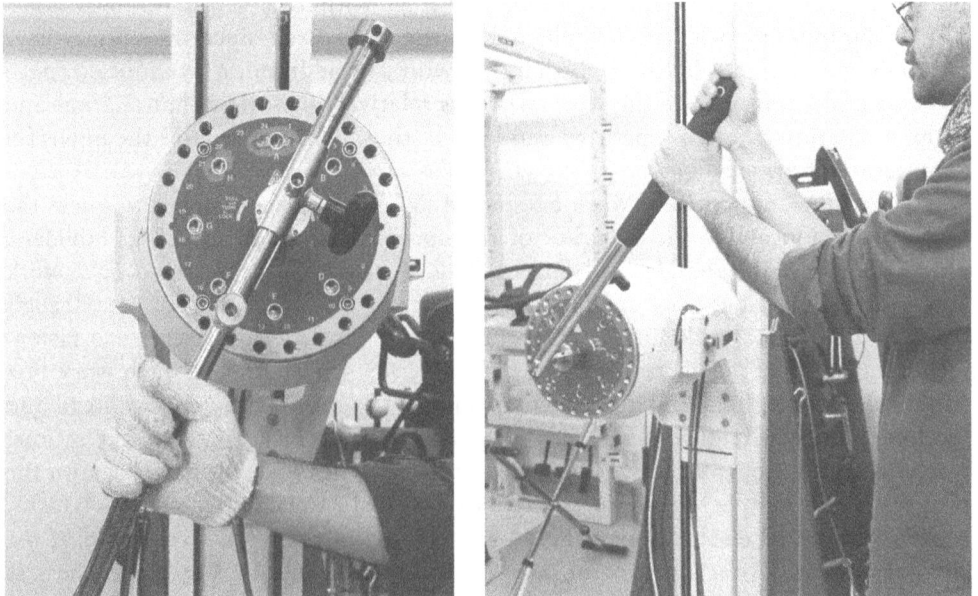

Figure 8.6 Assessment of pushing and pulling rebars (left: attachment #701; right: attachment #802)

and his elbow in flexion around 90°. Mr. Cheng then gripped the handle and performed pushing and pulling as much as he could tolerate. Multiple planes of movement were included to simulate all common actions he had to perform in his job duties. Again, the PIS of each hand was assessed. This was then followed by a dynamic strength test set at 80% of the PIS with 3 sets of 10 repetitions.

Evaluation of lifting and carrying

Mr. Cheng had to frequently lift and carry steel bars or rebars on the construction site, with their weights ranging from 10 to 40 kg. Sometimes, he might also be required to carry multiple steel bars or rebars at shoulder or waist level together with other colleagues. To determine Mr. Cheng's lifting and carrying ability, ARCON's NIOSH ST lifting tests were conducted first (Figure 8.7). The tests were used to evaluate his isometric lifting strength in comparison with his job requirements and to determine if it was safe for him to return to his previous work regarding the demands of the job. First,

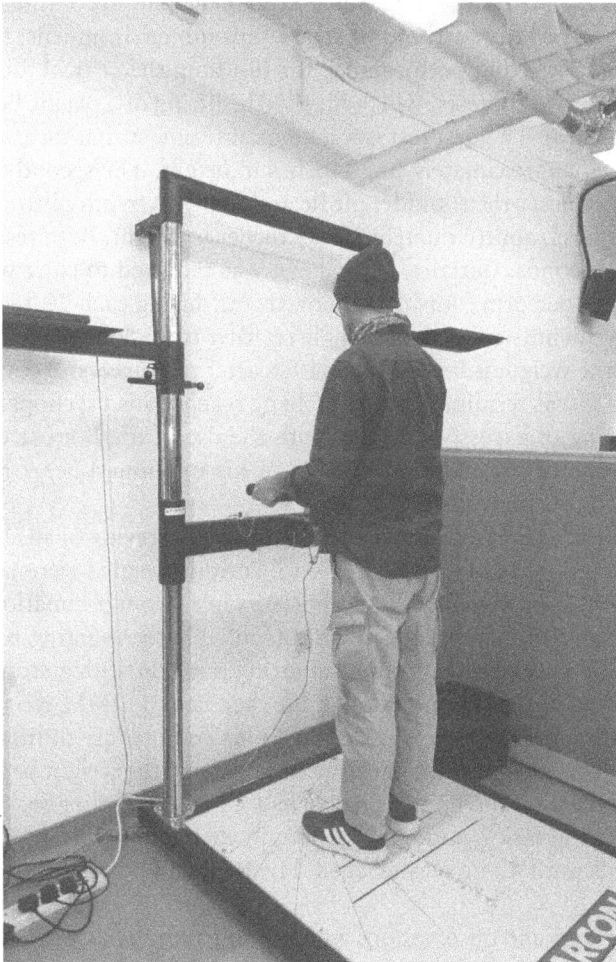

Figure 8.7 Assessment of isometric lifting strength using ARCON's NIOSH ST lifting tests

a leg lift was performed, with the narrow handle at 15 inches on the vertical scale. Mr. Cheng stood on the ST platform with his feet parallel and ankle bones over the 0 inch measurement on the platform scale. For all four subtests, he gripped and slowly lifted up the handles, holding them for five seconds, repeating this three times. A 15-second rest was allowed between each trial. After one subtest, the RPE was determined to assess his perceived physical exertion. A wide handle in the upright position would be used from the second to the fourth subtests. A torso lift was the second subtest, where the height of the ST crossbar remained unchanged, and Mr. Cheng stood with his feet parallel over the 15 inches measurement. The third subtest was an arm lift, with the height of the ST crossbar set at around 90° or slightly lower than his elbow. The fourth subtest was a high near lift, with the handle set at 60 inches on the vertical scale, and Mr. Cheng stood over the 10 inches measurement. In each subtest, he was instructed to lift up the handles and hold them for five seconds.

After ARCON's NIOSH ST lifting tests, the progressive isoinertial lifting evaluation (PILE) was used to assess Mr. Cheng's ability to perform repetitive lifting within a set time limit as quickly as possible. Since Mr. Cheng had to continually perform the lifting and carrying of heavy structural steel in his job environment, it was crucial to evaluate his repetitive lifting performance for fulfilling the critical job demands. The PILE is divided into two subtests, which involve the lifting of a plastic box with increasing weight (Figure 8.8). The first test is a lumbar assessment that measures lifting from floor to waist level, approximately 0–30 inches in height. The second test is a cervical assessment that evaluates the shoulder girdle and upper extremity lifting capacity from waist to shoulder level, approximately 30–54 inches in height. Both tests must be completed within 20 seconds. Initially, Mr. Cheng was required to start with a weight of 13 lb. He needed to perform four lifting movements during each 20-second interval. A single lifting movement is defined as a single transfer from floor to waist or from waist to shoulder, and the weight is increased by 10 lb after the successful completion of each lift cycle. The PILE was terminated if Mr. Cheng reached his psychophysical endpoint, such as complaining of excessive fatigue (with the use of the Borg scale for perceived exertion), his physiological endpoint at 85% of his maximum heart rate, or the safe limit of 55–60% of his body weight.

Last but not least, to further simulate the lifting and carrying of steel bars from floor to shoulder level, weight bars (Figure 8.9) with various weights were used. During the process, Mr. Cheng applied manual handling principles from occupational biomechanics to perform lifting and carrying assessments aimed at preventing back sprains. He was required to lift a weight bar from a squatting position with a straight back in the first trial, with 10 kg as the starting weight. He then had to lift the weight bar to shoulder level with both hands, which was similar to his end posture of lifting steel bars or rebars at work. He needed to stand up straight and carry the weight bar for one minute and then place it back on the floor using correct manual handling techniques. He was required to repeat the task by adding 5–10 kg in each trial, with a two-minute break between two trials until 40 kg was reached. His RPE and posture were recorded.

Specific considerations and observations when conducting the assessments
The following are a number of specific considerations and observations that were made when conducting Mr. Cheng's WCE.

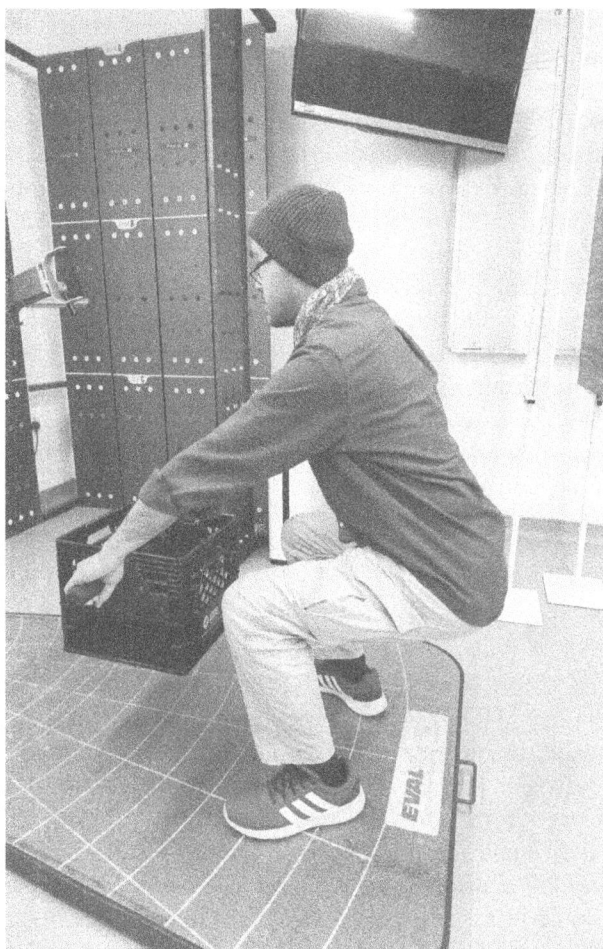

Figure 8.8 A PILE box with two side handles

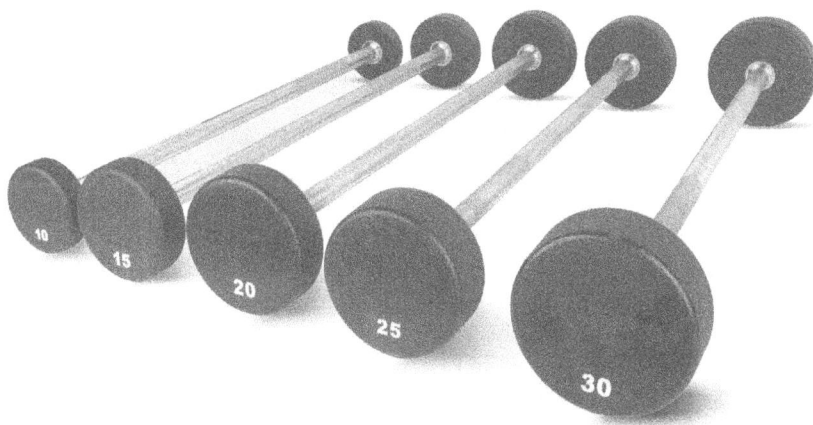

Figure 8.9 Weight bars

(1) First, any fracture complications had to be assessed. Complications such as carpal instability and residual pain are commonly present. When analyzing the graphs produced by either ARCON or BTE Primus RS, it was important to look for any sharp decreases as these may indicate the presence of sharp pain.

(2) Second, occupational biomechanics also needed to be observed, particularly Mr. Cheng's posture when performing the assessments. For example, the therapist had to ensure that Mr. Cheng's back remained straight when he was squatting to pick up heavy objects. Alternatively, Mr. Cheng could squat with a large base of support to prevent injuries such as back sprains. Some common manual handling techniques, such as holding the weight as close as possible to the body, had to be observed. Any awkward posture needed to be corrected immediately if found.

(3) Lastly, it was important to observe Mr. Cheng's imitativeness and motivation. If he displayed excessive avoidance behavior or exaggerated complaints about the task's difficulty, this could provide the therapist with insights into Mr. Cheng's perception of his own ability and readiness to RTW.

Possible limitations of the assessments

Possible limitations in job analysis

In common clinical practice, job analysis is done with reference to well-established databases such as O*NET or, in Mr. Cheng's case, the Construction Workers Registration Ordinance. However, employees with the same job title might have different job demands in various companies or under different employers or supervisors. For instance, the division of labor varies among companies. In organizations with more colleagues in similar roles, task delegation tends to be more flexible. Additionally, some companies have employers and co-workers who are more supportive and willing to assist employees RTW after an injury. The physical and psychological coping by injured workers would be much easier in such companies. Even for employees with the same job post, if some work in a more favorable work environment (either physically or socially), their stress and strain could be lower than those working in a poor work environment. Therefore, relying solely on existing databases for job analysis may not account for the individual differences among workers. Occupational therapists should focus on understanding and exploring the unique variations of their clients.

Possible limitations in work capacity evaluation

Although the WCE is comprehensive, objective, popular, and widely used internationally in work rehabilitation services, it has some well-known shortcomings, such as being time-consuming and expensive to administer. Taking Mr. Cheng's case as an example, a full WCE set required multiple professional and advanced assessments, such as the BTE Primus RS, ARCON, VALPAR Work Samples, PILE, and other clinical assessment tools. The cost of such equipment is high compared with other OT assessments. Moreover, the WCE assessment is usually conducted individually, meaning that one therapist or trained technician delivers the WCE for one client at a time. The manpower cost is also high. Besides, as the tests are primarily used to measure a client's physical and work abilities in the clinical setting, real-world environmental factors such as temperature, distractions, and interactions with colleagues, which might have a significant influence on a worker's performance, could not be included. This may undermine the predictive ability of the WCE in making an RTW decision.

In summary, Mr. Cheng was identified as having the following problems by the WCE:

■ An ambivalent attitude toward RTW as a structural steelworker.
■ Decreased right-hand power and pinch grip strength, which affected the ability of his right hand to use resistive tools.
■ Fair endurance in repeated gripping against resistance.
■ Handling and fingering ability of the right hand being below the job requirement level.
■ Bilateral and right unilateral lifting and carrying strengths being unable to meet the job demands.

Intervention

After the assessments, a work-hardening program was designed to develop the work feasibility and then employability of Mr. Cheng according to his work readiness. This comprised the following two stages.

Stage one: Work feasibility development

Since Mr. Cheng was still contemplating his own abilities and strongly identifying with the sick role or patient role, the overall objective of this work-hardening program was to help him acquire sufficient worker role behaviors. The program included the following components:

■ Stretching activities to improve the flexibility of the shoulder girdle and upper limbs.
■ Low-resistance and short-duration (ten minutes) strengthening activities, repeated two to four times daily, concentrating on the static strength and endurance of the upper back and the dynamic strength and endurance of the upper extremities.
■ Use of graded, simulated, and sedentary-to-light functional tasks to build basic functional tolerances, promote a sense of productivity and competence, enhance self-esteem, and provide experiences of success.
■ Instruction and practice in methods for active control of symptoms, including self-pacing, basic body mechanics, and work simplification, to promote the development of effective strategies to control pain while improving sustained activity tolerance.
■ Value clarification to assist Mr. Cheng in rediscovering positive values associated with being a worker.

After six weeks of training, Mr. Cheng's functional condition was significantly improved. He was more conscientious and aware of the importance of returning to work.

Stage two: Employability development

When Mr. Cheng had developed a worker's role and the motivation to RTW, he was upgraded to the next stage of the work-hardening program, which developed his work employability. The overall objective of this stage was to help Mr. Cheng match the critical demands of being a structural steelworker so that he could RTW. It consisted of the following content:

- Stretching activities to improve the flexibility of the shoulder girdle and upper limbs.
- Intensive and continually reinforced training in body mechanics and proper posture for manual handling operations through simulated work activities.
- Use of the BTE Primus RS attachment #181 and VALPAR Work Sample #9 to simulate overhead pulling and reaching, respectively.
- Use of the BTE Primus RS attachment #701 and attachment #802 to simulate pulling and pushing, the VALPAR Work Sample #4 and BTE Primus RS attachment #400 to simulate complicated movements (including wrist circumduction and finger dexterity) during rebar wire tying with a twister, and the ARCON two-handed crate to simulate bilateral lifting and the carrying of rebars.
- Practice in work efficiency techniques as indicated above to control symptoms and maximize sustained activity tolerance.

Outcome and follow-up data

Throughout the entire program, Mr. Cheng paced his work activities and maintained symptom levels that allowed for good work productivity. His main symptom complaints, including muscle weakness in the right upper limb, decreased power and pinch grip, a dull ache in the fracture site, and stabbing pain from the right upper limb to the neck and upper back, were much improved. After three months of the work-hardening program, he made consistent and gradual improvements in the following areas:

- Positive attitude toward RTW as a structural steelworker.
- Hand grip strength was improved, with the dominant right hand measuring 32 kg compared to 34 kg on the left.
- Right pinch grip was the same as left side.
- Handling and fingering ability of the right hand was improved, which was reflected by the speed of tool use demonstrated through the BTE Primus RS attachment #400.
- The ability of the right hand to use resistive tools showed good improvement, as indicated by both isometric and isotonic force measurements on the BTE Primus RS attachments #162, #701, and #802.
- Bilateral and right unilateral lifting capacities increased to 35 kg and 20 kg, respectively.
- Duration of repeated gripping against resistance increased to 45 minutes.
- Bilateral carrying ability increased to 30 kg for 20 feet using a box in a standard two-handed front-body carry. Right unilateral carrying ability increased to 15 kg for 20 feet using a toolbox in a right-handed carry.

Mr. Cheng returned to work on a one-month trial basis and was seen again by the occupational therapist to reassess his condition after the work trial. As there was no complaint of deterioration in his condition and he was observed to have good adaption to his pre-injury duties, he then returned to his usual and customary job duties.

Cultural elements in the occupational therapy process

Work rehabilitation has been available in Hong Kong for many years. Localization of the assessments and interventions has been done in the last two decades. A number of validations of clinical instruments related to vocational rehabilitation have been published. For instance, researchers have explored the applicability of the Dictionary of Occupational Titles (DOT) in Hong Kong, using the formwork carpenter as a case study. It was found that the DOT was somewhat relevant to local practice. However, several discrepancies attributable to the specificity of the job nature of formwork carpentry between the US and Hong Kong were identified. Local researchers also validated self-reported assessments such as the Chinese versions of the Oswestry Disability Index (CODI), the Lam Assessment of Employment Readiness (C-LASER), and the Fear-Avoidance Beliefs Questionnaire (FABQ-CHI) (Kwok et al., 2011). There are also studies that evaluated the efficacy of interventional programs designed for injured workers in order to develop evidence-based practice in work rehabilitation in Hong Kong. For example, a randomized controlled trial was conducted to investigate the effect of a workplace-based rehabilitation program on the RTW outcome of injured workers. This program investigated the effect of the therapeutic use of actual work facilities, the work environment, and the functions of a job coach on facilitating the RTW process of injured workers (Cheng & Hung, 2007). The results of this study showed that the workplace-based rehabilitation program appeared to be more effective in reducing psychosocial workplace factors related to separation from the work routine and in restoring occupational bondage with co-workers.

However, there is still a lack of a standard model of practice in managing local work injury cases. In the majority of clinical settings, a "biomedical" model is followed, where the medical doctor is the ultimate decision-maker when it comes to determining the treatment and RTW process. This process is not purely physical; it also involves many psychological, social, and economic factors. In an ideal scenario, injured workers would follow a uniform RTW trajectory consisting of a series of evolving phases, including seeking medical care, recovery, and sustained work re-entry. In many cases, however, the RTW process is nonlinear and a proportion of injured workers experience a variable and often undesirable RTW course, including extended (e.g., staying out of work for a longer period of time than expected) or intermittent work disability (e.g., alternating between being able and being unable to perform work tasks). The RTW process is influenced by the motivation, interests, and concerns of various stakeholders. Unfortunately, communication among various stakeholders, such as employers, insurance companies, case managers, and injured workers, is either non-effective or poor. Case managers in Hong Kong have recently gained popularity in work rehabilitation services. They serve as facilitators to promote the RTW of injured workers by acting as a connection and communication channel among various parties, ensuring that timely and appropriate treatment is delivered. In light of this, a new work injury management model was proposed by Chong and Cheng in 2010 (Chong & Cheng, 2010).

With advances in the application of artificial intelligence (AI) and machine learning, a Smart Work Injury Management (SWIM) system was introduced. It employs AI to perform in-depth analyses using text-mining techniques to extract both dynamic and static data from work injury case files to create unsupervised and supervised machine learning algorithms. When fully developed, this system will be able to provide a more accurate prediction model for the cost of work injuries according to local jurisdictional-level workers' compensation policies. More importantly, it will also predict the RTW trajectory and provide advice on medical care and RTW interventions to all RTW stakeholders (Cheng et al., 2020; Ng et al., 2023).

Summary

Work injuries represent a significant cost to the industry and productive capacity of both developed and developing countries. Absence due to illness and work disability constitutes a common and substantial public health problem that has major economic consequences worldwide. When a person is injured at work, there are changes in all aspects of the person's function, whether the injury is short-term or long-term, permanent or temporary, serious or minor. The ultimate goal of work rehabilitation is to allow workers to keep their jobs or return to gainful employment after work injury so as to prevent work disability. It is a work-oriented treatment program that has an outcome measured in terms of improvement in the injured worker's productivity. This is achieved through increased work tolerance, improved work rate, mastery of pain (through the effective use of symptom control techniques), improved work habits, increased confidence, and proficiency with work adaptations or assistive devices.

A work rehabilitation program involves an injured worker performing highly structured, simulated work tasks in an environment where expectations for basic worker behaviors (e.g., timeliness, attendance, and dress) are in line with workplace standards. It helps the injured worker achieve a level of productivity that is acceptable in the competitive labor market.

Appendix 8.1 The Physical Activity Readiness Questionnaire (PAR-Q)

Physical Activity Readiness
Questionnaire - PAR-Q
(revised 2002)

PAR-Q & YOU

(A Questionnaire for People Aged 15 to 69)

Regular physical activity is fun and healthy, and increasingly more people are starting to become more active every day. Being more active is very safe for most people. However, some people should check with their doctor before they start becoming much more physically active.

If you are planning to become much more physically active than you are now, start by answering the seven questions in the box below. If you are between the ages of 15 and 69, the PAR-Q will tell you if you should check with your doctor before you start. If you are over 69 years of age, and you are not used to being very active, check with your doctor.

Common sense is your best guide when you answer these questions. Please read the questions carefully and answer each one honestly: check YES or NO.

YES	NO		
☐	☐	1.	Has your doctor ever said that you have a heart condition <u>and</u> that you should only do physical activity recommended by a doctor?
☐	☐	2.	Do you feel pain in your chest when you do physical activity?
☐	☐	3.	In the past month, have you had chest pain when you were not doing physical activity?
☐	☐	4.	Do you lose your balance because of dizziness or do you ever lose consciousness?
☐	☐	5.	Do you have a bone or joint problem (for example, back, knee or hip) that could be made worse by a change in your physical activity?
☐	☐	6.	Is your doctor currently prescribing drugs (for example, water pills) for your blood pressure or heart condition?
☐	☐	7.	Do you know of <u>any other reason</u> why you should not do physical activity?

Appendix 8.2 The Ransford Pain Drawing

Pain Drawing Chart	Name:	
	Sex/Age:	HKID No.:
	Reference No.:	

Diagnosis: Date of ☐ Injury / ☐ Onset:

Occupation:

Distribution:

Remarks:

		OT:
		Date:

References

Barton, N. J. (2004). The late consequences of scaphoid fractures. *The Journal of Bone and Joint Surgery (British Volume)*, 86-B(5), 626–630. https://doi.org/10.1302/0301-620x.86b5.15413

Chan, H., Li-Tsang, C. W. P., Chan, C., Lam, C. S., Hui, K. L., & Bard, C. (2006). Validation of Lam Assessment of Employment Readiness (C-LASER) for Chinese injured workers. *Journal of Occupational Rehabilitation*, 16(4), 697–705. https://doi.org/10.1007/s10926-006-9050-3

Cheng, A. S. K., & Hung, L. K. (2007). Randomized controlled trial of workplace-based rehabilitation for work-related rotator cuff disorder. *Journal of Occupational Rehabilitation*, 17(3), 487–503. https://doi.org/10.1007/s10926-007-9085-0

Cheng, A. S. K., Ng, P. H. F., Sin, Z. P. T., Lai, S. H. S., & Law, S. W. (2020). Smart Work Injury Management (SWIM) system: Artificial intelligence in work disability management. *Journal of Occupational Rehabilitation*, 30(3), 354–361. https://doi.org/10.1007/s10926-020-09886-y

Chong, C. S., & Cheng, A. S. (2010). Work injury management model and implication in Hong Kong: A literature review. *Work*, 35(2), 221–229.

Department of Justice, Hong Kong SAR Government. (2021). *Cap. 583 Construction Workers Registration Ordinance*. Hong Kong e-Legislation. https://www.elegislation.gov.hk/hk/cap583

Incel, N. A., Ceceli, E., Durukan, P. B., Erdem, H. R., & Yorgancioglu, Z. R. (2002). Grip strength: Effect of hand dominance. *Singapore Medical Journal*, 43(5), 234–237.

Kwok, H. K. H., Szeto, G. P. Y., Cheng, A. S. K., Siu, H., & Chan, C. C. H. (2011). Occupational rehabilitation in Hong Kong: Current status and future needs. *Journal of Occupational Rehabilitation*, 21(Suppl. 1), S28–S34. https://doi.org/10.1007/s10926-011-9286-4

Matson, A. P., Garcia, R. M., Richard, M. J., Leversedge, F. J., Aldridge, J. M., & Ruch, D. S. (2017). Percutaneous treatment of unstable scaphoid waist fractures. *Hand*, 12(4), 362–368. https://doi.org/10.1177/1558944716681948

Ng, P. H. F., Chen, P. Q., Sin, Z. P. T., Lai, S. H. S., & Cheng, A. S. K. (2023). Smart Work Injury Management (SWIM) system: A machine learning approach for the prediction of sick leave and rehabilitation plan. *Bioengineering*, 10(2), 172. https://doi.org/10.3390/bioengineering10020172

Puopolo, S. M., & Rettig, M. E. (2003–2004). Management of acute scaphoid fractures. *Bulletin of the Hospital for Joint Diseases*, 61(3 & 4), 160–163. https://hjdbulletin.org/files/archive/pdfs/681.pdf

CHAPTER 9

Stroke

*Kenneth Nai-Kuen Fong, Sharon Fong Mei Toh,
Phyllis Liang, and Ching-Yi Wu*

Introduction

This chapter includes the following sections:

1 Stroke
- Definition and prevalence
- Risk factors of stroke
- Description of stroke and stroke syndromes
- Medical investigations following stroke
- Most relevant areas affected after stroke
2 Role of occupational therapists in stroke rehabilitation
- Goal of occupational therapy
- Areas of occupational therapy assessment
- Common treatment approaches in stroke rehabilitation
3 Community integration after stroke
- Community integration
- Cultural factors and environmental influence
- Challenges in community integration after stroke
- Role of occupational therapists in community integration
4 Caregiving and stroke
- Importance of caregiving
- Challenges in transitioning back into the community
- Supporting stroke survivors, their families, and caregivers
5 Case studies

DOI: 10.4324/9781032721170-13

Stroke

Definition and prevalence

A stroke is an acute focal injury to the central nervous system (CNS) due to a vascular issue which disrupts the supply of oxygen to the brain leading to ischemic damage and death (Gillen & Nilsen, 2020; Sacco et al., 2013).

Globally, stroke is the second leading cause of death and the main cause of acquired disability among adults (Feigin, 2007; Katan & Luft, 2018; Strong et al., 2007). In China, stroke poses a significant health challenge and is ranked the third leading cause of death behind cancer and heart disease (Wang et al., 2020). Compared to Western countries such as Europe, America, and Australia, stroke is a severe problem in Asia as it has a higher average mortality rate (Abduboriyevna & Yusufjonovich, 2018). Within the next 15 years, the burden of stroke due to illness, disability, and mortality is set to double worldwide (Feigin et al., 2014).

Epidemiology studies on stroke revealed various levels of mortality, incidence, prevalence, and burden in Asian countries (Turana et al., 2021). For instance, mortality rate and stroke burden were ranked lowest in Japan, at 43.3 per 100,000 person-years (burden 706.6/100,000 people), and Singapore at 47.9 per 100,000 person-years (burden 804.2/100,000 people). In contrast, Indonesia and Mongolia ranked the highest with a rate of 193.3 per 100,000 person-years (burden 3382.2/100,000 people) and 222.6 per 100,000 person-years (burden 4409.8/100,000 people), respectively (Venketasubramanian et al., 2017).

Besides mortality, stroke incurs a substantial economic burden, which varies in Asian countries (Evers et al., 2004). A recent review revealed that stroke management costs varied in three Southeast Asian countries, namely Indonesia, Malaysia, and Singapore (Wijaya et al., 2019). The stroke cost was $135.55 per daycare (3.88% of GDP per capita) in Indonesia, $227.53 per daycare (2.11% of GDP per capita) in Malaysia, and $366.76 per daycare (0.65% of GDP per capita) in Singapore (Wijaya et al., 2019). An evidence-based clinical stroke pathway helps to optimize the healthcare finance system (Wijaya et al., 2019) and reduce unnecessary stroke expenditure. In addition, to reduce stroke-related disabilities, stroke prevention and effective rehabilitation play a pivotal role. Apart from stroke, a transient ischemic attack (TIA) is another condition that warrants medical emergency. TIA is defined as a transient disruption of the tissue blood supply causing ischemia, showing clinical symptoms of stroke with a subsequent resolution within 24 hours (Edmans, 2010; Gillen & Nilsen, 2020). TIA is not considered a stroke but indicates a vital warning of an impending stroke (Panuganti et al., 2022; Solenski, 2004). After TIA, the 90-day risk is estimated to be 10%, with the highest risk of up to 50% occurring within 48 hours (Panuganti et al., 2022; Solenski, 2004). Therefore, rapid evaluation and early intervention of TIA are critical for future stroke prevention (Solenski, 2004).

Risk factors of stroke

Close to three-quarters of stroke risk is attributable to modifiable risk factors (Eastwood et al., 2015; Kim et al., 2016). These modifiable risk factors are hypertension, smoking, hyperlipidemia, and diabetes mellitus (O'Donnell et al., 2010). In the last two decades, reducing these modifiable risk factors reduced the incidence of stroke and disability-adjusted life-years (DALYs) (Katan & Luft, 2018).

Description of stroke and stroke syndromes

Strokes can be classified into two broad categories: ischemic and hemorrhagic. 80% of all strokes are ischemic, while the remaining 20% are caused by hemorrhagic stroke (Roth, 2007).

Ischemic stroke

Ischemic stroke occurs when there is an interruption of the cerebral blood supply to part of the brain, resulting in dysfunction initially and then tissue anoxia or death (infarct) (Edmans, 2010; Gillen & Nilsen, 2020). The Circle of Willis (Figure 9.1) is the vascular network that provides constant and regular blood flow to the brain and protects the brain from ischemia (Oumer et al., 2021). An ischemic stroke occurs when there is an occlusion of the blood vessels of the Circle of Willis that disrupts cerebral blood circulation. It is critical to identify the location of the occlusion to understand the potential areas of brain tissue damage as a result of the ischemia.

The Oxfordshire Community Stroke Project (OCSP) clinical classification is commonly used to classify ischemic stroke based on the signs and symptoms that clients experience (Bamford et al., 1991). This classification tool is used to predict the clinical outcomes of stroke and recommend management decisions (Yang et al., 2016). Table 9.1 outlines each subtype under the OCSP.

Apart from clinically classifying stroke with the OCSP, the causes of the cerebral infarct are classified using the Trial of Org 10172 in Acute Stroke Treatment (TOAST; see Table 9.2).

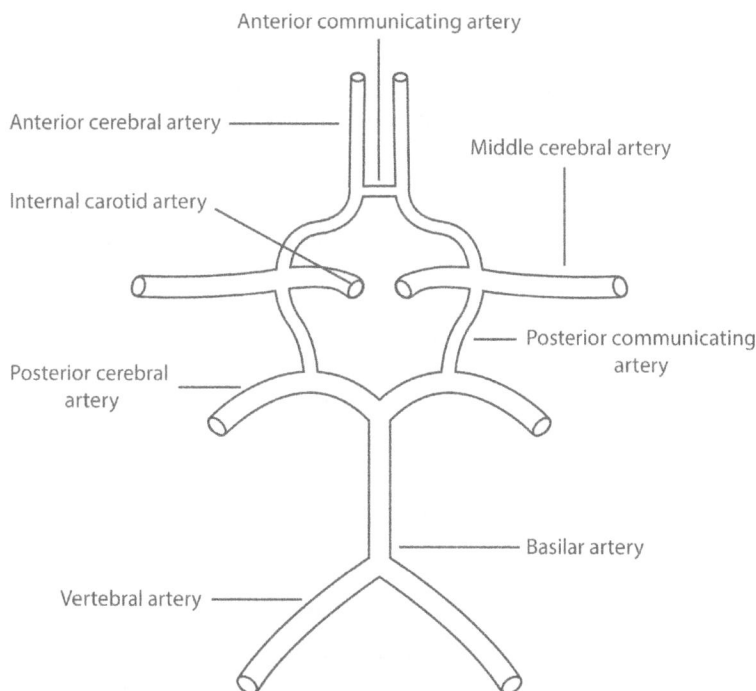

Figure 9.1 The Circle of Willis and cerebral circulation, where occlusion of the vessels can occur in an ischemic stroke

Table 9.1 Description of each subtype under the OCSP (Edmans, 2010; Warlow, 2006)

OCSP classification

Type	*Feature*	*Usual cause and prognosis*
Total anterior circulation infarct (TACI)	Presents with higher cortical dysfunction* (i.e., dysphasia), neglect, homonymous visual field deficit (hemianopia), and motor or sensory loss affecting more than two-thirds of the face, arms, and legs.	Infarct involving the large middle cerebral artery due to embolism or thrombosis with a high chance of mortality and severity of the disability.
Partial anterior circulation infarct (PACI)	Presents two out of three components of TACI, with higher cortical dysfunction alone or more restricted motor or sensory deficit (i.e., confined to one limb or hand and face).	Smaller infarct with similar causes as TACI. Have a better prognosis for recovery but a high risk of early recurrence.
Lacunar infarct (LACI)	Consists of four syndrome types: (1) Pure motor hemiparesis due to infarct in the posterior limb of internal capsule or pons; (2) Pure sensory stroke due to infarct in the ventrolateral of the thalamus; (3) Ataxic hemiparesis due to infarct in the base of the pons or genu of the internal capsule; and (4) Sensorimotor due to infarct at the junction of internal capsule and thalamus.	Small deep infarct related to small vessel disease. Have a relatively good prognosis in recovery.
Posterior circulation infarct (POCI)	Presents brainstem signs or cerebellar dysfunctions with any of the following: ■ Ipsilateral cranial nerve palsy with contralateral motor or sensory deficit; ■ Bilateral motor or sensory deficit; ■ Disorder of conjugate eye movement; ■ Cerebellar dysfunction without ipsilateral long-tract deficit (i.e., ataxic hemiparesis); and ■ Isolated homonymous visual field deficit.	Infarct in the posterior cerebral hemisphere, brainstem, or cerebellum due to small or large vessel diseases or embolism. Prognosis varies depending on causes and location.

Note: *Disorders of higher cortical dysfunction refer to aphasia, decreased level of consciousness, neglect, apraxia, and agnosia syndromes (Edmans, 2010).

Table 9.2 Types of TOAST classification (Adams et al., 1993; Warlow, 2006)

Type	Description	Occurrence
(1) Large artery atherosclerosis	Involves occlusion of the internal carotid or middle cerebral arteries by embolus or thrombus.	35%
(2) Cardioembolism	Clots originating from the heart migrate to the cerebral arteries causing blockage and stroke.	24%
(3) Small vessel occlusion	Refers to lacunar infarct caused by a thrombus or embolus in the smaller cerebral arteries.	18%
(4) Stroke of other determined etiology	Includes rare causes such as vasculopathy, hypercoagulable states, or hematologic disorder.	18%
(5) Stroke of undetermined etiology	Involves either of the following: ■ Two or more causes identified; ■ Negative evaluation; and ■ Incomplete evaluation.	5%

In ischemic stroke, three common subtypes include:

■ Embolic stroke;
■ Thrombotic stroke; and
■ Lacunar.

Cerebral embolic stroke

Cerebral embolic stroke is caused by an embolism of a clot in the cerebral arteries coming from other parts of the arterial system (Thomas et al., 2000). Emboli originating from cardiac lesions account for the most common types of embolic stroke (Gillen & Nilsen, 2020). The cardiac lesions can occur at the heart valves or cavities or due to rhythm disturbances causing a blood clot to form blood clotting within the heart, often seen in atrial fibrillation (Thomas et al., 2000).

Thrombotic cerebral infarct

This type of stroke results from occlusion at the main atherosclerotic lesion or embolism from this site to more distal cerebral arteries (Thomas et al., 2000). Another cause is arterial dissection (Gillen & Nilsen, 2020). For instance, a small tear develops in the artery's wall, allowing a thrombus to form, and the thrombus can be a source of emboli or large enough to occlude the whole vessel. Infarct of the large vessels is commonly involved in arterial dissections and is a common cause of stroke among the younger population (e.g., under 50 years old) (Gillen & Nilsen, 2020).

Hemorrhagic conversion is a complication after an ischemic cerebral infarct. It occurs when thrombi migrate, lyse, and reperfuse into the ischemic area, leading to small hemorrhages as the damaged capillaries and vessels lose their integrity (Gillen & Nilsen, 2020). These damaged areas coalesce and form a hemorrhage into ischemic tissue (Kistler et al., 1994).

Lacunar infarct

This infarct refers to small deep infarcts that occur in small perforating branches of the Circle of Willis, the middle cerebral artery stem, or the vertebral or basilar arteries. Occlusion in these vessels is due to a local disease of these vessels mainly related to chronic hypertension and diabetic microvascular disease (Thomas et al., 2000).

Hemorrhagic stroke

There are four common types of hemorrhagic stroke:

■ Deep hypertensive intracerebral hemorrhage;
■ Ruptured saccular aneurysm;
■ Bleeding from an arteriovenous malformation (AVM); and
■ Spontaneous lobar hemorrhage.

(Kistler et al., 1994)

Hypertensive cerebral hemorrhage

This type of stroke refers to a hemorrhage developing from penetrating arteries in the brain's deep structures, which have been damaged by hypertension (Gillen & Nilsen, 2020). Four common sites where hypertensive cerebral hemorrhage occurs are the putamen and internal capsule, pons, thalamus, and cerebellum (Gillen & Nilsen, 2020). Table 9.3 describes the syndromes of the four major types of hypertensive intracerebral hemorrhage.

Table 9.3 Description of the syndromes of the four major types of hypertensive intracerebral hemorrhage (adapted from Gillen & Nilsen, 2020)

Type	Structure involved	Clinical syndrome
Putamen	Internal capsule and basal ganglia	■ Contralateral hemiplegia ■ Eyes deviate away from the lesion ■ In severe cases, it leads to decerebrate rigidity, coma, or stupor
Thalamic	Thalamus and internal capsule	■ Contralateral hemiplegia ■ Prominent contralateral sensory deficit ■ Aphasia if the dominant (left) thalamus is involved ■ Homonymous hemianopia ■ Gaze palsy ■ Horner syndrome ■ Eyes deviate downward
Pontine	Pons, brainstem, and midbrain	■ May lead to locked-in syndrome and quadriplegia ■ In severe cases, it leads to coma, decerebrate rigidity, severe acute hypertension, and death
Cerebellar	Cerebellum	■ Nausea and vomiting ■ Ataxia ■ Vertigo or dizziness ■ Occipital headache ■ Gaze toward the lesion ■ Occasional dysarthria and dysphagia

Ruptured saccular aneurysm

Subarachnoid hemorrhage (SAH) is usually due to rupturing of the saccular aneurysm at the large arteries' bifurcations on the brain's inferior surface and is most commonly found in the anterior portion of the Circle of Willis (Kistler et al., 1994; Thomas et al., 2000). SAH is characterized by an acute, abrupt onset of atypical severe headache, brief loss of consciousness, nausea and vomiting, focal deficits, and a stiff neck at onset (Gillen & Nilsen, 2020; Mayberg et al., 1994).

Spontaneous intracerebral hemorrhage due to arteriovenous malformation

AVM is present at birth, and bleeding occurs in the second and third decades of life (Gillen & Nilsen, 2020). Larger AVMs in the brain are commonly found in the posterior portions of the cerebral hemispheres (Gillen & Nilsen, 2020). Common symptoms of spontaneous intracerebral hemorrhage include hemiplegia, headache, and seizures (Gillen & Nilsen, 2020).

Spontaneous lobar intracerebral hemorrhage

This is an intracerebral hemorrhage that occurs outside the basal ganglia and thalamus in the white matter of the cerebral cortex in the brain (Gillen & Nilsen, 2020). AVM is commonly associated with the cause of this type of hemorrhage, and other associated conditions include brain tumors, aneurysms, and bleeding diatheses (Fisher, 1975).

Medical investigations following stroke

After a stroke or TIA, medical investigations are performed to diagnose the stroke, determine the site and type of stroke, establish the cause(s) of stroke, and guide treatment to prevent further recurrent stroke (Edmans, 2010). Table 9.4 describes the types of medical investigation, and Figure 9.2 summarizes the pathways for ischemic stroke investigation after ruling out hemorrhage from a brain scan.

Table 9.4 Description of the types of medical investigation

Medical investigation	*Structure involved*	*Purpose*
(1) Computerized tomography (CT) and magnetic resonance imaging (MRI)	Brain	■ Diagnose stroke. ■ Determine site and type of stroke.
(2) Magnetic resonance angiography (MRA)	Blood vessels in the brain	■ Determine causes and site of stroke.
(3) Electrocardiography (ECG) and echocardiography	Heart	■ Determine causes of stroke. ■ Identify and rule out other medical complications.
(4) Transcranial and carotid Doppler	Blood vessels in the brain and neck	■ Determine causes and site of stroke. ■ Guide treatment for further prevention, such as reducing stenosis.
(5) Blood tests	–	■ Serve as standard evaluation to rule out other causes of stroke-like symptoms to aid in diagnosis. ■ Guide treatment.

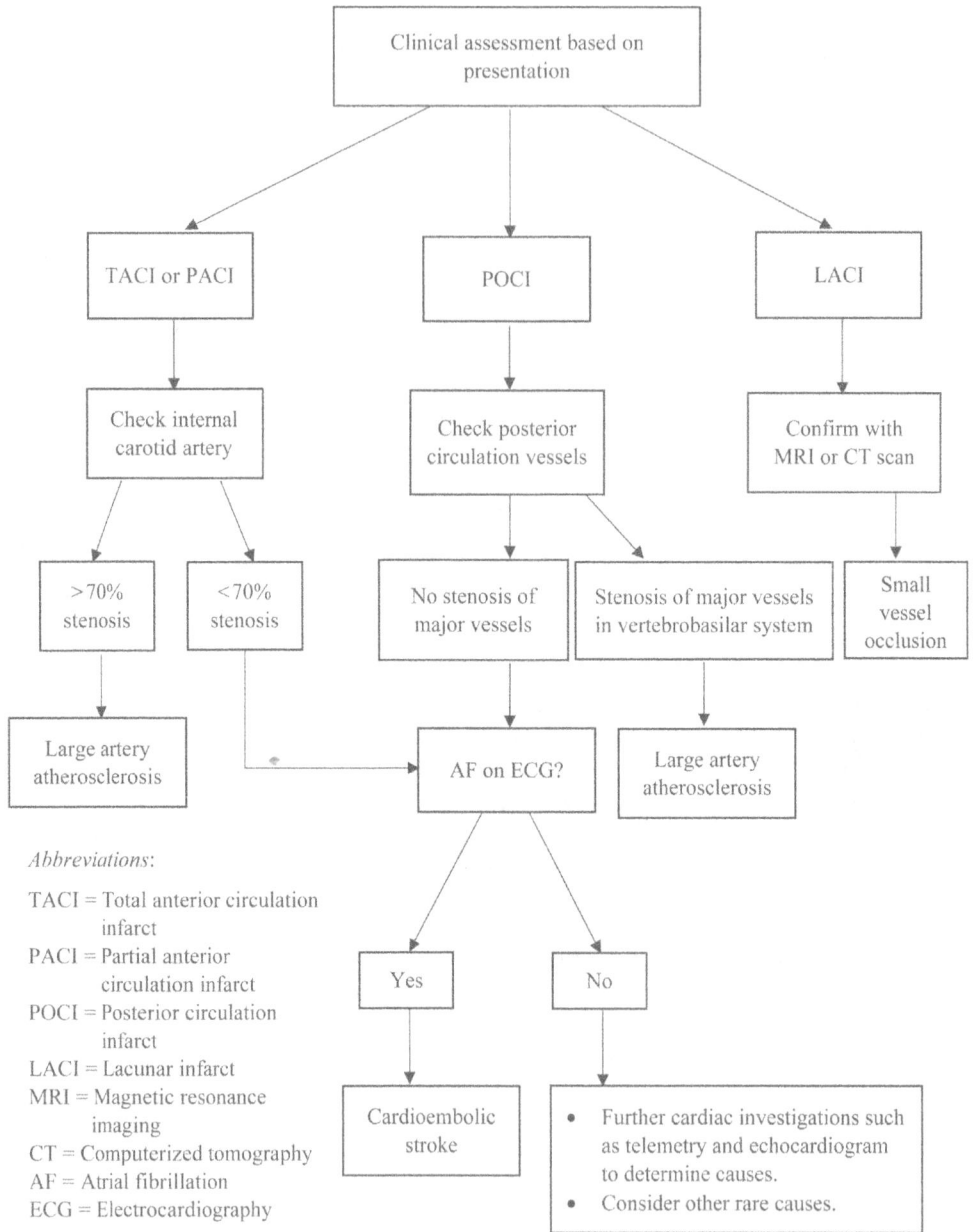

Figure 9.2 Summary of the pathways for ischemic stroke investigation after ruling out hemorrhage from a brain scan (adapted from Warlow, 2006)

Description of medical investigations following stroke

Computerized tomography and magnetic resonance imaging
Radiological imaging techniques such as computerized tomography (CT) and magnetic resonance imaging (MRI) are used to determine the site of the stroke and detect if the stroke is caused by a cerebral infarct or hemorrhage. It is critical to distinguish if the

stroke is ischemic or hemorrhagic in nature. The medical treatment differs between these two types of stroke. For instance, the use of antiplatelets (i.e., aspirin) or anti-coagulants is indicative for ischemic stroke but is a contraindication for hemorrhage. The Intercollegiate Stroke Working Party (2008) recommended performing a CT scan for all clients within 24 hours of stroke. A CT scan is useful to identify intracranial hemorrhages and rule out other intracranial pathologies that mimic strokes, such as tumors and subdural hematoma (Edmans, 2010). Stroke caused by large vessel occlusion can usually be detected by a CT scan, but this is not sensitive enough to detect smaller infarcts (Edmans, 2010). MRI is more sensitive to detecting earlier and smaller infarcts (Gillen & Nilsen, 2020) and is more suitable than a CT scan for scanning the brainstem and cerebellum surrounded by dense, bony structures (Edmans, 2010). In addition, MRI is also used to estimate the extent of ischemic penumbra, which is essential information to determine if the client is a suitable candidate for a mechanical thrombectomy (Gillen & Nilsen, 2020).

Magnetic resonance angiography

Magnetic resonance angiography (MRA) is used to detect any vascular abnormalities that may cause stroke or look for alteration of cerebral blood flow caused by an embolus or thrombus (Gillen & Nilsen, 2020). This procedure displays 3D reconstructions of arterial and venous cerebral circulations that help to identify if the stroke is caused by a thrombus, arterial stenosis resulting in occlusion, or dissection (Edmans, 2010).

Electrocardiography and echocardiography

Electrocardiography (ECG) is used to detect cardiac arrhythmia (i.e., atrial fibrillation) or myocardial infarct related to stroke (Gillen & Nilsen, 2020). The cardiac arrhythmia could account for the source of an embolism resulting in a stroke (Gillen & Nilsen, 2020). Cardiac diseases that might cause an embolic stroke include congestive heart failure, valvular disease, atrial fibrillation, and a recent myocardial infarct (Gillen & Nilsen, 2020). Echocardiography may be performed when an intracardiac thrombus or structural disease of the heart is suspected (Edmans, 2010).

Transcranial and carotid Doppler

Carotid Doppler ultrasound is usually performed to screen for any stenosis of the internal carotid Doppler. This technique involves imaging the artery and measuring blood flow velocity to estimate the degree of vessel stenosis (Edmans, 2010). It is recommended that clients with posterior circulation stroke should be tested with a transcranial Doppler scan to examine the vertebrobasilar system (Gillen & Nilsen, 2020).

Blood tests

Blood test screening constitutes part of a standard acute evaluation of a client with stroke. The blood tests aim to rule out other causes of stroke-like symptoms, diagnose complications, and allow a baseline analysis before initiating therapies such as anticoagulation (Gillen & Nilsen, 2020). The tests include full blood count, erythrocyte sedimentation rate (ESR), blood sugar, fasting lipids, clotting, and thrombophilia (Edmans, 2010). Table 9.5 describes the purposes of each blood test.

Table 9.5 Purposes of each blood test (adapted from Edmans, 2010)

Blood test	Purpose
Full blood count	■ Rule out any systematic infection such as aspiration pneumonia reflected from the raised white blood cells. ■ Investigate blood abnormalities that may predispose to stroke, such as polycythemia (increased red blood cells), thrombocytosis (increased platelets), and thrombocytopenia (reduced number of platelets).
Erythrocyte sedimentation rate	■ If this marker is raised, this may indicate infection, vasculitis, or carcinoma, which warrants further investigation.
Blood sugar	■ Screen for diabetes mellitus, which is a risk factor for stroke.
Fasting lipids	■ Screen for hyperlipidemia, which is one of the stroke risk factors.
Clotting screening	■ Coagulation tests are necessary for clients with hemorrhagic stroke. ■ For stroke clients who take warfarin, titration of the medication requires the international normalized ratio (INR) to be checked regularly.
Thrombophilia screen	■ The hereditary tendency toward blood clotting should be checked for clients who present with venous sinus thrombosis. ■ For young clients with arterial thrombosis with no other stroke risk factors identified, this screening should be considered (Hankey et al., 2001).

Most relevant areas affected after stroke

The World Health Organization's International Classification of Functioning, Disability and Health (ICF) model (World Health Organization, 2001) is used to explain the effect of stroke on an individual in areas such as pathology (disease or diagnosis), impairment (symptoms and signs), activity limitations (disability), and participation restriction (handicap). Figure 9.3 describes the relevant areas affected after the stroke.

Role of occupational therapists in stroke rehabilitation

Goal of occupational therapy

The World Federation of Occupational Therapists (2012) defines occupational therapy (OT) as "a client-centred health profession concerned with promoting health and well-being through occupation". Occupational therapists work with individuals to enhance their ability to engage in purposeful activities they want, need, or are expected to do by modifying the activities or environment to better support their engagement (World Federation of Occupational Therapists, 2012).

In stroke rehabilitation, the occupational therapist plays an integral role and is usually part of the multidisciplinary team that provides stroke care. OT treatment starts after a comprehensive assessment with treatment goal setting, which provides the treatment direction. In addition, both short-term and long-term goals in terms of priority

Pathology

Ischemic stroke (80%)
- Syndromes classified under the Oxfordshire Community Stroke Project (OCSP)

Hemorrhagic stroke (15%)
- Intracerebral bleed
- Subarachnoid hemorrhage

Not specific (5%)

Body function and impairment

Bodily functions affected
- Conscious level
- Cognition and perceptual
- Sensation and proprioception
- Muscle power, tone, and control
- Mobility
- Voice and articulation
- Balance and coordination
- Bladder and bowel control
- Sleep and personality

Structures affected
- Brain
- Cardiovascular system
- Upper and lower limbs
- Trunk

Activities (limitation)

Activities affected
- Communication
- Reading, writing, and calculation
- Self-care such as transfer, showering, toileting, dressing, and grooming
- Mobility
- Eating and feeding
- Driving and taking transportation
- Hand and arm use
- Recreation and leisure
- Instrumental ADL (IADL) such as housekeeping, meal preparation, and taking medication
- Work

Participation (restriction)

Restriction to participation
- Social interaction
- Participation in religious activities
- Participation in social and community activities
- Employment

Environmental factors

Personal factors

Contextual factors

Contextual factors (personal and environmental)
- Health professionals, services, system, and policies
- Home environment
- Support and relationship
- Assistive devices

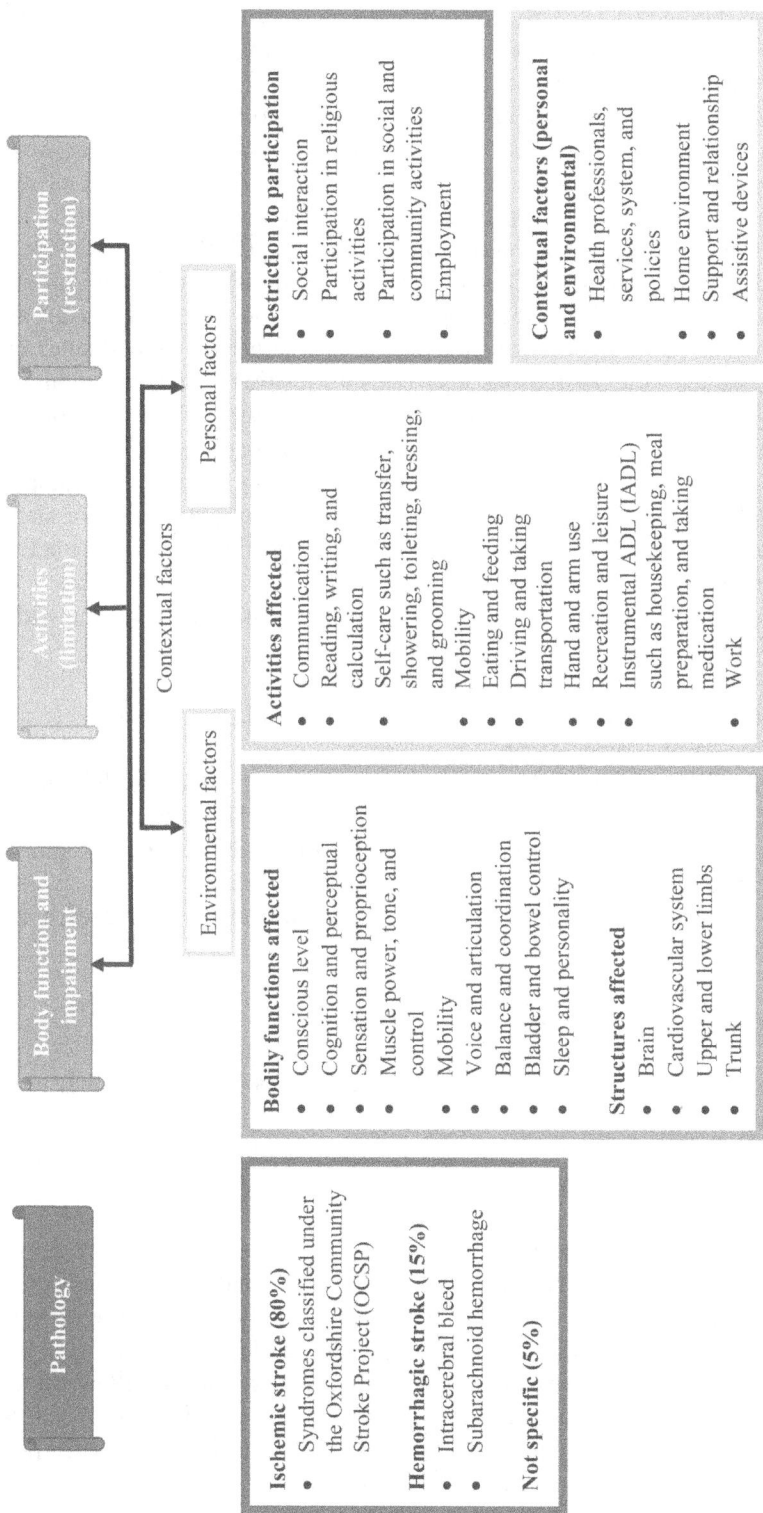

Figure 9.3 Relevant areas affected after stroke (adapted from Langhorne et al., 2011)

are included. The goals need to be completed in collaboration with the clients or caregivers – this is crucial because they need to understand what the OT goals are and why they are being asked to engage in certain activities.

There are commonly two general approaches in OT treatment for stroke: (1) using a top-down or bottom-up approach, or both, and (2) using restoration/maintenance (by means of practice, training, education) or compensation (by means of modification, prevention), or both. The top-down approach focuses on the deficits of the components of function, such as strength, range of motion (ROM), balance, etc., which are believed to be prerequisites to successful occupations. The bottom-up approach starts with inquiry into role competency, meaning, and purpose of the tasks, and then determines which particular tasks define each role, whether the individual can now do those tasks, and, if not, the reasons why (Trombly, 1993). The restoration approach holds that the individual has the potential to restore or establish the previous skills or abilities and resume his/her life routine and habits, or preserve his/her residual skills and abilities from further deterioration in terms of maintenance. The compensation approach makes use of adapting the environment, modifying the object, or altering the task demands and activity methods to allow the individual to perform the activity and task independently (American Occupational Therapy Association, 2014).

To be more specific, the goals of occupational therapists when working with clients with stroke are to (Rowland et al., 2008):

■ Facilitate and improve functional recovery, particularly the motor control and function of the hemiplegic arm;
■ Maximize the client's capability to perform functional tasks in both basic activities of daily living (BADL) and instrumental activities of daily living (IADL);
■ Teach clients with stroke to learn strategies to manage the motor, cognitive, perceptual, and behavioral problems associated with stroke;
■ Prepare and modify the home and work environment for clients with stroke to return to life and work.

In addition, occupational therapists should also:

■ Identify the meaningful and purposeful occupations of the client that need to be addressed; and
■ Help the client return home safely after hospitalization and eventually gain independence from caregivers or family.

Areas of occupational therapy assessment

To achieve these goals, the occupational therapist will conduct assessments to understand how changes in motor, cognitive, and sensory functions affect the client's ability to perform daily tasks after a stroke (Rowland et al., 2008). Based on the findings, the occupational therapist can develop a goal-focused intervention to allow the client to develop skills for participation in daily activities (Rowland et al., 2008). Table 9.6 lists the core areas of OT assessment according to the World Health Organization's ICF framework (World Health Organization, 2001).

Table 9.6 Core areas of OT assessment according to the World Health Organization's ICF framework

ICF dimension	Body function and structure	Activity	Participation	Environment and context
OT assessment areas	■ Vision ■ Visual perception ■ Cognition such as memory, executive skills, and attention ■ Sensorimotor, such as upper limb function, balance, and mobility ■ Psychosocial adjustment	■ Personal self-care or basic activities of daily living (BADLs) ■ Instrumental activities of daily living (IADLs) ■ Leisure ■ Driving ■ Work	■ Occupational roles ■ Community integration ■ Social participation (e.g., community-based activities or spiritual activities) ■ Employment	■ Physical (e.g., home, work) ■ Social (e.g., family, caregiver, friends, or other community support groups) ■ Cultural
Examples of commonly used assessment tools		BADL: ■ Modified Barthel Index (http://functionalpathways.com/intranet-files/Modifet_Barthel_Index.pdf) ■ Functional Independence Measure (https://www.health.wa.gov.au/~/media/Files/Corporate/general-documents/Data-collection/WORD/SANADC_Form_FIM-Medical-Record-Form.docx) IADL: ■ Lawton Instrumental Activities of Daily Living Scale (https://www.alz.org/careplanning/downloads/lawton-iadl.pdf) ■ Frenchay Activities Index (https://www.sralab.org/sites/default/files/2017-06/Frenchay%20Activities%20Index.pdf) Leisure: ■ MOHO Modified Interest Checklist (https://moho-irm.uic.edu/productDetails.aspx?aid=38) ■ Activity Card Sort (https://strokengine.ca/en/assessments/acs/)		

Common treatment approaches in stroke rehabilitation

Adapted one-handed method
This technique is based on the compensation approach, with the overall aim being to improve the independence of the client in his/her BADL and IADL. It involves (1) using the less affected arm or sound side to compensate for the hemiplegic side in performing functional tasks, (2) performing functional tasks in an alternative manner, and (3) finding new and efficient ways of performing functional tasks. Examples include wringing a towel using the less affected hand when grooming, sitting up in bed from the sound side with the support of the less affected arm, transferring to the non-hemiplegic side with less effort, dressing upper and lower garments with the affected side first and then the less affected side, and vice versa when taking off the garments.

Task-specific training
According to recent guidelines for adult stroke rehabilitation and recovery, task-specific training, also known as functional task training, is highly recommended. This approach involves tailoring tasks to challenge individual abilities, practicing them repeatedly, and increasing their difficulty. This recommendation is classified as Class I with Level of Evidence A (Winstein et al., 2016). A careful triage of the upper limb functions should be carried out by the occupational therapist to customize which tasks should be carried out according to the levels of arm impairment. A common tool for this is the Functional Test for the Hemiplegic Upper Extremity (FTHUE), which classifies the level of hemiparetic arm impairment due to stroke from 1 to 7 (Wilson et al., 1984), or, more broadly, into two categories: lower functioning (levels 1–4) and higher functioning (levels 5–7). The FTHUE was developed originally according to Brunnstrom's developmental stages of stroke recovery and has been validated locally in Hong Kong and used extensively for stratification of hemiplegic upper extremities in recent studies (Fong et al., 2004). The advantage of using this scale for task-specific training is that treatment for the arm and hand is considered as one, and that the ultimate treatment goal is to resume arm and hand functions. Repetition is a key element in task-specific training (Waddell et al., 2014). Once the upper limb functions have been stratified, training is customized or tailored individually based on the level of impairment for the training, with repetitions, continuous upgrading or downgrading according to the progress, and generalization to other functional tasks with similar task demands (Jin et al., 2019). However, there is a ceiling effect for this kind of functional scale on clients with higher upper extremity functioning in which the major difficulties are hand clumsiness and reduced finger coordination and manipulation due to hemiparesis. A standardized test on in-hand manipulation (IHM) has been developed to assess fine motor skills required in daily tasks such as writing and money handling since IHM has not been widely represented in upper extremity assessments for stroke (Klymenko et al., 2018). With advances in technology, robotic therapies including the use of end-effectors or exoskeletons incorporated with virtual reality are widely used as an adjunct to task-specific training in order to provide a high dosage of movement practice or intensity of training through repetitive, controllable guided movement with optimal sensory feedbacks (Krebs et al., 2009). Robotic therapies can reduce the time needed for supervising the therapy process, and clients can also learn to practice using the equipment independently at home or in a rehabilitation center (Figure 9.4).

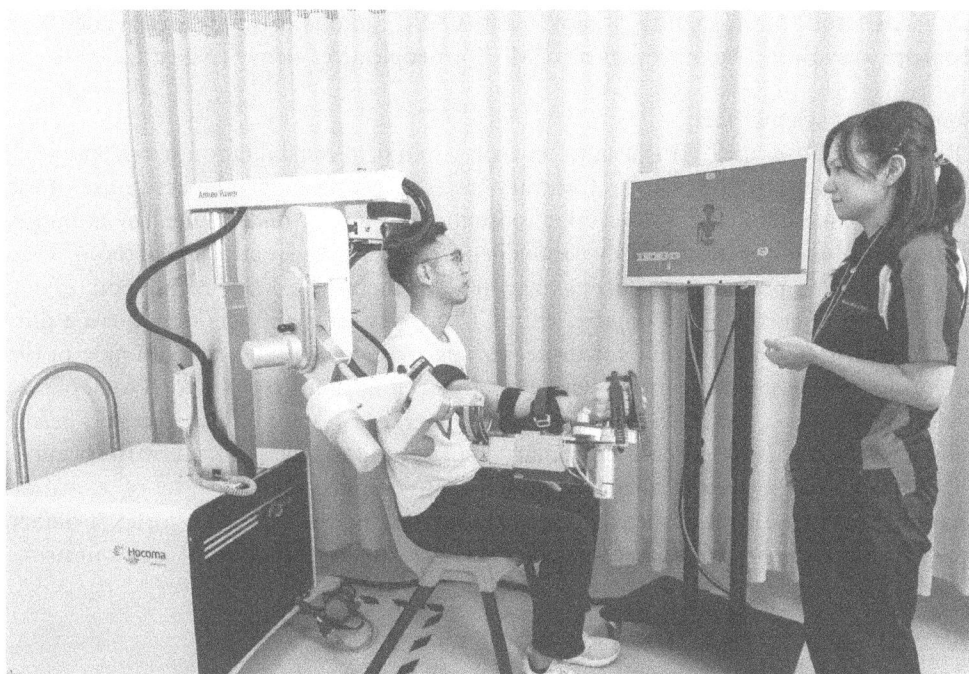

Figure 9.4 An occupational therapist supervising a client during a robotic therapy session in which the client uses an arm exoskeleton to practice virtual reality tasks shown on a screen

Constraint-induced movement therapy

Constraint-induced movement therapy (CIMT) is based on the restoration approach and emphasizes the forced use and intensive practice of the affected arm after hemiplegia, which is opposite to the adapted one-handed method. It is practiced by restraining the less affected arm to allow the individual to overcome "non-use", partly because of the learned or behavioral suppression or pathological neglect of using the hemiplegic arm in ADL (Leung et al., 2009). CIMT involves three elements: (1) repetitive, task-specific training or shaping through successive task approximation step by step with increasing difficulty which can be in the form of individualized or small-group training supervised by occupational therapists, (2) adherence-enhancing behavioral strategies by means of daily administration of the motor activity log (MAL), use of a behavioral contract, home diary, home skill assignment, etc., and (3) a restraint method for the less affected arm using a hand mitt or arm sling for at least five hours per day and a total of two weeks. A local randomized controlled study for CIMT was carried out in Hong Kong, with the results showing that there was significant improvement in hand function after CIMT in subacute stroke clients, which was maintained up to 12 weeks after treatment (Myint et al., 2008). However, CIMT has faced criticism for being primarily suitable for those with higher functioning of the affected arm, and there are safety concerns regarding an increased fall risk due to the restraint used. The MAL is the most representative measure for hand use in real life. It is a questionnaire administered through either a proxy interview or a self-rating by clients that asks how frequently and how well the clients use their impaired upper extremities in 30 ADL tasks over a certain period of time (Uswatte et al., 2006). It can be divided into two subscores: (1) the amount of use (AOU) and (2) the quality of movement (QOM), and is highly recommended as a measure to evaluate the outcomes of CIMT for people after stroke (Ng et al., 2008).

Remind-to-Move method

"Remind-to-Move" (RTM) is a new concept in physical rehabilitation for people with hemiplegia resulting from stroke. Contrary to CIMT, it promotes the active use of the hemiplegic arm following non-use due to hemiplegia and is underpinned by attention theory. RTM involves the use of a wearable sensory cueing device attached to the affected arm designed to promote the client's awareness of the affected side of the body (Fong et al., 2011) (Figure 9.5). Compared with CIMT, it is safer and less odd-looking during outdoor use and is suitable for those with either higher or lower functioning of the affected arm. The client wears the device for about three hours per day for a total of two weeks, and upon a vibration at a fixed-time interval (e.g., ten-minute interval), he/she must move according to a set of customary upper limb tasks determined by the occupational therapist. Previous studies have found that it elicited a higher level of activation than the sham treatment in the contralateral somatosensory association cortex, primary motor cortex, primary somatosensory cortex, and dorsolateral prefrontal cortex in stroke

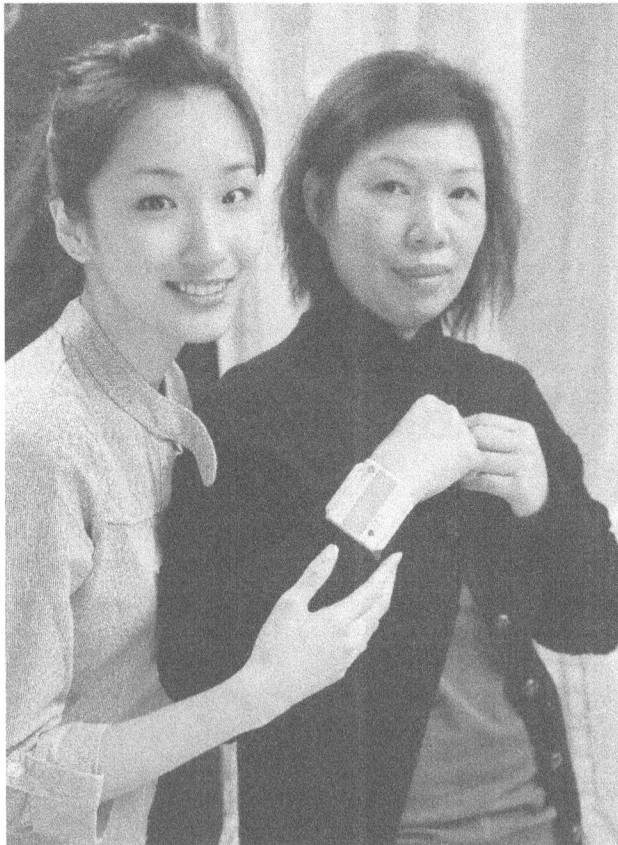

Figure 9.5 An occupational therapist supervising a client dressing upper garment with the use of a sensory cueing device worn over the client's affected arm

participants. In addition, the effect appeared to be associated with increased attention allocation toward moving the hands upon sensory cueing (Bai & Fong, 2020). A sham treatment is like a placebo, where participants experience the same incidental effect as the experimental group (i.e., wearing a wearable device) (Simpson & Weiner, 1989) but do not experience the actual therapeutic benefits (i.e., the wearable device which the sham group wore did not emit any sensory cues). A local randomized controlled trial using RTM in subacute stroke clients demonstrated that RTM via wearable devices used for the hemiplegic upper extremities could promote more arm recovery than the sham or control, and hence produced optimal functional improvement for subacute stroke clients (Wei et al., 2019). This wearable device has been further designed and translated to a telerehabilitation platform called "Smart Reminder" to be used in stroke clients for home-based training by means of reminding clients to follow graded ROM exercises customized by occupational therapists (Toh et al., 2023; Toh et al., 2025).

Bimanual arm training

Bimanual arm training (BAT) is defined as a training approach where the two upper limbs are moved simultaneously and symmetrically (i.e., following similar spatiotemporal trajectories). This approach varies from both CIMT and RTM, which encourage clients to use the affected arm more. The BAT hypothesis is that during unilateral movement, the ipsilateral hemisphere is inhibited through the corpus callosum between the two hemispheres. However, there is an interhemispheric disinhibition in the CNS when both arms are moved simultaneously, meaning that less attention or energy is allocated for executing a simultaneous bilateral movement, which allows for activation of the undamaged hemisphere to facilitate the activation of the damaged hemisphere (Hayner et al., 2010). Although recent studies show that BAT is no more effective than unilateral training in terms of overall improvement in the dexterity of the affected arm, it is more useful for improving the power of the affected arm, particularly in clients with lower arm function (Morris et al., 2008; Wu et al., 2011).

Mental imagery

Mental imagery (MI) is a top-down training method that makes use of mentally practicing the body movement required for specific bodily actions during functional tasks when field practice is not feasible. More importantly, it does not require actual motor practice. This method has been proven to provide additional benefits to conventional OT (Zimmermann-Schlatter et al., 2008). It is commonly used in combination with the actual motor practice of functional tasks to improve overall functional recovery and achieve faster generalization. For people with stroke who cannot physically move their limbs, MI offers the benefit of activating brain regions similar to actual movement (Kho et al., 2014). There are two approaches of practicing MI: (1) first-person motor imagery (FPMI) – a person imagines performing the movement from inside their body, and (2) third-person motor imagery (TPMI) – a person imagines performing the movement from the outside of their body or imagines someone else performing the movement (Welage et al., 2023). Both approaches are feasible for hemiparetic upper extremity and ADL training in people with stroke, but individuals may feel more motivated to learn when they visualize a successful task completion from a third-person perspective (Welage et al., 2023). MI comprises three steps: task analysis enhancement, problem identification, and task performance. The process involves getting the client to identify the task steps by mentally imagining the task, visualizing his/her own performance with the help of visual feedback (video recording), and repeating the task until he/she completes it using the proper method (Liu et al., 2004). Visualization or action observation has been hypothesized to prime the motor cortex to elicit the mirror neuron system even without overt movement execution, thereby promoting motor relearning and contributing to stroke motor recovery (Zhang et al., 2018). A local randomized controlled trial demonstrated that MI intervention was effective in improving clients' ability to perform tasks for which they had not previously trained and in environments that differed from their training settings. This involved the generalization of skills learned at the task performance level (Liu et al., 2009).

Community integration after stroke

Community integration

Community integration after stroke is considered a sign of progressive recovery (Lindsay et al., 2014) and an essential goal of rehabilitation (Tipnis et al., 2021). Poor community integration has been associated with depression, reduced quality of life (Wood et al., 2010), and life satisfaction (Aström et al., 1992) among individuals with stroke. While it is important to address issues related to ADL, mobility, and communication as soon as possible after stroke, there is also a need for continued rehabilitation in terms of community integration, which includes social competency and participation, community mobility, self-management of health, employment, and education (Duncan et al., 2005; Tipnis et al., 2021).

McColl et al. (2001) define community integration as "being happily situated, productively occupied and effectively supported in the community". Successful community integration involves active participation in the community, having independence, maintaining relationships, and engaging in meaningful activities (Tipnis et al., 2021). Community reintegration refers to "returning to the community following an absence due to illness, injury or traumatic event" (Scaffa & Reitz, 2013). According to McColl et al. (1998), there are four components of community integration: assimilation, social support, occupation, and independent living. Table 9.7 describes these components.

Cultural factors and environmental influence

From the OT perspective, an individual's occupation is shaped by his/her environments and contexts, which include human or non-human, physical, social, and cultural environments. People make choices about their occupations, which reflect their circumstances and perceived occupational opportunities at that particular time and in the context of one's physical and social environments (Schell et al., 2014). In stroke recovery, the manner of caregiving (social environment) and the form of environmental support are two key factors determining whether the client is able to return home safely and successfully. In a recent study of an early supported discharge program for mild-to-moderate subacute stroke clients in Singapore, it was found that having social problems was a negative predictor of long-term return-to-work, while being the breadwinner was a positive predictor of return-to-work at five-year follow-up (Teo et al., 2022). The facilitators of a successful return-to-work at five-year follow-up for stroke clients of working age are: support from

Table 9.7 Four components of community integration

***

Assimilation

- Conformity: Fitting in with other people; knowing the rules.
- Orientation: Knowing how to navigate the community; being familiar with one's surroundings.
- Acceptance: Being comfortable in the community; feeling understood and acknowledged.

Social support

- Close relationships: Feeling connected and in close proximity with family and friends; engaged in relationships that are important, meaningful, intimate, reciprocal, and mutual.
- Diffuse relationships: Interacting with others in the community, neighbors, service providers, and co-workers.

Occupation

- Leisure: Participating in social and recreational activities with others in the community.
- Productivity: Contributing to society or family, having a sense of purpose, engaged in employment, education, or volunteer work.

Independent living

- Personal independence: Experiencing autonomy; having some control over one's life and choices.
- Satisfaction with the living situation: Living in a place where they can be autonomous; living independently outside an institution.

***

family and friends, financial factors such as having to support the family, and support from employers and co-workers (Teo et al., 2022). Another key concern for stroke clients successfully returning to the home and community is the cultural factor. Cultural influences shape our beliefs, attitudes, values, and goals, etc. In terms of caregiving, people of East Asian culture tend to reach a state of interdependence among their family members rather than reaching a goal of independence for health and well-being. This means they value connections with others in the family, which are shaped by intra-family relationships (Kitayama et al., 2010; Ng et al., 2015). In East Asia, individuals and groups shape their communities. Indeed, it is common practice in East Asian families for the client to be taken care of by one of the family members, and that being a caregiver seems to be an obligatory role for them in big families. On the contrary, Western culture is more individualized, and clients aim to either reach their independence goals at home without caregivers' support or eventually resettle in residential care institutions.

Challenges in community integration after stroke

Community integration has been deemed challenging for most stroke survivors. Nearly two-thirds of individuals with stroke reported having restrictions in reintegrating into the community at six months after stroke (Mayo et al., 2002). Another study found that 83% of stroke participants faced restrictions in participating in daily occupations such as work, housework, leisure, and social activities three to six months after stroke (Bergström et al., 2015). Previous research suggests that environmental limitations in the community influence stroke survivors' willingness to go outdoors (Barnsley et al., 2012; Lennon et al., 2013), and individuals with stroke will consciously adapt their participation in valued activities according to these limitations (Robison et al., 2009).

The following shows the physical environmental barriers faced by stroke survivors in the literature.

At home

- Narrow doorways
- Stairs and steps
- Absence of handrails
- Heavy doors
- Limited space to move around
- Poorly designed shower and toilet (i.e., bathtub or curbs)
- Squat toilet

(Brookfield et al., 2015; Reid, 2004; Schulz et al., 2012)

Outdoors

- Uneven surfaces
- Absence of handrails
- Stairs and steps
- Narrow walkways
- Absence of lifts or narrow lift doors

(Reid, 2004)

The occurrence of falls is another major complication after stroke (Tilson et al., 2012) that impedes community integration. Prevalence of falls during the first six months post-hospitalization is high, ranging from 36% to 73% (Alemdaroğlu et al., 2012; Forster & Young, 1995; Mackintosh et al., 2006). A study in Hong Kong showed that the prevalence of falls among people suffering from chronic stroke with mild-to-moderate disabilities who had been discharged from hospital for over one year was 52.6%, of which 58% of falls occurred indoors and 42% occurred outdoors. The activities preceding the fall in order of priority were walking, transitioning body posture, and going upstairs or downstairs (Chan & Fong, 2013). Those who had visual acuity impairment were more likely to have multiple falls. In contrast, those living with spousal support and better balance were less likely to have multiple falls (Chan & Fong, 2013). A study in Singapore showed that the risk factors of falls in community stroke survivors were balance, mobility problems, the need for self-care assistance, taking sedative or psychotropic medications, cognitive impairment, depression, and a history of previous falls (Xu et al., 2018). Screening for falls should be a component of routine clinical care for individuals with stroke (Xu et al., 2018). In addition to home safety, fall prevention programs should address self-care activities and participation in the community (Xu et al., 2018). According to the updated international guidelines on falls, evidence for home environment assessment and intervention by occupational therapists as part of a multifactorial fall prevention program for older people is considered very strong, i.e., grade A evidence (Panel on Prevention of Falls in Older Persons, American Geriatrics Society and British Geriatrics Society, 2011; Montero-Odasso et al., 2022). A meta-analysis study found that environmental interventions had a significant effect on reducing 39% falls among older people at high risk (Clemson et al., 2008).

Other than physical environmental limitations and risk of falls, individuals with stroke and their caregivers face several issues relating to community integration. These are described in Table 9.8.

Table 9.8 Difficulties faced during community integration

Components of community integration (McColl et al., 1998)	Issues and difficulties faced by stroke survivors and their families

Assimilation
 	
■ Conformity to the social environment
■ Orientation to one's surroundings
■ Acceptance within the community
	■ Limitation in community mobility[a]:
	  ■ Difficulty in using previously used public transport and need to change the mode of public transport used.
	  ■ Driving disruption.[b]
	  ■ Need for assistive devices such as a walking aid, manual or motorized wheelchair to commute in the community.
	  ■ Negotiating environmental barriers such as steps, narrow walkways, and a lack of ramps (Figure 9.6).
	  ■ Reliance on others for outdoor mobility and when taking public transport.
	  (Liang et al., 2017b; Stahl & Lexell, 2018)
	■ Reduced participation in community-based activities (i.e., wellness center, social club, support group).

Social support ■ Close relationships with families, friends, and caregivers ■ Diffuse relationships with service providers, neighbors, and co-workers	■ Difficulty in coping with support care by caregivers, risk of burnout, and loss of autonomy. ■ Managing changes in service providers during the transition phases of various stages of recovery. ■ Navigating community-based health services to address ongoing rehabilitation needs. ■ Reduced social interaction with friends.
Occupation ■ Leisure ■ Productivity	■ Inability to return to previous work or return to gainful employment. ■ Reduced participation in leisure and social activities.
Independent living ■ Personal independence ■ Satisfaction with current living arrangement	■ Reliance on others' assistance in self-care and IADL due to residual impairment and low self-efficacy (Korpershoek et al., 2011), resulting in reduced social and community participation. ■ Changes in living arrangements, such as living with a foreign domestic worker (FDW) (as caregiver). ■ Participation in community rehabilitation services dependent on caregiver's or family's availability to accompany.

Notes:

[a] Community mobility refers to "moving around in the community using public or private transportation such as driving, walking, taking buses, taxis or other transportation" (American Occupational Therapy Association, 2008, p. 631).

[b] Driving disruption refers to a temporary interruption or permanent driving cessation that occurs following an acquired brain injury (Liang et al., 2017a).

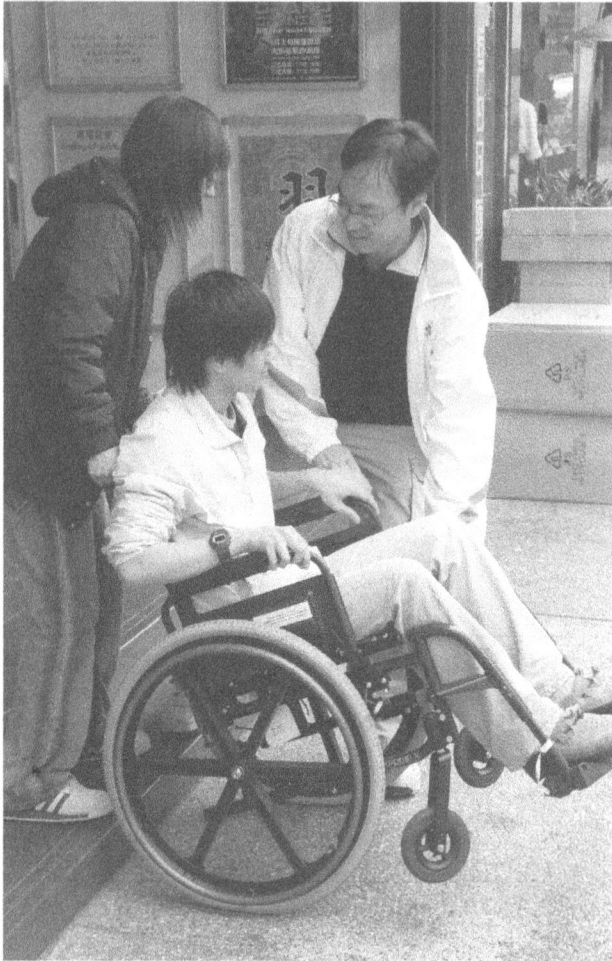

Figure 9.6 An occupational therapist educating a caregiver on how to negotiate a wheelchair up and down an outdoor curb

Role of occupational therapists in community integration

Before the stroke client is discharged back home, the occupational therapist needs to consider the home accessibility of the client. Stroke individuals with residual disability face environmental barriers to moving around in and outside their homes and performing ADL (Scaffa & Reitz, 2013). Based on the stroke client's home environment, the therapist may recommend home modifications (e.g., ramps, widened doorways, grab bar installation, and removal of steps and curbs) to increase accessibility and promote independence and quality of life (Scaffa & Reitz, 2013). The occupational therapist plays an important role in facilitating community integration, working with the stroke client to identify the appropriate context for daily living, work, leisure, and social participation (Scaffa & Reitz, 2013). In addition, the therapist conducts evaluations to determine the client's occupational history, goals, and current level of function to maximize his/her potential for successful community integration (Scaffa & Reitz, 2013).

Table 9.9 Role of occupational therapists in supporting stroke survivors to reintegrate back into the community

Community integration	What occupational therapists can do
(1) Assimilation	<ul><li>Train clients in community mobility to navigate their surroundings.</li><li>Prescribe mobility aids (e.g., a scooter, motorized wheelchair, etc.) if necessary.</li><li>Work with community service providers (e.g., befrienders, senior activity centers, or wellness centers) near clients' homes to support clients' social participation.</li></ul>
(2) Social support	<ul><li>Educate clients and their families on available community services, support groups, and other stroke-related resources.</li><li>Assess the psychosocial needs of clients and caregivers such as burnout. Provide timely intervention or referral to appropriate professionals to address these needs.</li></ul>
(3) Occupation	<ul><li>Assess and identify with clients the desired leisure and social activities to work on.</li><li>Rehabilitate clients to develop skills to engage in desired leisure and social activities.</li><li>Assess the vocational needs of clients and rehabilitate them to return to work or school.</li></ul>
(4) Independent living	<ul><li>Conduct home assessments and modifications to improve accessibility.</li><li>Work with clients to identify and use alternative public transportation if clients are unable to resume using the previous mode of transportation (e.g., driving).</li><li>Conduct community mobility training in using public transport.</li><li>Educate clients and caregivers on the risk factors of falls, including cognitive and psychosocial aspects (Xu et al., 2018).</li></ul>

Table 9.9 outlines the role of occupational therapists in supporting stroke survivors to reintegrate back into the community.

In conclusion, occupational therapists play a vital role in helping stroke survivors regain functional skills and adapt to long-term impairments, facilitating their reintegration back into their communities (Scaffa & Reitz, 2013). They work with stroke clients, families, agencies, and communities to promote independent living and active participation of clients and conduct accessibility assessments in the clients' living spaces.

Caregiving and stroke

Importance of caregiving

Over half of individuals with stroke face residual impairments in their physical, cognitive, and sensory functions after being discharged from the hospital (Langhorne et al., 2009; Thom et al., 2006). These individuals require assistance in managing their ADL and with follow-up medical and rehabilitation services after being discharged. Often, they are reliant on their caregivers and families to provide personal and medical-orientated care. Hence, caregivers play a significant role in the support of stroke survivors. Hermanns and Mastel-Smith (2012) defined caregiving as "the process of helping another person who is unable to do for themselves in a 'holistic' (physically, mentally, emotionally, and socially) manner".

There are various types of caregiving, such as paid, unpaid, or both. Unpaid caregiving usually comprises families, friends, and community (e.g., faith-based and informal peer support) (Tyagi et al., 2021). There are two common types of unpaid caregiving: spouse and adult–child caregivers (Tyagi et al., 2021). Other types include sibling and distant relative caregivers. Paid caregiving refers to foreign domestic workers (FDW) or professionally trained personal care assistants who receive a fixed monthly salary to provide services within the household that employs them (Tyagi et al., 2021). Ha et al. (2018) defined an FDW as "a full-time, live-in migrant worker who is typically a female, being employed to provide domestic duties". The FDW may assist the stroke survivors with their personal care and household chores.

Challenges in transitioning back into the community
After a stroke, the clients, their families, and their caregivers face multiple challenges and changes during care transition at various stages of recovery (Cameron et al., 2016). Navigating the continuum of care following a stroke is particularly challenging for stroke survivors and their caregivers when transitioning home after being discharged from the hospital (Cameron et al., 2008). Stroke clients and their caregivers move from a well-supported inpatient setting, with care services provided by a multidisciplinary team, to an unstructured community setting where they need to manage the care arrangements for the stroke survivors on their own (Tyagi et al., 2020). Some families and caregivers feel unsupported and are unaware of the available community services (Cameron et al., 2008; Pindus et al., 2018). Others mentioned that they often felt unprepared to manage the care at home and believed that they were not adequately trained to provide personal care assistance, rehabilitation, and administer medication for the stroke survivors (Kerr & Smith, 2001; Tyagi et al., 2020). Family caregivers must provide assistance beyond BADL, as well as handle other complex needs such as driving stroke survivors to various locations (Liang, 2017a). This could be a source of stress and burden that could evolve over time (Liang, 2017b).

Supporting stroke survivors, their families, and caregivers
Healthcare professionals play an essential role in supporting stroke survivors and their caregivers to smoothly transition back to their homes after being discharged from the hospital. Box 9.1 describes the recommendations made by the Canadian Stroke Best Practice Guidelines (Cameron et al., 2016) for healthcare professionals to consider when supporting clients, families, and caregivers.

Occupational therapists play a vital role in educating caregivers and equipping them with the necessary skills to enhance the quality of life of stroke survivors and help them smoothly transition into the home environment after being discharged (Wolf et al., 2015). During the inpatient period, occupational therapists prepare stroke clients to return home through various interventions, including:

- Retraining of ADL skills;
- Initiating home assessment and modification to optimize the environment to support clients' safety and function;

Box 9.1 Recommendations made by the Canadian Stroke Best Practice Guidelines (Cameron et al., 2016)

1 Adequate assessment and preparation for care transition and changes in setting through comprehensive and timely education.

Patients, families, and caregivers should be assessed and prepared for transitions between different care stages and settings through education on stroke management, support services in the community, skill training, and psychosocial support.

1.1.1 Stroke service providers should screen patients, their families, and caregivers for their level of coping, risk of depression or burnout, and other physical and psychological issues.

1.1.2 Supporting patients, families, and caregivers is crucial in all care transition stages. The use of telemedicine modalities should be considered to increase access to such support services.

2 Consistent and continuous stroke education at all stages of the continuum of care.

Stroke education must be an integral part of stroke care which addresses all stages and settings across the continuum of care.

2.1 Assessment of the patients, their families, and caregivers' learning needs should be considered prior to stroke education.

2.2 A process for delivering education should be implemented once the learning needs are assessed. Education should include information sharing, the teaching of self-management skills, and training of caregivers and families to provide safe stroke care.

2.3 Patients and families should be provided information, support, and access to services when transiting back to the community. Awareness and access to the available community services are vital for the patients and their caregivers to be well-supported after hospital discharge.

2.4 Stroke education should empower patients, families, and caregivers to self-manage stroke care. Patient education should promote self-efficacy through the mastering of self-management skills. Patients should be encouraged to participate in rehabilitation related to vocational, leisure, and social reintegration needs.

- Prescribing assistive devices to aid clients and their caregivers in managing ADL;
- Prescribing exercises; and
- Educating and training caregivers to help stroke clients manage their BADL and IADL, as well as improve their functional performance and fall prevention skills.

Table 9.10 outlines the caregiver education provided by occupational therapists.

Table 9.10 Caregiver education provided by occupational therapists

Content	Mode of training
(1) Train caregivers in how to assist clients in performing their care, including transfers, dressing, toileting, personal hygiene, and bathing.	Hands-on practice and observation for skill-based tasks such as transfers and ADL tasks.
(2) Educate caregivers on how to use prescribed assistive devices when assisting clients in their ADL.	Hands-on practice and observation.
(3) Home safety and fall prevention education.	Verbal and visual (e.g., handouts).
(4) Exercises for clients to perform after discharge.	Verbal and visual (e.g., handouts and demonstration).
(5) Educate caregivers about available rehabilitation and community support group services.	Verbal and visual (e.g., brochures).

Case study 1: Philip

Acute phase

Philip is a 45-year-old man who used to work as an optician in a local retail shop. On December 22, 2018, he experienced a severe pounding headache on the left side of his head and a sudden onset of weakness in his right arm and right leg. Suspecting that Philip had a stroke, his colleague helped him call an ambulance and sent him to the nearby acute hospital. He arrived at the Emergency Department (ED) two hours after the acute onset of weakness. On admission to the ED, he was found to have an elevated blood pressure of 190/110 mmHg. Philp remained alert and orientated. During an initial physical examination by the ED doctor, he presented with loss of body movement in the right upper limb and sensory loss on the right side of his body. Besides the physical weakness, his speech was observed to be slurred. He reported to the doctor that he was a heavy smoker and smoked 20 cigarettes daily for the past 20 years. His past medical history included hypertension, hyperlipidemia, and diabetes mellitus. The ED doctor suspected an acute stroke and ordered an emergency CT scan, initial blood workup, and ECG. The initial blood workup and ECG were unremarkable. The emergency CT scan showed no intracranial hemorrhage, internal bleeding, or other abnormalities. The neurologist ordered an MRI after reviewing the CT scan report and Philp's clinical presentation. The MRI finding showed an acute infarct on the left side of his pons with mild cerebral edema. Aspirin was given to him and he was admitted to the acute stroke unit for further monitoring. Upon reviewing the medical and radiological findings, the neurologist diagnosed his condition as left pontine lacunar infarct with a TOAST classification of small vessel disease. He was placed on telemetry in the acute stroke unit to check for any heart arrhythmia and sent for various workups such as carotid Doppler and echocardiogram. The carotid Doppler images, telemetry, and echocardiogram results were normal. During his stay in the stroke unit, he was referred to the rehabilitation team comprising a physiotherapist, occupational therapist, and speech therapist. Both the physiotherapist and occupational therapist reviewed his condition and recommended him for inpatient rehabilitation as he was considered to have good rehabilitation potential. The speech therapist did not find abnormality with his swallowing but noted issues concerning his expressive communication. The speech therapist found that he had moderate dysarthria.

Understanding clients' performance in ADL is crucial because it reflects the consequences of impairment, i.e., disabilities or what clients can or cannot do (e.g., cannot move about by walking and are dependent on a wheelchair) (World Health Organization, 1980). Occupational therapists assess clients' BADL and IADL for the purposes of obtaining a baseline as the starting point for treatment planning, communicating with other healthcare professionals about clients' existing abilities and rehabilitation potential, and evaluating before and after treatment to obtain the evaluation outcome. BADL consists of personal care (e.g., feeding, dressing, grooming, personal hygiene, going to the toilet, bathing, etc.) and getting around (e.g., transfer, mobility, etc.), among others. They are tasks necessary for survival, dignity, and personal care. IADL refers to activities that require more advanced skills in all performance areas (e.g., communicating, problem-solving and social skills, interaction with environments, etc.). They are complex daily tasks to be carried out in a safe manner within a reasonable amount of time. Both BADL and IADL are measured in the form of the client's ADL ability (what a person can do in a standardized or controlled environment), ADL capability (what a person can do in his/her real environment, using his/her own potential), actual performance (what a person will do in his/her daily environment), and perceived difficulties (what a person feels about his/her difficulty in performance in his/her environment by means of self-reporting). Measurement of the level of assistance is the most common in most of ADL scales because the amount of assistance needed is closely related to the manpower resources, i.e., the number of helpers necessary to take care of the client. The common levels of assistance can be broadly divided into three categories, with sublevels for each category: (1) independence: complete/total independence, modified independence, (2) dependence: complete/total dependence, near dependence, and (3) assistance: supervision or stand-by assistance, manual assistance. Manual assistance can be further classified into minimal assistance (the client pays about 75% or above ability), moderate assistance (the client pays 50% or above ability), and maximal assistance (the client pays 25% or below ability) (Pendleton & Schultz-Krohn, 2013).

The Barthel Index (BI) was developed in 1965 and adopts the levels of assistance for ADL measurement. It consists of ten variables describing BADL, including (1) fecal incontinence, (2) urinary incontinence, (3) grooming, (4) going to the toilet, (5) feeding, (6) transfers, (7) walking, (8) dressing, (9) climbing stairs, and (10) bathing (Mahoney & Barthel, 1965). It has a total score of 20, with a higher number representing a greater likelihood of being able to live at home with a degree of independence following discharge from the hospital (Mahoney & Barthel, 1965). The Modified Barthel Index (MBI) was developed in 1989 to improve the sensitivity of the scale by expanding the total score from 20 to 100 (Shah et al., 1989a; Shah et al., 1989b). A Hong Kong-Chinese version of the MBI was developed in 2007 for local use (Leung et al., 2007).

During the hospitalization, Philip found that his right-side function was greatly restricted. He was unable to move his right arm, get up from bed, or walk independently. Therapists conducted a functional assessment using the MBI as shown in Table 9.11.

His BI showed that he had severe dependence in BADL and required a wheelchair to get around.

Though his right upper limb retained some movement on day two, it was still significantly weak. The manual muscle testing (MMT) chart for the upper and lower limbs is shown in Table 9.12.

Table 9.11 MBI during the inpatient period

Index item	Score					Remarks
Bowel	0	2	5	8	10	
Bladder	0	2	5	8	10	Wear diapers.
Feeding	0	2	5	8	10	
Personal hygiene	0	1	3	4	5	
Dressing	0	2	5	8	10	
Going to the toilet	0	2	5	8	10	
Bathing	0	1	3	4	5	
Ambulation	0	3	8	12	15	
Wheelchair mobility (if cannot walk)	0	1	3	4	5	
Climbing stairs	0	2	5	8	10	
Chair transfer	0	3	8	12	15	Maximum assist by 1.
Total	50					

Note: The shaded boxes refer to Philip's MBI scores.

MBI score interpretation

Total score	Interpretation
0–20	Total dependence
21–60	Severe dependence
61–90	Moderate dependence
91–99	Slight dependence
100	Independence

Table 9.12 MMT chart for the upper and lower limbs

	Right	Left
Shoulder flexion	–	2–
Elbow flexion/extension	–	2–/0
Fingers flexion/extension	5/5	0/0
Hip flexion/extension	–	2/2–
Knee flexion/extension	–	2+/2
Ankle dorsiflexion/plantarflexion	–	0/0

The sudden loss of function and independence caused Philip to become depressed during his hospitalization. He reported thoughts of "helplessness" and "uselessness" with his current ability. Nevertheless, Philip remained motivated to engage in therapy sessions to regain his physical function and mobility. He developed a good rapport with his therapists but became overly reliant on them. Philip stayed in the rehabilitation hospital for three months and was discharged to the outpatient clinic for further rehabilitation.

Discussion questions

1. Can you list the types of medical investigations conducted for Philip and the reasons for those investigations?
2. What do you think are the possible inpatient goals the occupational therapist would set for Philip after a discussion with him?
3. Based on the ICF model, can you list the possible areas that would be affected by the stroke in Philip?
4. If you were Philip's occupational therapist, what types of intervention would you recommend?

Community phase

One year after the stroke, Philip still had residual deficits in his physical function, such as limitations in the functional use of his right upper limb and reduced dynamic standing balance and mobility. As reflected in his MBI (Table 9.13), he required moderate assistance in self-care, such as bathing and stair climbing. Philp was able to walk with an aid for a short distance (not more than 50 m) within his house. However, he needed to be accompanied by his caregiver when out in the community, such as when taking public transport. He stayed in a four-room private flat with his wife, son, and a maid. His flat is on a lift-landing floor, and there are two toilets in his house. He sleeps in the master bedroom with an ensuite bathroom. There is no curb at the main door entrance but a three-inch high curb at both toilet entrances.

After the stroke, his cognitive function was assessed after reporting having brain fog. The occupational therapist performed a cognitive assessment using the Montreal Cognitive Assessment (MoCA), and he scored a normal range of 28 out of 30. Although Philp's speech was still slightly slurred, his dysarthria had improved with more precise articulation. He had intact comprehension ability and could follow complex instructions, such as three-step instructions. Philip demonstrated a good understanding of his medical condition and physical limitations. However, he had reduced self-efficacy in his physical ability to perform self-care and IADL.

Philp was diagnosed with post-stroke depression, and he mentioned that he had insomnia frequently. He often reported that he felt sad and discouraged about his current disability one year after his stroke. He enjoyed the therapy and was highly motivated every session. However, he was not compliant to perform his prescribed home exercises on his own despite requesting more intensive sessions.

Prior to the stroke, Philip worked as an optician and was the sole breadwinner in the family. His previous work required a high competence in bimanual fine motor skills,

Table 9.13 MBI after one year

Index item	Score					Remarks
Bowel	0	2	5	8	10	
Bladder	0	2	5	8	10	
Feeding	0	2	5	8	10	
Personal hygiene	0	1	3	4	5	
Dressing	0	2	5	8	10	
Going to the toilet	0	2	5	8	10	
Bathing	0	1	3	4	5	Need assistance from helper to clean his back; sit on a chair to take shower.
Ambulation	0	3	8	12	15	Ambulate independently, but for not more than 50 m.
Wheelchair mobility (if cannot walk)	0	1	3	4	5	
Climbing stairs	0	2	5	8	10	
Chair transfer	0	3	8	12	15	
Total	88					

and he could not resume his previous work due to his right hemiparesis. Philip was not optimistic about returning to work or taking up another employment. He maintained a fixed view that his mobility and hemiplegic hand needed to recover fully before returning to gainful employment.

Philip was a regular churchgoer. He maintained a good relationship with his church friends and would join the church activities. He used to enjoy playing badminton and traveling before his stroke. Due to his current disability, he did not resume any of his previous interests. Philip found solace and comfort from his religion as a Christian whenever he felt depressed about his current state of life after the stroke.

Discussion questions

1 Based on the Person-Environment-Occupation (PEO) model, can you frame your understanding of Philip?
2 What are the issues you identify that affect Philip's integration back into the community?
3 What are the goals you will set for Philip as a community occupational therapist?
4 What interventions will you recommend as his community occupational therapist to help him reintegrate successfully into the community?

Case study 2: Ah Kuan

Acute phase

Ah Kuan had been a taxi driver for 15 years. Eight years ago, he suffered a stroke while driving. Since then, his right-side function has been greatly restricted. It has now been eight years since his stroke, and Ah Kuan has stated that he ceased his exercises three years after the stroke. He looked puzzled and frustrated. His mother said that he was very lethargic after the stroke and that he would always eat or sleep. He was not used to the change at first and refused to take medicine. For over three years after the onset, he only took medicine occasionally; thus, he continued to have high blood pressure (HBP) after the stroke. He complained that only he had had a stroke and that society was unfair to him. Ah Kuan got angry with his occupational therapists soon after the stroke because he thought they did not understand his real needs. He was very upset and dissatisfied with himself at the time, mainly because his children were not beside him. He also had several unhappy disputes with his ex-wife. He had thought of suicide before, but then chose to think about his life positively.

After four weeks of medical treatment and rehabilitation, Ah Kuan's medical condition was stabilized. He could walk outdoors independently with a quadripod, including climbing up and down stairs, though with a mild right-foot drop due to an increase in extensor tone during stepping. His affected upper limb was at functional level 3 out of 7 in the FTHUE. There was an increase in flexor tone of his right arm during exertion and manual facilitation was necessary. He was independent when dressing his upper body and lower body, although he had difficulty with the zips on his jackets, tying shoe laces, and fastening belts. The results of the Berg Balance Test (BBT) showed that he had difficulty alternately stepping up and down curbs. A cognitive screening by the MoCA showed that he had normal cognition, except being slow in expressive speech. He had no everyday memory deficits, as shown from the results of the Rivermead Behavioural Memory Test - Third Edition (RBMT-3). He was now living alone and able to take care of himself independently. He was independent in terms of hygiene and grooming at the sink and showering in the bathroom, but required extra time finishing kitchen tasks in the rehabilitation unit's kitchen. He particularly had difficulty in bimanual tasks such as cutting food and opening zipper bags. A home visit was done by an occupational therapist, and he was found to have adapted to his environment at home, except that he was told to remove loose rugs from the kitchen and toilet entrances to prevent falls.

Discussion questions

1 Can you list the types of OT assessments conducted for Ah Kuan and the reasons for these assessments?
2 What IADL tasks will Ah Kuan need to master to be more independent and return home safely?
3 Based on the ICF model, can you list the possible areas that would be affected by the stroke in Ah Kuan?
4 What is the role of OT in helping Ah Kuan to return home safely and eventually reach his goal of independence?

Community phase

Ah Kuan's attitude toward occupational therapists has changed. He stressed that mutual communication was crucial so that a rapport could be built and treatment by the therapist could be more effective and tailored to his needs. After resuming his morning exercises, he was more active and felt that everything was changing. His exercises included stretching his tendons every day. He was independent in the community and could eat out, taking the Mass Transit Railway (MTR) and public buses to and from his home and workplace independently. He could go shopping at a nearby supermarket, except that he still had difficulty in carrying things and was unable to do some bimanual tasks. He walked slowly and carefully in the wet market because it was usually crowded, and the floor was often wet and slippery. He had found a job in a shelter workshop, where his main role was to operate an assembly machine. Ah Kuan joined a client-led support organization last year and began to participate in group activities. He liked to go there because all group members were stroke survivors. The members supported each other and gave him confidence.

Discussion questions

1   Based on the PEO model, can you frame your understanding of Ah Kuan?
2   What are the issues you identify that affect Ah Kuan's integration back into the community?
3   Can you identify all the meaningful occupations of Ah Kuan that need to be addressed? How can an occupational therapist prioritize the areas to address?
4   What further interventions will you recommend as his community occupational therapist to help Ah Kuan reintegrate successfully into the community?

Summary

The disabilities after stroke are multiple, and stroke recovery is a complex process involving spontaneous recovery, restitution (restoring the lost abilities through remediation), and substitution (relearning the lost functions through compensation). OT plays an essential role in both restoration and compensation approaches in stroke rehabilitation – task-specific training and task-based treatment are of the highest levels in published clinical evidence for stroke rehabilitation. Occupational therapists are responsible for educating and facilitating stroke survivors about how to manage their BADL and IADL, prescribing assistive devices, conducting home visits and modifications, and supporting stroke survivors to return to the home and community safely with their families, eventually becoming independent. The role of OT in stroke rehabilitation also includes addressing the return-to-work issues for stroke survivors, helping them to identify and attain meaningful occupations in the course of their recovery.

References

Abduboriyevna, R. K., & Yusufjonovich, N. S. (2018). Stroke burden in Asia: To the epidemiology in Uzbekistan. *European Science Review*, (7–8), 156–161.

Adams, H. P. Jr, Bendixen, B. H., Kappelle, L. J., Biller, J., Love, B. B., Gordon, D. L., & Marsh 3rd, E. E. (1993). Classification of subtype of acute ischemic stroke. Definitions for use in a multicenter clinical trial. TOAST. Trial of Org 10172 in Acute Stroke Treatment. *Stroke*, *24*(1), 35–41. https://doi.org/10.1161/01.STR.24.1.35

Alemdaroğlu, E., Uçan, H., Topçuoğlu, A. M., & Sivas, F. (2012). In-hospital predictors of falls in community-dwelling individuals after stroke in the first 6 months after a baseline evaluation: A prospective cohort study. *Archives of Physical Medicine and Rehabilitation*, *93*(12), 2244–2250. https://doi.org/10.1016/j.apmr.2012.06.014

American Occupational Therapy Association. (2008). Occupational therapy practice framework: Domain and process (2nd ed.). *American Journal of Occupational Therapy*, *62*(6), 625–683.

American Occupational Therapy Association. (2014). Occupational therapy practice framework: Domain and process (3rd ed.). *American Journal of Occupational Therapy*, *68*(Suppl. 1), S1–S48.

Aström, M., Asplund, K., & Aström, T. (1992). Psychosocial function and life satisfaction after stroke. *Stroke*, *23*(4), 527–531. https://doi.org/10.1161/01.STR.23.4.527

Bai, Z., & Fong, K. N. K. (2020). "Remind-to-Move" treatment enhanced activation of the primary motor cortex in patients with stroke. *Brain Topography*, *33*(2), 275–283. https://doi.org/10.1007/s10548-020-00756-7

Bamford, J., Sandercock, P., Dennis, M., Warlow, C., & Burn, J. (1991). Classification and natural history of clinically identifiable subtypes of cerebral infarction. *The Lancet*, *337*(8756), 1521–1526. https://doi.org/10.1016/0140-6736(91)93206-O

Barnsley, L., McCluskey, A., & Middleton, S. (2012). What people say about travelling outdoors after their stroke: A qualitative study. *Australian Occupational Therapy Journal*, *59*(1), 71–78. https://doi.org/10.1111/j.1440-1630.2011.00935.x

Bergström, A. L., von Koch, L., Andersson, M., Tham, K., & Eriksson, G. (2015). Participation in everyday life and life satisfaction in persons with stroke and their caregivers 3-6 months after onset. *Journal of Rehabilitation Medicine*, *47*(6), 508–515. https://doi.org/10.2340/16501977-1964

Brookfield, K., Fitzsimons, C., Scott, I., Mead, G., Starr, J., Thin, N., Tinker, A., & Ward Thompson, C. (2015). The home as enabler of more active lifestyles among older people. *Building Research & Information*, *43*(5), 616–630. http://dx.doi.org/10.1080/09613218.2015.1045702

Cameron, J. I., O'Connell, C., Foley, N., Salter, K., Booth, R., Boyle, R., Cheung, D., Cooper, N., Corriveau, H., Dowlatshahi, D., Dulude, A., Flaherty, P., Glasser, E., Gubitz, G., Hebert, D., Holzmann, J., Hurteau, P., Lamy, E., & LeClaire, S., on behalf of the Heart and Stroke Foundation Canadian Stroke Best Practice Committees. (2016). Canadian Stroke Best Practice Recommendations: Managing transitions of care following stroke, guidelines update 2016. *International Journal of Stroke*, *11*(7), 807–822. https://doi.org/10.1177/1747493016660102

Cameron, J. I., Tsoi, C., & Marsella, A. (2008). Optimizing stroke systems of care by enhancing transitions across care environments. *Stroke*, *39*(9), 2637–2643. https://doi.org/10.1161/STROKEAHA.107.501064

Chan, K. S., & Fong, K. N. K. (2013). Accidental falls among community-dwelling people with chronic stroke in Hong Kong. *Asian Journal of Gerontology and Geriatrics*, *8*(2), 61–67. http://hdl.handle.net/10397/21346

Clemson, L., Mackenzie, L., Ballinger, C., Close, J. C. T., & Cumming, R. G. (2008). Environmental interventions to prevent falls in community-dwelling older people: A meta-analysis of randomized trials. *Journal of Aging and Health*, *20*(8), 954–971. https://doi.org/10.1177/0898264308324672

Duncan, P. W., Zorowitz, R., Bates, B., Choi, J. Y., Glasberg, J. J., Graham, G. D., Katz, R. C., Lamberty, K., & Reker, D. (2005). Management of adult stroke rehabilitation care: A clinical practice guideline. *Stroke*, *36*(9), e100–e143. https://doi.org/10.1161/01.STR.0000180861.54180.FF

Eastwood, S. V., Tillin, T., Chaturvedi, N., & Hughes, A. D. (2015). Ethnic differences in associations between blood pressure and stroke in South Asian and European men. *Hypertension*, *66*(3), 481–488. https://doi.org/10.1161/HYPERTENSIONAHA.115.05672

Edmans, J. (Ed.). (2010). *Occupational therapy and stroke* (2nd ed.). Wiley-Blackwell.

Evers, S. M., Struijs, J. N., Ament, A. J., van Genugten, M. L., Jager, J. C., & van den Bos, G. A. (2004). International comparison of stroke cost studies. *Stroke*, *35*(5), 1209–1215. https://doi.org/10.1161/01.STR.0000125860.48180.48

Feigin, V. L. (2007). Stroke in developing countries: Can the epidemic be stopped and outcomes improved? *The Lancet Neurology*, *6*(2), 94–97. https://doi.org/10.1016/S1474-4422(07)70007-8

Feigin, V. L., Forouzanfar, M. H., Krishnamurthi, R., Mensah, G. A., Connor, M., Bennett, D. A., Moran, A. E., Sacco, R. L., Anderson, L., Truelsen, T., O'Donnell, M., Venketasubramanian, N., Barker-Collo, S., Lawes, C. M. M., Wang, W., Shinohara, Y., Witt, E., Ezzati, M., & Naghavi, M., on behalf of the Global Burden of Diseases, Injuries, and Risk Factors Study 2010 (GBD 2010) and the GBD Stroke Experts Group. (2014). Global and regional burden of stroke during 1990-2010: Findings from the Global Burden of Disease Study 2010. *The Lancet*, *383*(9913), 245–255. https://doi.org/10.1016/S0140-6736(13)61953-4

Fisher, C. M. (1975). Clinical syndromes in cerebral thrombosis, hypertensive hemorrhage, and ruptured saccular aneurysm. *Neurosurgery*, *22*, 117–147.

Fong, K. N., Lo, P. C., Yu, Y. S., Cheuk, C. K., Tsang, T. H., Po, A. S., & Chan, C. C. (2011). Effects of sensory cueing on voluntary arm use for patients with chronic stroke: A preliminary study. *Archives of Physical Medicine and Rehabilitation*, *92*(1), 15–23. https://doi.org/10.1016/j.apmr.2010.09.014

Fong, K., Ng, B., Chan, D., Chan, E., Ma, D., Au, B., Chiu, V., Chang, A., Wan, K., Chan, A., & Chan, V. (2004). Development of the Hong Kong version of the Functional Test for the Hemiplegic Upper Extremity (FTHUE-HK). *Hong Kong Journal of Occupational Therapy*, *14*(1), 21–29. https://doi.org/10.1016/S1569-1861(09)70025-7

Forster, A., & Young, J. (1995). Incidence and consequences of falls due to stroke: A systematic inquiry. *BMJ*, *311*(6997), 83–86. https://doi.org/10.1136/bmj.311.6997.83

Gillen, G., & Nilsen, D. M. (2020). *Stroke rehabilitation: A function-based approach* (5th ed.). Elsevier.

Ha, N. H. L., Chong, M. S., Choo, R. W. M., Tam, W. J., & Yap, P. L. K. (2018). Caregiving burden in foreign domestic workers caring for frail older adults in Singapore. *International Psychogeriatrics*, *30*(8), 1139–1147. https://doi.org/10.1017/S1041610218000200

Hankey, G. J., Eikelboom, J. W., van Bockxmeer, F. M., Lofthouse, E., Staples, N., & Baker, R. I. (2001). Inherited thrombophilia in ischemic stroke and its pathogenic subtypes. *Stroke*, *32*(8), 1793–1799. https://doi.org/10.1161/01.str.32.8.1793

Hayner, K., Gibson, G., & Giles, G. M. (2010). Comparison of constraint-induced movement therapy and bilateral treatment of equal intensity in people with chronic upper-extremity dysfunction after cerebrovascular accident. *American Journal of Occupational Therapy*, *64*(4), 528–539.

Hermanns, M., & Mastel-Smith, B. (2012). Caregiving: A qualitative concept analysis. *Qualitative Report*, *17*(38), 75.

Intercollegiate Stroke Working Party. (2008). *National clinical guideline for stroke* (3rd ed.). Royal College of Physicians. https://www.strokeguideline.org/app/uploads/2023/03/2008-National-Clinical-Guideline-for-Stroke-3rd-edition.pdf

Jin, M., Zhang, Z., Bai, Z., & Fong, K. N. K. (2019). Timing-dependent interaction effects of tDCS with mirror therapy on upper extremity motor recovery in patients with chronic stroke: A randomized controlled pilot study. *Journal of the Neurological Sciences*, *405*, 116436. https://doi.org/10.1016/j.jns.2019.116436

Katan, M., & Luft, A. (2018). Global burden of stroke. *Seminars in Neurology*, *38*(2), 208–211. https://doi.org/10.1055/s-0038-1649503

Kerr, S. M., & Smith, L. N. (2001). Stroke: An exploration of the experience of informal caregiving. *Clinical Rehabilitation*, *15*(4), 428–436. https://doi.org/10.1191/026921501678310234

Kho, A. Y., Liu, K. P. Y., & Chung, R. C. K. (2014). Meta-analysis on the effect of mental imagery on motor recovery of the hemiplegic upper extremity function. *Australian Occupational Therapy Journal*, *61*(2), 38–48. https://doi.org/10.1111/1440-1630.12084

Kim, Y. D., Jung, Y. H., & Saposnik, G. (2016). Traditional risk factors for stroke in East Asia. *Journal of Stroke*, *18*(3), 273–285. https://doi.org/10.5853/jos.2016.00885

Kistler, J. P., Ropper, A. H., & Martin, J. B. (1994). Cerebrovascular diseases. In K. J. Isselbacher, E. Braunwald, J. D. Wilson, J. B. Martin, A. S. Fauci, & D. L. Kasper (Eds.), *Harrison's principles of internal medicine* (13th ed., pp. 2233–2256). McGraw-Hill.

Kitayama, S., Karasawa, M., Curhan, K. B., Ryff, C. D., & Markus, H. R. (2010). Independence and interdependence predict health and wellbeing: Divergent patterns in the United States and Japan. *Frontiers in Psychology*, 1, 163. https://doi.org/10.3389/fpsyg.2010.00163

Klymenko, G., Liu, K. P. Y., Bissett, M., Fong, K. N. K., Welage, N., & Wong, R. S. M. (2018). Development and initial validity of the in-hand manipulation assessment. *Australian Occupational Therapy Journal*, 65(2), 135–145. https://doi.org/10.1111/1440-1630.12447

Korpershoek, C., van der Bijl, J., & Hafsteinsdóttir, T. B. (2011). Self-efficacy and its influence on recovery of patients with stroke: A systematic review. *Journal of Advanced Nursing*, 67(9), 1876–1894. https://doi.org/10.1111/j.1365-2648.2011.05659.x

Krebs, H. I., Volpe, B., & Hogan, N. (2009). A working model of stroke recovery from rehabilitation robotics practitioners. *Journal of NeuroEngineering and Rehabilitation*, 6(6). https://doi.org/10.1186/1743-0003-6-6

Langhorne, P., Bernhardt, J., & Kwakkel, G. (2011). Stroke rehabilitation. *The Lancet*, 377(9778), 1693–1702. https://doi.org/10.1016/S0140-6736(11)60325-5

Langhorne, P., Coupar, F., & Pollock, A. (2009). Motor recovery after stroke: A systematic review. *The Lancet Neurology*, 8(8), 741–754. https://doi.org/10.1016/S1474-4422(09)70150-4

Lennon, O. C., Doody, C., Ni Choisdealbh, C., & Blake, C. (2013). Barriers to healthy-lifestyle participation in stroke: Consumer participation in secondary prevention design. *International Journal of Rehabilitation Research*, 36(4), 354–361. https://doi.org/10.1097/MRR.0b013e3283643d48

Leung, D. P. K., Ng, A. K. Y., & Fong, K. N. K. (2009). Effect of small group treatment of the modified constraint induced movement therapy for clients with chronic stroke in a community setting. *Human Movement Science*, 28(6), 798–808. https://doi.org/10.1016/j.humov.2009.04.006

Leung, S. O. C., Chan, C. C. H., & Shah, S. (2007). Development of a Chinese version of the Modified Barthel Index—Validity and reliability. *Clinical Rehabilitation*, 21(10), 912–922. https://doi.org/10.1177/0269215507077286

Liang, P., Fleming, J., Gustafsson, L., Griffin, J., & Liddle, J. (2017a). Family members' experiences of driving disruption after acquired brain injury. *Brain Injury*, 31(4), 517–525. https://doi.org/10.1080/02699052.2017.1283058

Liang, P., Gustafsson, L., Liddle, J., & Fleming, J. (2017b). Family members' needs and experiences of driving disruption over time following an acquired brain injury: An evolving issue. *Disability and Rehabilitation*, 39(14), 1398–1407. https://doi.org/10.1080/09638288.2016.1196397

Lindsay, P., Furie, K. L., Davis, S. M., Donnan, G. A., & Norrving, B. (2014). World Stroke Organization Global Stroke Services Guidelines and Action Plan. *International Journal of Stroke*, 9(SA100), 4–13. https://doi.org/10.1111/ijs.12371

Liu, K. P., Chan, C. C., Lee, T. M., & Hui-Chan, C. W. (2004). Mental imagery for promoting relearning for people after stroke: A randomized controlled trial. *Archives of Physical Medicine and Rehabilitation*, 85(9), 1403–1408. https://doi.org/10.1016/j.apmr.2003.12.035

Liu, K. P. Y., Chan, C. C. H., Wong, R. S. M., Kwan, I. W. L., Yau, C. S. F., Li, L. S. W., & Lee, T. M. C. (2009). A randomized controlled trial of mental imagery augment generalization of learning in acute poststroke patients. *Stroke*, 40(6), 2222–2225. https://doi.org/10.1161/STROKEAHA.108.540997

Mackintosh, S. F., Hill, K. D., Dodd, K. J., Goldie, P. A., & Culham, E. G. (2006). Balance score and a history of falls in hospital predict recurrent falls in the 6 months following stroke rehabilitation. *Archives of Physical Medicine and Rehabilitation*, 87(12), 1583–1589. https://doi.org/10.1016/j.apmr.2006.09.004

Mahoney, F. I., & Barthel, D. W. (1965). Functional evaluation: The Barthel Index. *Maryland State Medical Journal*, 14, 61–65.

Mayberg, M. R., Batjer, H. H., Dacey, R., Diringer, M., Haley, E. C., Heros, R. C., Sternau, L. L., Torner, J., Adams, H. P. Jr, & Feinberg, W. (1994). Guidelines for the management of aneurysmal subarachnoid hemorrhage: A statement for healthcare professionals from a special writing group of the Stroke Council, American Heart Association. *Stroke*, 25(11), 2315–2328. https://doi.org/10.1161/01.STR.25.11.2315

Mayo, N. E., Wood-Dauphinee, S., Côté, R., Durcan, L., & Carlton, J. (2002). Activity, participation, and quality of life 6 months poststroke. *Archives of Physical Medicine and Rehabilitation*, 83(8), 1035–1042. https://doi.org/10.1053/apmr.2002.33984

McColl, M. A., Carlson, P., Johnston, J., Minnes, P., Shue, K., Davies, D., & Karlovits, T. (1998). The definition of community integration: Perspectives of people with brain injuries. *Brain Injury, 12*(1), 15–30. https://doi.org/10.1080/026990598122827

McColl, M. A., Davies, D., Carlson, P., Johnston, J., & Minnes, P. (2001). The community integration measure: Development and preliminary validation. *Archives of Physical Medicine and Rehabilitation, 82*(4), 429–434. https://doi.org/10.1053/apmr.2001.22195

Montero-Odasso, M., van der Velde, N., Martin, F. C., Petrovic, M., Tan, M. P., Ryg, J., Aguilar-Navarro, S., Alexander, N. B., Becker, C., Blain, H., Bourke, R., Cameron, I. D., Camicioli, R., Clemson, L., Close, J., Delbaere, K., Duan, L., Duque, G., & Dyer, S. M., The Task Force on Global Guidelines for Falls in Older Adults. (2022). World guidelines for falls prevention and management for older adults: A global initiative. *Age and Ageing, 51*(9), afac205. https://doi.org/10.1093/ageing/afac205

Morris, J. H., van Wijck, F., Joice, S., Ogston, S. A., Cole, I., & MacWalter, R. S. (2008). A comparison of bilateral and unilateral upper-limb task training in early poststroke rehabilitation: A randomized controlled trial. *Archives of Physical Medicine and Rehabilitation, 89*(7), 1237–1245. https://doi.org/10.1016/j.apmr.2007.11.039

Myint, J. M. W. W., Yuen, G. F. C., Yu, T. K. K., Kng, C. P. L., Wong, A. M. Y., Chow, K. K. C., Li, H. C. K., & Wong, C. P. (2008). A study of constraint-induced movement therapy in subacute stroke patients in Hong Kong. *Clinical Rehabilitation, 22*(2), 112–124. https://doi.org/10.1177/0269215507080141

Ng, A. H., Steele, J. R., Sasaki, J. Y., Sakamoto, Y., & Williams, A. (2015). Culture moderates the relationship between interdependence and face recognition. *Frontiers in Psychology, 6*, 1620. https://doi.org/10.3389/fpsyg.2015.01620

Ng, A. K. Y., Leung, D. P. K., & Fong, K. N. K. (2008). Clinical utility of the Action Research Arm Test, the Wolf Motor Function Test and the Motor Activity Log for hemiparetic upper extremity functions after stroke: A pilot study. *Hong Kong Journal of Occupational Therapy, 18*(1), 20–27. https://doi.org/10.1016/S1569-1861(08)70009-3

O'Donnell, M. J., Xavier, D., Liu, L., Zhang, H., Chin, S. L., Rao-Melacini, P., Rangarajan, S., Islam, S., Pais, P., McQueen, M. J., Mondo, C., Damasceno, A., Lopez-Jaramillo, P., Hankey, G. J., Dans, A. L., Yusoff, K., Truelsen, T., Diener, H.-C., & Sacco, R. L., on behalf of the INTERSTROKE investigators. (2010). Risk factors for ischaemic and intracerebral haemorrhagic stroke in 22 countries (the INTERSTROKE study): A case-control study. *The Lancet, 376*(9735), 112–123. https://doi.org/10.1016/S0140-6736(10)60834-3

Oumer, M., Alemayehu, M., & Muche, A. (2021). Association between Circle of Willis and ischemic stroke: A systematic review and meta-analysis. *BMC Neuroscience, 22*(1), 3. https://doi.org/10.1186/s12868-021-00609-4

Panel on Prevention of Falls in Older Persons, American Geriatrics Society and British Geriatrics Society. (2011). Summary of the updated American Geriatrics Society/British Geriatrics Society Clinical Practice Guideline for Prevention of Falls in Older Persons. *Journal of the American Geriatrics Society, 59*(1), 148–157. https://doi.org/10.1111/j.1532-5415.2010.03234.x

Panuganti, K. K., Tadi, P., & Lui, F. (2022). Transient ischemic attack. In *StatPearls [Internet]*. StatPearls Publishing. https://www.ncbi.nlm.nih.gov/books/NBK459143/

Pendleton, H. M., & Schultz-Krohn, W. (Eds.). (2013). *Pedretti's occupational therapy: Practice skills for physical dysfunction* (7th ed.). Elsevier.

Pindus, D. M., Mullis, R., Lim, L., Wellwood, I., Rundell, A. V., Abd Aziz, N. A., & Mant, J. (2018). Stroke survivors' and informal caregivers' experiences of primary care and community healthcare services – A systematic review and meta-ethnography. *PLoS ONE, 13*(2), e0192533. https://doi.org/10.1371/journal.pone.0192533

Reid, D. (2004). Accessibility and usability of the physical housing environment of seniors with stroke. *International Journal of Rehabilitation Research, 27*(3), 203–208. https://doi.org/10.1097/00004356-200409000-00005

Robison, J., Wiles, R., Ellis-Hill, C., McPherson, K., Hyndman, D., & Ashburn, A. (2009). Resuming previously valued activities post-stroke: Who or what helps? *Disability and Rehabilitation, 31*(19), 1555–1566. https://doi.org/10.1080/09638280802639327

Roth, E. J. (2007). Rehabilitation in stroke syndromes. *Physical Medicine and Rehabilitation*, 1175–1209.

Rowland, T. J., Cooke, D. M., & Gustafsson, L. A. (2008). Role of occupational therapy after stroke. *Annals of Indian Academy of Neurology, 11*(Suppl. 1), S99–S107. https://www.ncbi.nlm.nih.gov/pmc/articles/PMC9204113/

Sacco, R. L., Kasner, S. E., Broderick, J. P., Caplan, L. R., Connors, J. J., Culebras, A., Elkind, M. S. V., George, M. G., Hamdan, A. D., Higashida, R. T., Hoh, B. L., Janis, L. S., Kase, C. S., Kleindorfer, D. O., Lee, J.-M., Moseley, M. E., Peterson, E. D., Turan, T. N., & Valderrama, A. L., Council on Nutrition, Physical Activity and Metabolism. (2013). An updated definition of stroke for the 21st century: A statement for healthcare professionals from the American Heart Association/American Stroke Association. *Stroke, 44*(7), 2064–2089. https://doi.org/10.1161/STR.0b013e318296aeca

Scaffa, M. E., & Reitz, S. M. (2013). *Occupational therapy in community-based practice settings* (2nd ed.). F.A. Davis Company.

Schell, B. A. B., Gillen, G., & Scaffa, M. E. (2014). *Willard & Spackman's occupational therapy* (12th ed.). Lippincott Williams & Wilkins.

Schulz, C. H., Hersch, G. I., Foust, J. L., Wyatt, A. L., Godwin, K. M., Virani, S., & Ostwald, S. K. (2012). Identifying occupational performance barriers of stroke survivors: Utilization of a home assessment. *Physical & Occupational Therapy in Geriatrics, 30*(2), 109–123. https://doi.org/10.3109/02703181.2012.687441

Shah, S., Vanclay, F., & Cooper, B. (1989a). Predicting discharge status at commencement of stroke rehabilitation. *Stroke, 20*(6), 766–769. https://doi.org/10.1161/01.STR.20.6.766

Shah, S., Vanclay, F., & Cooper, B. (1989b). Improving the sensitivity of the Barthel Index for stroke rehabilitation. *Journal of Clinical Epidemiology, 42*(8), 703–709. https://doi.org/10.1016/0895-4356(89)90065-6

Simpson, J., & Weiner, E. (Eds.). (1989). *The Oxford English dictionary* (2nd ed.). Oxford University Press.

Solenski, N. J. (2004). Transient ischemic attacks: Part I. Diagnosis and evaluation. *American Family Physician, 69*(7), 1665–1674. https://www.aafp.org/pubs/afp/issues/2004/0401/p1665.html

Stahl, A., & Lexell, E. M. (2018). Facilitators for travelling with local public transport among people with mild cognitive limitations after stroke. *Scandinavian Journal of Occupational Therapy, 25*(2), 108–118. https://doi.org/10.1080/11038128.2017.1280533

Strong, K., Mathers, C., & Bonita, R. (2007). Preventing stroke: Saving lives around the world. *The Lancet Neurology, 6*(2), 182–187. https://doi.org/10.1016/S1474-4422(07)70031-5

Teo, S. H., Fong, K. N. K., Chen, Z., & Chung, R. C. K. (2022). Predictors of long-term return-to-work at five-year follow-up for mild-to-moderate subacute stroke patients enrolled in an early supported discharge program. *Work, 73*(3), 1001–1010.

Thom, T., Haase, N., Rosamond, W., Howard, V. J., Rumsfeld, J., Manolio, T., Zheng, Z.-J., Flegal, K., O'Donnell, C., Kittner, S., Lloyd-Jones, D., Goff, D. C. Jr, Hong, Y., Members of the Statistics Committee and Stroke Statistics Subcommittee, Adams, R., Friday, G., Furie, K., Gorelick, P., Kissela, B., & Wolf, P. (2006). Heart disease and stroke statistics – 2006 update: A report from the American Heart Association Statistics Committee and Stroke Statistics Subcommittee. *Circulation, 113*(6), e85–e151. https://doi.org/10.1161/CIRCULATIONAHA.105.171600

Thomas, T., Stephen, B., & Colin, M. (2000). The global burden of cerebrovascular disease. *Cerebrovascular Disease, 67*.

Tilson, J. K., Wu, S. S., Cen, S. Y., Feng, Q., Rose, D. R., Behrman, A. L., Azen, S. P., & Duncan, P. W. (2012). Characterizing and identifying risk for falls in the LEAPS study: A randomized clinical trial of interventions to improve walking poststroke. *Stroke, 43*(2), 446–452. https://doi.org/10.1161/STROKEAHA.111.636258

Tipnis, S. S., Pawar, V. V., Shinde, R. A., Kumari, D., Padmashali, L., & Mehrotra, S. (2021). Community integration among individuals with stroke: A scoping review protocol. *Journal of Public Health, 31*, 993–997. https://doi.org/10.1007/s10389-021-01603-0

Toh, S. F. M., Cruz Gonzalez, P., & Fong, K. N. K. (2023). Usability of a wearable device for home-based upper limb telerehabilitation in persons with stroke: A mixed-methods study. *Digital Health, 9*, 1–15. https://doi.org/10.1177/20552076231153737

Toh, F. M., Lam, W. W. T., Cruz Gonzalez, P., & Fong, K. N. K. (2025). Effects of a wearable-based intervention on the hemiparetic upper limb in persons with stroke: A randomized controlled trial. *Neurorehabilitation and Neural Repair*, 39(1), 31–46. https://doi.org/ 10.1177/15459683241283412

Trombly, C. (1993). Anticipating the future: Assessment of occupational function. *American Journal of Occupational Therapy*, 47(3), 253–257.

Turana, Y., Tengkawan, J., Chia, Y. C., Nathaniel, M., Wang, J.-G., Sukonthasarn, A., Chen, C.-H., Minh, H. V., Buranakitjaroen, P., Shin, J., Siddique, S., Nailes, J. M., Park, S., Teo, B. W., Sison, J., Soenarta, A. A., Hoshide, S., Tay, J. C., & Sogunuru, G. P., on behalf of the HOPE Asia Network. (2021). Hypertension and stroke in Asia: A comprehensive review from HOPE Asia. *Journal of Clinical Hypertension*, 23(3), 513–521. https://doi.org/10.1111/jch.14099

Tyagi, S., Koh, G. C., Luo, N., Tan, K. B., Hoenig, H., Matchar, D. B., Yoong, J., Chan, A., Lee, K. E., Venketasubramanian, N., Menon, E., Chan, K. M., De Silva, D. A., Yap, P., Tan, B. Y., Chew, E., Young, S. H., Ng, Y. S., Tu, T. M., & Tan, C. S. (2020). Dyadic approach to supervised community rehabilitation participation in an Asian setting post-stroke: Exploring the role of caregiver and patient characteristics in a prospective cohort study. *BMJ Open*, 10(4), e036631. https://doi.org/10.1136/bmjopen-2019-036631

Tyagi, S., Luo, N., Tan, C. S., Tan, K. B., Tan, B. Y., Menon, E., Venketasubramanian, N., Loh, W. C., Fan, S. H., Yang, K. L. T., Chan, A. S. L., Farwin, A., Lukman, Z. B., & Koh, G. C. (2021). Support system diversity among family caregivers of stroke survivors: A qualitative study exploring Asian perspectives. *BMC Geriatrics*, 21(1), 594. https://doi.org/10.1186/ s12877-021-02557-4

Uswatte, G., Taub, E., Morris, D., Light, K., & Thompson, P. A. (2006). The Motor Activity Log-28. *Neurology*, 67(7), 1189–1194. https://doi.org/10.1212/01.wnl.0000238164.90657.c2

Venketasubramanian, N., Yoon, B. W., Pandian, J., & Navarro, J. C. (2017). Stroke epidemiology in South, East, and South-East Asia: A review. *Journal of Stroke*, 19(3), 286–294. https://doi.org/10.5853/jos.2017.00234

Waddell, K. J., Birkenmeier, R. L., Moore, J. L., Hornby, T. G., & Lang, C. E. (2014). Feasibility of high-repetition, task-specific training for individuals with upper-extremity paresis. *American Journal of Occupational Therapy*, 68(4), 444–453.

Wang, Y.-J., Li, Z.-X., Gu, H.-Q., Zhai, Y., Jiang, Y., Zhao, X.-Q., Wang, Y.-L., Yang, X., Wang, C.-J., Meng, X., Li, H., Liu, L.-P., Jing, J., Wu, J., Xu, A.-D., Dong, Q., Wang, D., & Zhao, J.-Z., on behalf of China Stroke Statistics 2019 Writing Committee. (2020). China Stroke Statistics 2019: A report from the National Center for Healthcare Quality Management in Neurological Diseases, China National Clinical Research Center for Neurological Diseases, the Chinese Stroke Association, National Center for Chronic and Non-communicable Disease Control and Prevention, Chinese Center for Disease Control and Prevention and Institute for Global Neuroscience and Stroke Collaborations. *Stroke and Vascular Neurology*, 5(3), 211–239. https://doi.org/10.1136/svn-2020-000457

Warlow, C. (Ed.). (2006). *The Lancet handbook of treatment in neurology*. Elsevier Health Sciences.

Wei, W. X. J., Fong, K. N. K., Chung, R. C. K., Cheung, H. K. Y., & Chow, E. S. L. (2019). "Remind-to-Move" for promoting upper extremity recovery using wearable devices in subacute stroke: A multi-center randomized controlled study. *IEEE Transactions on Neural Systems and Rehabilitation Engineering*, 27(1), 51–59. https://doi.org/10.1109/TNSRE.2018.2882235

Welage, N., Bissett, M., Coxon, K., Fong, K. N. K., & Liu, K. P. Y. (2023). Development and feasibility of first- and third-person motor imagery for people with stroke living in the community. *Pilot and Feasibility Studies*, 9, 33. https://doi.org/10.1186/s40814-023-01263-9

Wijaya, H. R., Supriyanto, E., Salim, M. I. M., Siregar, K. N., & Eryando, T. (2019). Stroke management cost: Review in Indonesia, Malaysia and Singapore. *AIP Conference Proceedings*, 2092(1), 030022. https://doi.org/10.1063/1.5096726

Wilson, D. J., Baker, L. L., & Craddock, J. A. (1984). Functional test for the hemiparetic upper extremity. *American Journal of Occupational Therapy*, 38(3), 159–164.

Winstein, C. J., Stein, J., Arena, R., Bates, B., Cherney, L. R., Cramer, S. C., Deruyter, F., Eng, J. J., Fisher, B., Harvey, R. L., Lang, C. E., MacKay-Lyons, M., Ottenbacher, K. J., Pugh, S., Reeves, M. J., Richards, L. G., Stiers, W., & Zorowitz, R. D., on behalf of the American Heart Association Stroke Council, Council on Cardiovascular and Stroke Nursing, Council on Clinical Cardiology, and Council on Quality of Care and Outcomes Research. (2016). Guidelines for adult stroke rehabilitation and recovery: A guideline for healthcare professionals from the American Heart Association/American Stroke Association. *Stroke*, *47*(6), e98–e169. https://doi.org/10.1161/STR.0000000000000098

Wolf, T. J., Chuh, A., Floyd, T., McInnis, K., & Williams, E. (2015). Effectiveness of occupation-based interventions to improve areas of occupation and social participation after stroke: An evidence-based review. *American Journal of Occupational Therapy*, *69*(1), 6901180060p1–6901180060p11.

Wood, J. P., Connelly, D. M., & Maly, M. R. (2010). 'Getting back to real living': A qualitative study of the process of community reintegration after stroke. *Clinical Rehabilitation*, *24*(11), 1045–1056. https://doi.org/10.1177/0269215510375901

World Federation of Occupational Therapists. (2012). *About occupational therapy*. WFOT. http://www.wfot.org/AboutUs/AboutOccupationalTherapy/DefinitionofOccupational Therapy.aspx

World Health Organization. (1980). *International Classification of Impairments, Disabilities, and Handicaps: A manual of classification relating to the consequences of disease*. World Health Organization. https://iris.who.int/bitstream/handle/10665/41003/9241541261_eng. pdf?sequence=1

World Health Organization. (2001). *International classification of functioning, disability and health (ICF)*. World Health Organization. https://www.who.int/standards/classifications/ international-classification-of-functioning-disability-and-health

Wu, C., Chuang, L., Lin, K., Chen, H., & Tsay, P. (2011). Randomized trial of distributed constraint-induced therapy versus bilateral arm training for the rehabilitation of upper-limb motor control and function after stroke. *Neurorehabilitation and Neural Repair*, *25*(2), 130–139. https://doi.org/10.1177/1545968310380686

Xu, T., Clemson, L., O'Loughlin, K., Lannin, N. A., Dean, C., & Koh, G. (2018). Risk factors for falls in community stroke survivors: A systematic review and meta-analysis. *Archives of Physical Medicine and Rehabilitation*, *99*(3), 563–573.e5. https://doi.org/10.1016/j. apmr.2017.06.032

Yang, Y., Wang, A., Zhao, X., Wang, C., Liu, L., Zheng, H., Wang, Y., Cao, Y., & Wang, Y. (2016). The Oxfordshire Community Stroke Project classification system predicts clinical outcomes following intravenous thrombolysis: A prospective cohort study. *Therapeutics and Clinical Risk Management*, *12*, 1049–1056. https://doi.org/10.2147/TCRM.S107053

Zhang, J. J. Q., Fong, K. N. K., Welage, N., & Liu, K. P. Y. (2018). The activation of the mirror neuron system during action observation and action execution with mirror visual feedback in stroke: A systematic review. *Neural Plasticity*, *2018*(1), 2321045. https://doi.org/ 10.1155/2018/2321045

Zimmermann-Schlatter, A., Schuster, C., Puhan, M. A., Siekierka, E., & Steurer, J. (2008). Efficacy of motor imagery in post-stroke rehabilitation: A systematic review. *Journal of Neuroengineering and Rehabilitation*, *5*, 8. https://doi.org/10.1186/1743-0003-5-8

CHAPTER 10

Developmental disorders

*Chi-Wen Chien, Johnny Wai Hon Lam, and
May Sok Mui Lim*

Introduction

Developmental disorders (DD) are a heterogeneous group of functional impairments attributed to physical, learning, language, or cognitive deficiencies that begin in early childhood (Bornstein & Hendricks, 2013). These disorders can affect a person's ability to learn, communicate, socialize, and engage in daily occupations. Examples of DD include attention-deficit/hyperactivity disorder, autism spectrum disorder (ASD), cerebral palsy, intellectual disability, learning disorders, communication disorders, and other developmental delays. While the exact causes of DD are not fully understood, they are thought to result from a complex interplay of genetic, environmental, and biological factors. Published reports indicated that about 6–15% of children aged 0–6 in Oriental regions (e.g., Taiwan, Hong Kong, etc.) were diagnosed with one or more DD (Tang et al., 2008).

The clinical conditions of DD can vary depending on the specific disorder. There are some common features of DD, including delayed or atypical development, communication difficulties (e.g., producing speech sounds incorrectly), social difficulties (e.g., unwillingness to take turns), emotional difficulties (e.g., expressing feelings inappropriately), behavioral difficulties (e.g., performing repetitive behaviors), cognitive and learning difficulties (e.g., easily being distracted and inability to learn information), and sensory processing difficulties (e.g., over- or under-responsiveness to specific sensory input). Of these conditions, delayed or atypical development is the one most frequently cited reason for referral to pediatric occupational therapy (OT) services (Chien & Lo, 2009; Tang et al., 2008). The aim of these services is to facilitate children's fundamental performance components, including motor, cognitive, self-care, or social skills. When assessing and intervening with children with DD, occupational therapists must follow several general principles (Case-Smith, 2015), including (1) an individualized approach tailored to each child's unique needs, (2) a family-centered approach involving caregivers/parents in the assessment and intervention processes, and (3) a play-based approach using fun activities to target developmental goals. It is

DOI: 10.4324/9781032721170-14

also important to use evidence-based interventions that are proven effective, as well as to collaborate with other healthcare professionals involved in the child's care.

In this chapter, we present a DD case to illustrate how occupational therapists use the abovementioned principles in the assessment or intervention processes. Students are expected to understand the information therapists would collect to analyze this case by using the Person-Environment-Occupation (PEO) model. We also present the related assessments that are administered to the case and the interventions provided. Specifically, the OT assessments and interventions in three Oriental regions (Taiwan, Hong Kong, and Singapore) are described separately to illustrate the similarities and differences if the case were seen in these regions. Finally, we include important considerations for service provision to children with DD to help prepare students for future clinical practice in pediatric settings.

Case study: A child with autism spectrum disorder who has limited social interaction at preschool

Background

Teddy is a four-year-old boy diagnosed with ASD (code 6A02), psychomotor retardation (code MB23.N), and developmental speech or language disorders, unspecified (code 6A01.Z), based on the International Classification of Diseases 11th Revision (ICD-11). He was referred to OT because his kindergarten teacher noticed some problems with him and suggested his parents bring him for a developmental evaluation. For example, the child was not focused in class and often walked around. He had difficulty maintaining eye contact with the teacher. At home, his mother also noticed that Teddy had a short attention span, avoided eye contact with others, and often refused to eat. Below are the child's medical, family, educational, and developmental histories.

Medical history

When Teddy was about one year old, he was hospitalized for a week due to a fever. About four months ago, Teddy's mother brought him to a child psychiatric service for consultation. The doctor conducted clinical observations with Teddy and interviewed his parents using the Childhood Autism Rating Scale (Wu et al., 2014). Teddy's score was 32, signifying mild autism. Two months ago, the child psychiatrist prescribed 10 gm Tofranil, an antidepressant, per day for Teddy to sleep better at night. A month ago, the dose was increased to 20 gm and the medicine is still being taken.

Family history

Teddy's parents are middle-class and both work full-time. He has a five-year-old sister who attends upper kindergarten. The family currently lives in a two-story apartment with three bedrooms in a large metropolitan area. However, before the age of three, Teddy lived with his grandparents while his parents lived in another city and visited him about once a week. His grandfather often left him to play alone in his room, while his grandmother spent more time looking after him. Due to his grandparents' caregiving style, he had little stimulation and exposure to music, stories, and interaction with other children. Although he now lives with his parents, he can be headstrong and demanding, frequently wanting to be carried by his mother. Outside of kindergarten hours, he enjoys playing with his sister and only specific children that he knows. His favorite activities at home are arranging his mother's books neatly in a row or pulling out the tape from cassette tapes. On weekends, Teddy's parents sometimes take him and his sister to the park nearby.

Educational and developmental history
Teddy has been attending full-day middle kindergarten at the same public preschool as his sister since he was three years old. As mentioned in the background information, his teacher has expressed concern that Teddy is not attentive during class and often plays alone. He is not proactive in asking other children to play and is also afraid of new situations and strangers, which interferes with the learning activities conducted outside or by people not known to him. Additionally, he fails to make eye contact with his classmates and teachers. Despite these issues, his classmates still like Teddy and greet him when they meet.

Teddy was born at 38 weeks with a birth weight of 3.4 kilograms. His mother reported that Teddy was clumsy when he first started learning to walk, and he might still lose his balance when engaging in gross motor activities such as jumping on a toy horse. In terms of fine motor and play skills, he enjoys playing with Lego blocks and toy figurines alone at home. Teddy has a short attention span and cannot sit quietly in a chair while waiting during group games. He often crawls around or spins in place, seeking self-stimulation, and requires reminders at the beginning of activities and when it is his turn. In terms of speech and oral motor skills, he has recently started to understand simple instructions and can make short sentences with four to five words. He has been extremely reluctant to eat meat and has only been willing to eat sandwiches, rice balls, and snacks since the age of three. He learned how to go to the toilet on his own after attending kindergarten but still needs assistance in wiping. Teddy is dependent on others for help in dressing and undressing.

Preliminary analysis
Teddy's background information and related histories were analyzed through the PEO model. The PEO model, as introduced in Chapter 1, was developed by Prof. Mary Law and her colleagues (1996), and emphasizes that occupational performance is the outcome of the transaction of three major components: person, environment, and occupation. Defined as the dynamic experience of a person engaging in purposeful activities and tasks within an environment, occupational performance has been viewed as the central focus of OT. In the PEO model, the extent of a client's occupational performance is dependent on the congruence of fit among the person, environment, and occupation in which the person engages. The more closely the three components overlap or fit, the more harmonious the occupational performance is assumed to be. This harmony could indicate a higher level of independence, satisfaction, safety, efficiency, or acceptability in occupational performance. Occupational therapists can utilize the PEO model to identify factors that support or hinder clients' occupational performance at the beginning of the assessment and intervention processes.

Figure 10.1 summarizes Teddy's PEO analysis, his environment, and the occupations in which he engages. In the *Person* component, Teddy was diagnosed with ASD and displays relevant behaviors, such as limited verbal expression, lack of eye contact

	Strengths	Weaknesses
Client factors	Being born full-term. Acceptable birth weight.	Having ASD, developmental speech or language disorders, and psychomotor delay.
Body structures and functions	No bodily impairment.	Having difficulties in sustaining attention. Appearing to have sleep problems. Appearing to be introverted and shy.
Values and beliefs	Value on constructive play such as Lego.	Limited value on engagement in classroom activities.
Performance skills	Appearing to have adequate gross motor skills.	Limited balance. Poor oral motor, verbal expression, and social interaction skills. Seeking sensory stimulation.
Performance patterns	Habit of playing in playgrounds on weekends. Regular weekday routine for preschool. Roles of student, sibling, and classmate.	Habits of eating specific types of food.

Person

Occupational performance

Environment   Occupation

	Afford	Press		Whether client engages in, and, if yes, describe his occupational form
Natural environment and human-made changes to environment	Living in a three-bedroom apartment.	Living within a large metropolitan area.	**BADL**	Independence in eating food using fingers. Dependence in (un)dressing. Partial independence in going to the toilet.
Products and technology	Access to playgrounds in parks.	Nil	**IADL**	Nil
Support and relationships	A sister who plays with client at home. Parents who are available on the weekends.	Nil	**Health management**	Taking Tofranil on a routine basis.
			Rest and sleep	Falling asleep with the assistance of medicine.
			Education	Limited participation in classroom activities.
Attitudes	Classmates who like client.	Teachers' attitude about client's classroom behavior. Grandparents' style of caregiving.	**Work**	Nil
			Play	Playing with blocks and dolls alone at home.
Services, systems, and policies	Access to public preschool education system.	Nil	**Leisure**	Playing in playgrounds on the weekends.
			Social participation	Lack of social interaction with teachers and classmates at preschool.

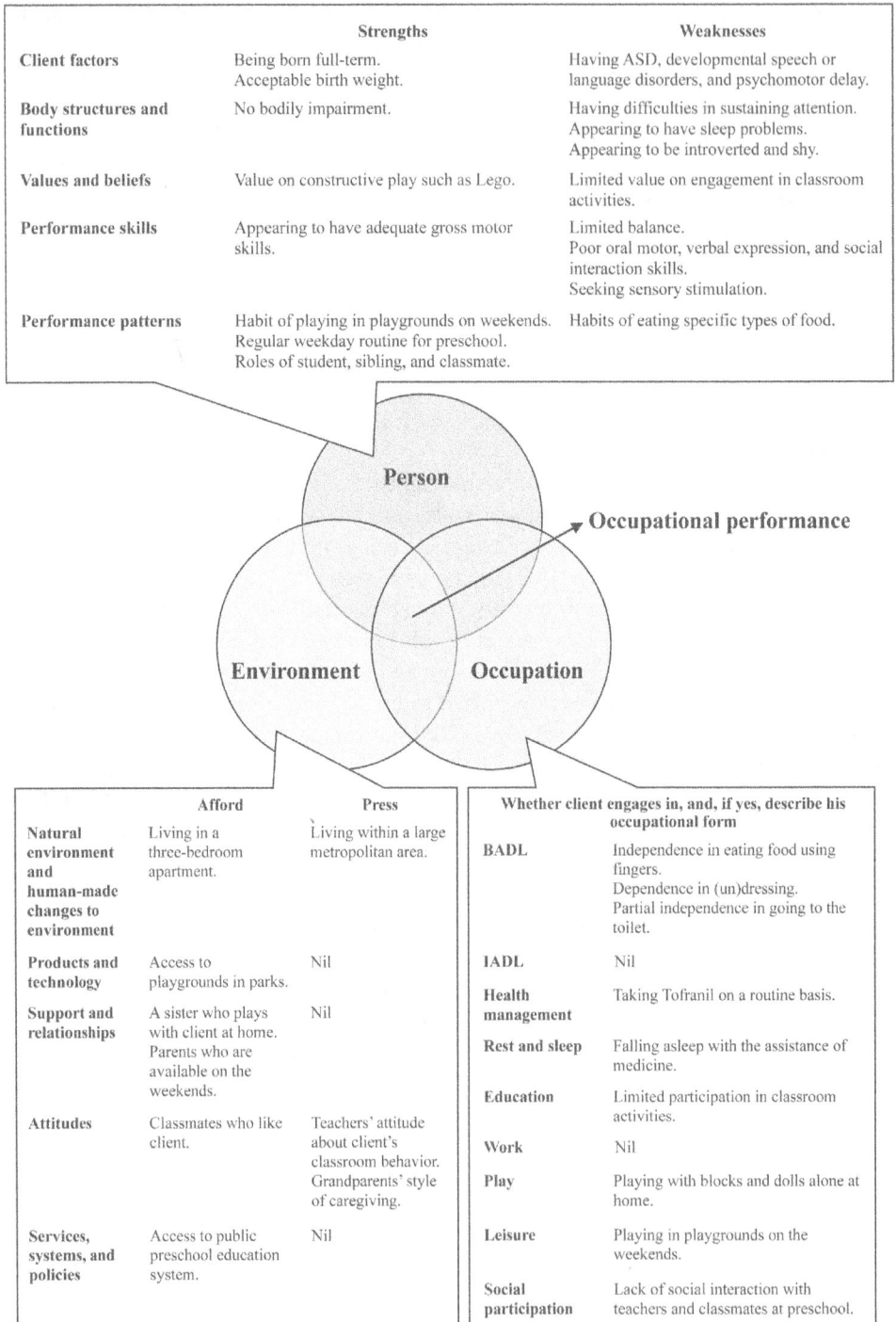

Figure 10.1 Analysis of the case background through the PEO model

and social interaction, repetitive sensory self-stimulation, and limited food choices. He also appears to exhibit delayed development in balance and oral motor skills, but he is affectionate toward his sister and mother and enjoys playing with toy cars. There is limited information on his fine motor ability from the background information. In the *Environment* component, there are some social and attitudinal factors that support Teddy's engagement in occupations. For example, his classmates are friendly and accepting of his behaviors during class. Teddy has an older sister who plays with him, and his parents take him to nearby playgrounds to play with other children over the weekend. In the *Occupation* component, several limited areas of occupational engagement are noted for Teddy. These include education (in which his inattention, lack of social interaction, and sensory self-stimulation interfere with his participation), play and leisure (in which parallel play is reported mostly), and social participation (in which he has limited interaction with teachers and classmates at preschool).

Occupational therapists can use the PEO analysis of Teddy's background information to develop an initial understanding of how ASD and related behaviors impact his occupational performance. For example, Teddy's parallel play and self-stimulation behaviors may hinder his participation in classroom learning activities due to the mismatch between his behavior and the teachers' expectations of students' educational engagement. This profile provides a foundation for the detailed assessment, problem identification, and intervention implementation that therapists will follow. The next section will describe the OT assessment and intervention processes in detail, using the hypothetical scenario for Teddy if he were in Taiwan, Hong Kong, or Singapore.

Occupational therapy assessments and interventions in Taiwan

Context

If Teddy were in Taiwan, he would be referred to a Joint Child Development Assessment Center for a comprehensive developmental assessment and subsequent treatment. These centers are commonly affiliated with local hospitals and employ an interdisciplinary or transdisciplinary approach involving various child-related professionals (including occupational therapists). The establishment of these centers is supported by the Early Intervention for Infants and Young Children with Developmental Delays or Disabilities Act. This was enacted by the Ministry of Health and Welfare to ensure that children with DD aged 0–6 receive timely assessment and developmental services. Additionally, the National Health Insurance system provides financial support for medical treatment and rehabilitation for children with DD.

Assessments

In the center that Teddy and his family visited, the case manager referred Teddy to Rachel, who is an occupational therapist. In the first session, Rachel and the whole early intervention (EI) team conducted joint clinical observations, in which two team members engaged with Teddy and observed his behavior and performance. Each professional focused on a different aspect of Teddy's performance and made notes accordingly. Rachel was responsible for Teddy's fine motor, sensory integration, and activities of daily living (ADL) functions, as required by the center. Some observational notes made by Rachel are shown in Table 10.1.

Later, Rachel separately interviewed the mother about Teddy's daily routine and self-care functions using the Chinese version of the Pediatric Evaluation of Disability Inventory (PEDI) (Tsang & Chen, 2012). This helped to describe Teddy's occupational patterns and problems in the domain of ADL, which is an important occupation for preschool-age children. As Teddy exhibited fine motor issues during the observation, Rachel conducted a standardized fine motor developmental test on him, i.e., the fine motor subscale of the Peabody Developmental Motor Scales – Second Edition (PDMS-2) (Folio & Fewell, 2000). The assessment results helped to understand Teddy's developmental milestones in terms of grasping and visual-motor integration abilities that are fundamental for everyday activities. Teddy was also diagnosed with ASD and might have atypical sensory processing patterns (Lane et al., 2014). Thus, Rachel asked Teddy's mother to complete the Chinese Sensory Profile (CSP) (Tseng, 1998). The CSP helps identify sensory processing strengths and challenges, as well as sensory preferences for subsequent interventions.

The following is a summary of Teddy's regular weekday routine according to his mother. At 8:00 am, Teddy wakes up and his mother has to carry him out of bed. At 8:30 am, Teddy eats only bread before going to preschool. When he returns home at 6:30 pm, he watches TV for a while before dinner. During dinner, at 7:00 pm, Teddy eats very slowly and often spills food onto the table or floor. He frequently asks his mother to feed him and struggles with self-feeding. At 9:00 pm, Teddy goes to bed. Before sleeping, his sister plays with him and his mother sometimes chats or listens to music with him. The mother expressed concern about Teddy's stubborn eating habits, lack of attention in the classroom, and limited social interaction with others at preschool and in playgrounds. The mother also reported that Teddy insisted on certain activities or materials (such as specific TV channels, specific clothes, and playing with toy cars) and had difficulty transitioning to other activities once engaged.

Table 10.1 presents the assessment results and interpretations. Overall, Teddy demonstrated delayed self-care ability compared to his same-age peers, requiring significant assistance from his mother. His fine motor skills, including grasping and visual-motor integration, were far below the expected developmental milestone for his age. Regarding his sensory processing, Teddy exhibited definite variations in oral sensory sensitivity, inattention/distractibility, and sensory sensitivity. He also had a tendency to seek sensory input, react emotionally, and exhibit fine motor/perceptual dysfunction.

Problem identification

Based on her assessments, Rachel identified three occupational performance problems using the PEO model. First, Teddy was inefficient in performing ADL (i.e., eating and dressing). Although these activities were age-appropriate, Teddy's performance was not congruent between this occupation and his personal factors (i.e., oral sensitivity, sensory sensitivity, and delayed fine motor skills) and environmental factors (i.e., his mother's tendency to over-assist without knowing facilitation strategies). Second, he had minimal and unacceptable involvement in classroom activities despite being a student, which is his primary occupation at this age. However, there was a low degree of congruence among the PEO components due to his short attention span and sensory-seeking behavior. The teachers also had negative attitudes toward Teddy's distractive behaviors and did not know how to address them during class. Third, Teddy did not

Table 10.1 Summary of OT assessments conducted in the Taiwanese context

Notes from joint clinical observations

- He was shy, did not make eye contact or have two-way interaction with others except for his mother, and was afraid of touching materials of various fabric textures.
- He had a short attention span and high activity level (e.g., often leaving his seat).
- After prompts, he stacked 3–4 blocks and fitted the shapes (a triangle, square, and diamond) into the correct places using a palmar grasp.
- He opened *The Three Little Pigs* book and looked at the pictures, followed by speaking a few words (e.g., pig, tree) and short sentences (e.g., it chases little piggy) after prompting.
- He grasped a spoon unstably to feed the doll.
- He enjoyed the vestibular stimuli when playing a slide.
- He used an immature tripod grasp to hold the markers and tried to draw pigs on the paper.

Measure	Scoring	Interpretation
PEDI self-care domain	Functional skills (normative standard scores: 38.5) Caregiver assistance (normative standard scores: 28.3)	The score for functional skills is below 1 standard deviation of the mean, indicating that his self-care abilities are lower than what is typically expected for his age. The score for caregiver assistance is below 2 standard deviations of the mean, indicating that he needs much more assistance in self-care activities than same-age children.
PDMS-2-FM	Grasping (percentile rank: 1) Visual-motor integration (percentile rank: 9) Fine motor composite (quotient: 67 and percentile rank: 1)	The percentile rank in the grasping subtest indicates that his grasping ability is very poor. The percentile rank in the visual-motor integration subtest indicates that his visual-motor integration ability is below average. The fine motor quotient indicates that his overall fine motor ability is very poor when compared to same-age children.
CSP	Sensory seeking (score: 55) Emotionally reactive (score: 52) Low endurance tone (score: 40) Oral sensitivity (score: 14) Inattention/distractibility (score: 20) Low registration (score: 31) Sensory sensitivity (score: 12) Sedentary (score: 14) Fine motor/perceptual (score: 7)	Based on the cut-off scores*, Teddy was classified as having probable variations in sensory seeking, emotionally reactive, and fine motor/perceptual factors. He exhibited definite variations in oral sensory sensitivity, inattention/distractibility, and sensory sensitivity.

Note: *The cut-off scores for the typical performance of a four-year-old are 62 for sensory seeking, 58 for emotionally reactive, 39 for low endurance tone, 32 for oral sensitivity, 26 for inattention/distractibility, 34 for low registration, 16 for sensory sensitivity, 12 for sedentary, and 9 for fine motor/perceptual factors.

Abbreviations: PEDI = Pediatric Evaluation of Disability Inventory; PDMS-2-FM = fine motor subscale of Peabody Developmental Motor Scales – Second Edition; CSP = Chinese Sensory Profile.

perform satisfactorily in social activities at preschool or in the playground. This occupational performance problem related to his limited social interaction skills in personal factors, lack of interest in socializing with others in occupational factors, and limited exposure to social activities within his relevant environment.

To address these occupational performance problems, Rachel suggested that Teddy receive OT at least once a week to improve the fundamental component skills in the report. She also recommended providing the mother with consultation or education, and conducting school visits or calls to facilitate Teddy's performance by creating a supportive environment.

Occupational therapy interventions

Teddy's mother agreed to attend one 50-minute OT session per week, and the intervention would be conducted by the other occupational therapist, Teresa, in the same hospital. Based on the child's developmental assessment report, Teresa worked with the mother to set the following goals:

Goal 1: Teddy will eat rice using a spoon through fine motor skill training, sensory activities, and parent education in one month. His performance is expected to improve from complete dependence to supervision and will be measured using parent reporting and observation. The progress will be reviewed fortnightly.

Goal 2: Teddy will interact with more children in playgrounds by receiving group-based play therapy and offering parent consultation within two months. His performance is expected to improve from not at all to playing together for ten minutes and will be measured using participation questionnaires. The progress will be reviewed monthly.

Goal 3: Teddy will engage in classroom activities by following teachers' instructions attentively through the provision of sensory activities and environmental modifications in two months. His engagement duration is expected to improve from 2 to 20 minutes and will be measured using teacher reporting. The progress will be reviewed monthly.

Group-based therapeutic play group

Teresa considered that Teddy had deficiencies in sensory processing and social skills, which were interfering with his performance in terms of meal eating, classroom activities, and social participation. She decided to place Teddy in an existing therapeutic play group that included two boys of the same age with similar problems. This therapeutic play group contained play-based sensory-motor activities designed to improve children's ability to process and integrate sensation using challenging activities of their interest that were of just the right difficulty. Specifically, Teresa used sensory integration therapy to increase Teddy's tolerance to various textual materials on his limbs and in his mouth. Sensory integration therapy has been shown to improve the adaptive responses to sensory experiences in children with ASD (Case-Smith et al., 2015). At the same time, group-based play could provide Teddy with a venue to understand social rules and improve social skills in simulated but playful contexts.

The procedure of the play group consisted of a 5-minute warm-up and 25 minutes of sensory-motor activities. To start, Teresa incorporated Robocar Poli as the play theme and allowed each child to choose a favorite ride-on vehicle to explore the therapeutic room. Although Teddy was initially shy, he became more comfortable after seeing the other children play and receiving comfort from his mother. Then, Teresa introduced the play idea that they were part of the Poli team and would be rescuing people in two scenes.

The first scene involved rolling a big bouncy ball up a hill and letting it roll down to hit a tumbler (representing the "bad guy") before saving people. Various textural mats were placed along the walking path, providing tactile stimuli for Teddy to adapt to as he walked on them with bare feet. The rationale for this activity was to facilitate his sensory processing function in reaction to disliked textures through proprioceptive play. The second scene involved blowing ping-pong balls using straws from one end of the floor to the other, pretending to rescue people to the safe zone. The straws were made of various textures (e.g., paper, silicone, bamboo, etc.) to facilitate Teddy's acceptance of different oral sensations through graded exposure and oral motor exercises (i.e., blowing the ping-pong balls in this case). During the play, Teddy needed to wait in line and take turns by giving the next child a high-five. This created opportunities for him to learn about turn-taking and interact with other children.

To keep the activities just challenging enough for Teddy, Teresa upgraded/downgraded the activity parameters during play. For example, she added more mats with disliked textures when Teddy's tolerance increased. She reduced the size of the bouncy ball when it became too heavy to be pushed up the hill. She changed the bamboo straws to silicone ones and added large plastic balls to make it harder. These changes were made to provide Teddy with a successful and enjoyable experience.

Individual fine motor training

After the group play session, Teresa helped each child to engage in fine motor activities individually in the remaining 20 minutes. Teddy was given a Mosaic Building Blocks Peg Drill Set to build a car on a peg board using pegs, screws, screwdrivers, and wrenches. Teresa showed him a picture of the finished product to help guide him. The purpose of this activity was to help train Teddy's three-jaw chunk grasp and in-hand manipulation skills. The motor skill acquisition frame of reference (Kaplan, 2010) was used to structure the activity as a closed task with constant feedback from himself or the therapist to facilitate his fine motor skill acquisition. Additionally, upgrades and downgrades were implemented by providing various tools and product pictures with varying levels of complexity.

Parent consultation and education

Following Teddy's direct treatment, Teresa spoke with his mother about training activities she could do at home to decrease his oral sensory sensitivity and improve mealtimes. She provided an information sheet developed by Planck and Bisognin (2016) that offered strategies and activities. For example, when introducing new foods, such as meat, she suggested mixing a small amount with foods that Teddy already liked, and to provide immediate, specific praise for his attempts. The goal was to extend the treatment effect to a real-world situation and help his mother improve Teddy's optimal performance. Two weeks later, Teddy's mother reported that he was gradually accepting high-moisture minced meat when mixed with rice. One month later, Teddy was able to use a spoon to eat rice with constant verbal prompts in order to receive post-meal rewards such as pudding.

Teddy's mother also observed that he was making progress in his social skills during the play group in the therapeutic room. After consulting with Teresa, she arranged to leave work early every Wednesday and took Teddy and his sister to the playground. Teresa advised her to use environmental resources to help Teddy interact with other kids better on the playground, such as bringing his toy cars to play with his sister and inviting other children to join in. At first, Teddy did not want to share his toy cars with other children. But as he went there more regularly, he became increasingly comfortable with other children and began to share his toys. He also played games such as chasing and kicking the ball with them, and took turns on the slide or swing, according to the mother's report.

School visits

Teresa arranged a visit to Teddy's school to observe his classroom performance and spoke with his kindergarten teacher. During the visit, the teacher mentioned that she had seen some small improvements in Teddy's attention since he began receiving OT. However, he still occasionally became distracted and spun around meaninglessly when doing table tasks during class. Teresa suggested environmental adaptation strategies to the teacher, such as reducing visual distractions in the classroom and at Teddy's desk. She also recommended some pre-class sensory-based activities to address Teddy's need for sensory input. For example, the teacher could guide all the children through warm-up activities such as shaking and wiggling their bodies to music to help them get ready to learn and then calm down. When Teddy became restless during class, the teacher could also allow him to ride on a hopper ball for five minutes to provide some sensory input. The teacher agreed to try these suggestions and would report on Teddy's performance to his mother through daily school notes.

Occupational therapy assessments and interventions in Hong Kong

Context

Based on the hypothetical scenario where Teddy lives in Hong Kong, after being diagnosed, he was referred to the Subsystem for Disabled Pre-schoolers of the Central Referral System for Rehabilitation Services. Under this referral system, Teddy was assigned to a waiting list of one of the preschool rehabilitation services, which is monitored by the Social Welfare Department. The preschool rehabilitation services available in Hong Kong include the Early Education and Training Centre (EETC), the Integrated Programme in Kindergarten-cum-Child Care Centre (IP), the On-site Pre-school Rehabilitation Services (OPRS), and the Special Child Care Centre (SCCC). The establishment of these services is supported by several acts and regulations, such as the Child Care Services Ordinance (Cap. 243/243A), which regulates the operation of early education and training centers, providing preschool education and rehabilitation services to children with special education needs. Another supporting act is the Rehabilitation Programme Plan (RPP), a government policy document that outlines the provision of rehabilitation services for people with disabilities, including a section on early childhood rehabilitation services.

Considering Teddy's conditions, he would most likely be assigned to either the EETC or OPRS. In this section, the OPRS is used as an example. It is a kindergarten-based rehabilitation service characterized by a multidisciplinary team that includes clinical/ educational psychologists, registered social workers, occupational therapists, speech therapists, physiotherapists, special childcare workers, and stakeholders of the kindergarten. This service aims to provide EI to children with special needs in classrooms and offer support to class teachers/childcare workers and caregivers/parents.

Assessments

Patrick, the occupational therapist responsible for Teddy's training, is one of the members of the OPRS team supporting the kindergarten in which Teddy studies. In the first OT session, Teddy's demographics, including his birth history, developmental history, and family background, were collected. A variety of non-standardized assessments were carried out to gather information on Teddy's occupational performance, which included clinical observations of his play performance, an interview with his parents, and the checklists/questionnaires on self-care skills performance, social participation, and school functioning, respectively (Figure 10.2). Some of the key points are noted in Table 10.2.

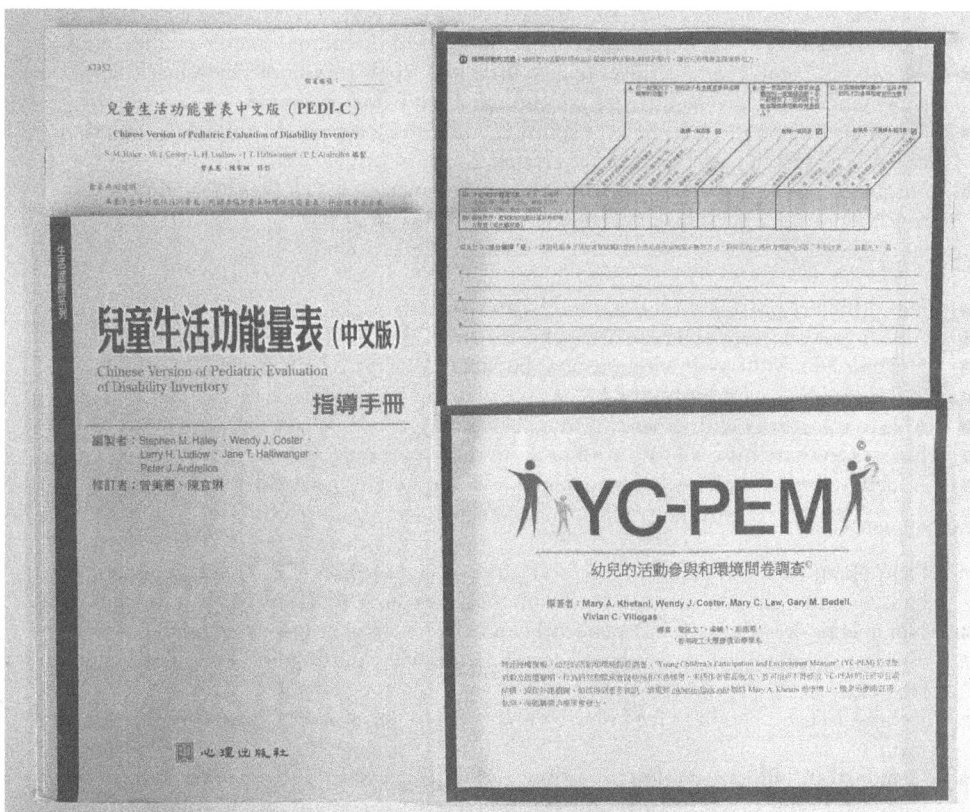

Figure 10.2 Two OT assessments, i.e., the Pediatric Evaluation of Disability Inventory (PEDI) and the Young Children's Participation and Environment Measure (YC-PEM), were used to evaluate Teddy's self-care skills, performance, and participation

Table 10.2 Summary of the information collected from Teddy's assessments conducted in the Hong Kong context

---

Information from the clinical observations, checklist, and interview

---

Clinical observations

- Passive and nervous; rarely initiating interaction with others.
- Avoided physical touch from the therapist, such as shaking hands, light touches on the shoulders, etc.
- Appeared to be clumsy and asynchronized when catching balls.
- Demonstrated poor acceptance to new challenges. For example, when the therapist gave him a therapy ball to support his climbing instead of a ladder, he refused the therapist's suggestion; when the therapist gave him therapeutic putty (or theraputty) instead of clay to play with for the first time, he also refused to touch the therapeutic putty.
- Preferred to stack blocks alone for most of the table time. Stacked blocks alone most of the time during free play at the table.
- Used the pincer grasp to hold pencils and spoons; unstable writing and scoping actions were observed.
- Lost attention quickly on table tasks that involved mainly higher cognitive functions, but did not make many physical movements (e.g., reading). He performed better and was able to concentrate for 2–3 minutes in other tasks that involved more physical movements with lower cognitive demands (e.g., bead threading, stacking cubes, etc.).
- Able to read aloud some phrases (e.g., a little pig) from story books by himself, and some short sentences (e.g., the little pig is running) upon being prompted.
- When playing on the mat, he kept spinning and rolling repeatedly to seek stimulation and was observed to get dizzy after around 20 spins.
- Disgusted by the texture of glue; he rubbed his hands on his clothes every time after touching the glue with his fingers.

Checklist

- Has difficulty putting on socks, jackets, and T-shirts.
- Able to put on shoes and take off socks, trousers, and T-shirts on his own.
- Not able to feed himself with a spoon, but able to eat with his fingers.
- Has difficulties with buttoning but is able to unzip his jacket.
- Able to take turns with other children during play.
- Refuses to share his own toys with peers in the classroom.
- Seldom interacts with his peers at school and plays on his own most of the time.

Interview

- Picky about his food. He only likes food with smooth textures (e.g., bread, gummies, rice balls, noodles, etc.); he spits out food with rough textures (e.g., minced meat, biscuits, etc.).
- Not able to dress himself independently and always asks for help from adults.
- Needs assistance with strength and coordination when putting on socks, T-shirts, and trousers.
- Refuses to use a spoon to feed himself and is fed by his mother or grandmother for every meal.
- Demonstrates short attention in reading and writing tasks. Once he is asked to sit on a chair for table tasks, he leaves his seat frequently to go spinning and rolling around the living room. The mother has received complaints from his teacher about the same problem, i.e., he fails to stay in his seat in the classroom.
- The primary concerns of Teddy's mother are his self-stimulating behaviors and difficulties in feeding and dressing.

By interpreting the above assessment findings, Patrick made the following hypotheses about the underlying causes of Teddy's occupational performance issues using the PEO model. Specifically, he identified several personal factors as fundamental components affecting Teddy's performance in ADL and play. For instance, Teddy's clumsiness in catching balls and performing dressing tasks is caused by a delay in upper limb coordination, while his difficulty in grasping and buttoning is linked to fine motor delay. His over-responsiveness to touching various textures in terms of objects and food, as well as his self-stimulating behaviors such as spinning and rolling, are caused by sensory processing dysfunction. To confirm these hypotheses and establish treatment goals, Patrick decided to administer several standard assessments. These included the Bruininks-Oseretsky Test of Motor Proficiency – Second Edition – Fine Motor Form (BOT-2-FM) (Bruininks & Bruininks, 2005), which was administered to assess Teddy's upper limb manual coordination and fine manual control. The Hong Kong Preschool Fine-Motor Developmental Assessment (HK-PFMDA) (Siu et al., 2011) was also conducted to evaluate Teddy's fine motor development, and the Sensory Processing and Self-regulation Checklist (SPSRC) (Lai et al., 2019) was used to assess his sensory processing and self-regulation performance. Table 10.3 summarizes the results of these standardized assessments.

Table 10.3 Summary of standardized assessment results in the Hong Kong context

Assessment	Scoring*	Interpretation
BOT-2-FM	Fine manual control (percentile rank: 12) Manual coordination (percentile rank: 16)	The percentile rank in fine manual control indicates a below-average performance in Teddy's fine motor precision skills and fine motor integration skills. The percentile rank in manual coordination indicates a below-average performance in his manual dexterity and upper limb coordination.
HK-PFMDA	Raw score: 126 Percentile rank: 10 Standard deviation: –1.12 SD	The percentile rank with –1.12 SD indicates an overall delay in his development of fine motor skills.
SPSRC	*Ability* Facing changes or challenges: –1.27 SD Tactile: –1.24 SD Vestibular: –1.57 SD *Latent factor* Emotional regulation–facing changes: –1.15 SD Sensory-seeking behavior: –1.36 SD Sensory over-responsivity: –1.13 SD	The results suggest that Teddy has problems regulating his emotions when facing challenges. There is a probable deviation in his sensory processing of tactile and vestibular stimuli. Sensory-seeking behaviors and over-responsive behaviors are also identified.

Note: *Only related figures are shown.

Abbreviations: BOT-2-FM = Bruininks-Oseretsky Test of Motor Proficiency – Second Edition – Fine Motor Form; HK-PFMDA = Hong Kong Preschool Fine-Motor Developmental Assessment; SPSRC = Sensory Processing and Self-regulation Checklist; SD = standard deviation.

Based on the above standardized assessment results, it was confirmed that Teddy had delayed development in his fine motor skills, and difficulties in the sensory processing of tactile and vestibular stimuli. Patrick formulated an individual education plan (IEP) for Teddy before the multidisciplinary meeting. The following aspects are involved in an IEP:

(1) The affected occupational performance (i.e., daily activities in self-care/learning/leisure);
(2) The underlying causes/reasons affecting the case's performance (i.e., sensory processing, fine motor skills, etc.);
(3) Considerations about the priority of the intervention (i.e., parent's/teacher's concerns, developmental needs, etc.);
(4) Recommendations on the intervention plan; and
(5) Treatment goals.

Using the PEO model, Patrick identified three major occupational performance problems that Teddy was facing. The first was his low participation in class and table tasks at home due to his repeated sensory-seeking behaviors. This was also associated with his avoidance in social and physical contact with others, and his anxiety in meeting strangers and adapting to new environments, which were highly related to his inadequate social interaction skills and problems in sensory processing. The second was his poor feeding and eating performance, which was related to his over-responsiveness to intra-oral tactile stimulation and poor fine motor skills. The third problem was his poor performance in dressing tasks, which was due to his delay in upper limb coordination and fine motor skills.

Under the OPRS, treatment sessions can be arranged in either the clinic or kindergarten by therapists, subject to administrative considerations. Therapists can decide to work with caregivers/parents or class teachers on specific goals depending on the children's needs. In this case, Patrick planned to provide biweekly follow-up sessions for Teddy, which included a monthly treatment session in the treatment room in his clinic involving the mother, and a monthly visit to the kindergarten to give Teddy classroom support and offer consultation to the teacher.

Occupational therapy interventions

First, Patrick arranged a meeting with Teddy's mother to explain the assessment results, problems identified, and treatment goals. All treatment goals in Teddy's IEP would be reviewed, and progress would be evaluated after three months. The three treatment goals are:

Goal 1: Teddy will stay in his seat for a longer time (from 30 seconds to 5 minutes) with less self-stimulating behaviors upon reduced frequency of prompting in three months. Sensory activities and gradual social support from peers will be provided to help Teddy concentrate and follow the classroom routine.
Goal 2: Teddy will feed himself with a spoon, with the assistance level changing from dependence to mild physical assistance in six months. Sensory activities targeting oral sensitivity and fine motor skills training on grasping will be introduced.

Goal 3: Teddy will pull up his socks and put on T-shirts and trousers with adequate upper limb and finger strength and appropriate coordination of the upper extremities in three months. He will be able to independently manage the pulling action in two out of three types of garments.

Afterward, Patrick created an individualized intervention plan for Teddy. To maximize its effectiveness, a variety of treatment activities were planned for both home-based and classroom-based training, while classroom routine-based activities and a home program were suggested to the teacher and mother, respectively. By adopting the PEO model in the intervention design, Teddy's occupational performance could be enhanced through interventions focused on the personal, environmental, and occupational factors, respectively. For example, to improve Teddy's school participation, modifications to the school environment were suggested, and peer support in the classroom was offered. Peer support has been proven to enhance the communication skills of young children with ASD (Chapin et al., 2018), making it an important environmental facilitator.

Considering Teddy's sensory processing, Patrick chose sensory integration therapy (Case-Smith et al., 2015) as the main intervention to improve his sensory processing function, which was a personal factor affecting his occupational performance in education and ADL. For Teddy's ADL performance, the intervention focused additionally on scaffolding the essential skills needed to perform ADL tasks using the acquisitional frame of reference (Luebben & Royeen, 2010).

Intervention in the kindergarten

Patrick interviewed the teacher during his school visit. It was reported by the teacher that there was a boy in the class called Anson, who liked Teddy very much. Anson actively approached and shared toys with Teddy when he saw Teddy playing on his own. Anson is a smart and caring boy who can follow instructions promptly when the teacher switches activities in class, and he is always willing to offer help to his classmates. Teddy responds to the interactions initiated by Anson occasionally, and was observed to be particularly responsive when they were engaged in gross motor activities.

After getting the teacher's consent, Patrick came up with an environmental facilitation idea where Anson was invited to be the peer helper and social partner for Teddy. The teacher then assigned Anson to sit next to Teddy when they were doing table tasks and encouraged Anson to offer help to enhance Teddy's engagement in class. The help could be in the form of reminding Teddy of the task instructions or asking Teddy to follow him and get back to the class activity when he was lost and performing self-stimulating behaviors. In addition, the teacher was advised to allow more opportunities for Anson to interact with Teddy, so that Teddy could learn some social skills and rules from Anson during their interactions. The same environmental strategy could also be applied to other cooperative games that involved taking turns. Teddy was motivated to learn these social rules by following what Anson did.

Concerning Teddy's self-stimulating behaviors, some sensory activities that could be incorporated into the class routines were recommended to the teacher. This could help to meet Teddy's sensory needs so as to reduce his sensory-seeking behaviors and improve his classroom participation. As an example, the teacher was advised to engage the whole class in physical movements like spinning three times upon hearing the instruction "spin, spin, spin, and we go to the green" before asking students to line up at the green line marked on the floor. These movements involved cognitive function in color recognition and offered sensory stimulation to Teddy and the rest of the class, who had been sitting at the table for a period of time. It was also suggested that the gross motor activity time for Teddy should be lengthened from 20 to 30 minutes every day to offer more sensory stimulations that were needed.

Patrick visited the kindergarten again after two weeks. It was reported by the classroom teacher that Teddy was getting along well with Anson. Teddy was relatively more engaged in class with help from Anson and was able to follow some instructions during table tasks when reminded by Anson. However, his self-stimulating behaviors persisted, particularly during prolonged tasks. Patrick further advised the teacher to break down the long sitting tasks into 15-minute intervals for Teddy, with small breaks of around three minutes for Teddy to go to the sensory corner, where a spinning chair was prepared for self-regulation. The teacher agreed with the adjustment and Teddy's progress would be reviewed again at the next visit.

Intervention in the clinic and home program

To address Teddy's hyper-responsivity to tactile stimulation, Patrick designed a face-painting activity for Teddy using edible paint, and the mother was also involved. The ingredients of the paint included cornstarch, flour, honey, food coloring, and water. Teddy was asked to mix all the ingredients in a bowl with his bare hands. While mixing the ingredients, Teddy was encouraged to put the sticky mixture on his hands, forearms, and face. Teddy refused to do so at the beginning, but when his mother started by gently touching only a small area of his hands with the mixture according to Patrick's guidance, Teddy accepted the touch and finally was willing to put the mixture all over his hands and face by himself.

Similarly, Patrick focused on enhancing Teddy's personal factors in the PEO model to promote his performance skills during fine motor skills and grasping training. He planned an assembly game using blocks and Velcro. Each block was prepared by putting double-sided Velcro on all six surfaces. 3 cm × 3 cm × 3 cm blocks that could be held, assembled, and disassembled easily using a tripod grasp were selected first. Teddy was allowed to build whatever he wanted (e.g., a robot, building, plane, etc.). The size of the blocks fitted Teddy's hands; so he could grasp them well with the tripod pattern. More strength was required to assemble and disassemble the blocks due to the resistance of the Velcro, which reinforced his tripod grasp pattern. At the end of this activity, Teddy built a robot and was allowed to bring it home when he asked.

To complete the training, a home program for training upper limb coordination was prescribed by engaging Teddy and his mother in a competition. Several therabands (large elastic bands) of various lengths were prepared. For each turn, the therabands were tied loosely over Teddy's and his mother's shoulders, upper forearms, and feet, and Teddy and his mother were required to pull the therabands into certain body positions. The one who could complete the tasks fastest would win. The target positions were carefully selected to simulate the action of putting on socks and T-shirts and managing the sleeves, which enhanced the coordination of the upper extremities in putting on various types of clothing.

All training objectives were achieved in the first session, supplemented by the home program, which included Teddy's acceptance of a sticky texture on his forearms and face in the painting activity, enhancing the tripod grasp pattern through assembling and dissembling the blocks, and enhancing upper limb coordination in dressing actions by using the therabands. At the same time, Teddy was observed to enjoy the session and the mother was reported to be happy with the progress made.

For the second session, Patrick decided to do similar activities with Teddy to minimize his anxiety over new activities. For the sensory activity, various new ingredients including mini jelly cubes and peanut crumbs were added to the face paint mixture, which provided more tactile stimuli. Teddy was also encouraged to try some peanut crumbs mixed with honey to increase his oral acceptance of rough textures. Teddy accepted the new ingredients and told Patrick that he liked the taste of the peanut crumbs. For the grasping activity, smaller 2 cm × 2 cm × 2 cm blocks were used to increase the difficulty in grasping with the tripod pattern. Teddy was observed to use a more stable tripod grasp with adequate strength in assembling and disassembling the blocks. For the home program, it was reported that Teddy was more coordinated in pulling the therabands into different positions on his body after training for two weeks. Therabands with slightly more resistance were used to further enhance the movement patterns before transitioning to real garments to promote Teddy's performance in dressing activities.

Occupational therapy assessments and interventions in Singapore

Context

If Teddy were in Singapore, he would be assessed by a pediatrician and referred to the Early Intervention Programme for Infants and Children (EIPIC), which uses the routine-based model (McWilliam et al., 2020). The EIPIC team includes EI professionals (e.g., teachers) and health professionals who work closely to design appropriate IEP goals and deliver interventions in the center to children with developmental needs from birth to six years old (Ministry of Social and Family Development, 2021). The team also provides caregiver support at home. EIPIC centers are supported by the Early Childhood Development Centers Act, which regulates the operation of early childhood development centers in Singapore. Additionally, the Development Support and Learning Program provides EI and support for children with mild to moderate developmental needs in mainstream preschool.

After the initial team screening of Teddy's functional performance, he was enrolled in an EI center-based program four days a week, with each session lasting for two hours. He attended his regular preschool after his EIPIC class, and took the school bus between the two settings.

Assessments

Teddy's occupational therapist, Fae, was part of the EIPIC team who worked closely with him. Teddy was placed in a class with two EIPIC teachers and five children. In the first week, Fae worked with the classroom teacher and observed Teddy within his classroom routine. She also paid attention to Teddy's interests, strengths, and behaviors. The teacher was concerned about Teddy's ability to follow instructions and complete table-top activities. Fae noticed that Teddy struggled with fine motor activities, got frustrated quickly, and would attempt to get out of his seat and walk away. Fae also observed Teddy during snack and playtime. Her observations are listed in Table 10.4.

The teacher conducted a routine-based interview (McWilliam et al., 2009) with the caregivers/parents and commented to the EIPIC team about the family's concerns over mealtime and play. Fae followed up with a phone interview with Teddy's mother to understand more about his occupations within the home environment. His mother reported her struggle in getting Teddy to feed himself and his limited food choices. Teddy was usually fed by an adult before the family meal. He was selective with food textures and would walk around during mealtime unless entertained by music videos on YouTube channels.

Besides gathering information from Teddy's mother on how he played at home, Fae also completed the Symbolic and Imaginative Play Developmental Checklist (SIPDC)

Table 10.4 Observations of Teddy's performance in the Singaporean EIPIC context

EIPIC class observations

- At circle time, Teddy preferred to stand instead of sit. He was interested when children's music videos were played on screen and would imitate actions in songs such as "Baby Shark" or "Wheels on the Bus". When the teacher read a story, he frequently looked away and was not interested.
- He displayed a short attention span and high activity level (e.g., often leaving his seat).
- He usually left his seat quickly after experiencing some difficulty, such as not being able to insert a puzzle piece.
- Teddy struggled to use two hands together. He had difficulty in threading beads.
- He used an immature tripod grasp to hold the markers. He was able to imitate circles but not squares. He could imitate drawing random straight lines but not lines to join dots.
- He did not understand the concept of coloring in a picture and would scribble over it.
- Teddy predominantly used his right hand when asked to do tasks but would switch to his left hand occasionally.
- When given *The Three Little Pigs* book, he opened it and looked at pictures, followed by speaking a few words (e.g., pig, tree) and short sentences (e.g., it chases little piggy) after prompting.
- During free play, he was interested in putting Duplo blocks together. He showed no interest in what his classmates were building.
- When given some cooking toys, his pretend play was very limited, restricting to random one-step actions such as stirring in a bowl.
- He performed well in most gross motor activities. He enjoyed the vestibular stimuli when playing on a slide in the playground outside the center.

Measure	Scoring	Interpretation
SIPDC	Play theme: 20 months Sequence of play action: 18 months Object substitution: 20 months Social interaction: 2 years Role play: 20 months Doll/Teddy play: 2 years	The results indicate that his pretend play level is at 20–24 months. This means that his attention to pretend play would be very short as he does not have many play ideas. He would also struggle with his classmates in pretend play, particularly with different play themes.

Abbreviation: SIPDC = Symbolic and Imaginative Play Developmental Checklist.

(Stagnitti, 1998) by asking about Teddy's play skills. Apart from playing with toy cars by pushing them around on the table, Teddy showed little interest in other toys. For a short period of time, he could imitate his sister's play actions, such as walking a toy teddy bear. His mother expressed hope that he could play better with other children or his sister.

After the assessment, Fae discussed with the EIPIC team and contributed to the IEP. The IEP sets out measurable goals for a child. After a month of attending EIPIC, the team met the caregivers/parents and shared the IEP goals, which were set to be achieved within 12 months. The EI team members would work together to monitor the child's progress for each goal.

Occupational therapy interventions within EIPIC

Helping a child develop age-appropriate self-care skills such as self-feeding can help the child develop a greater sense of independence (Lim & Jones, 2017). In addition to attending center-based EIPIC, Teddy's mother agreed to attend coaching sessions with Fae to work on the self-feeding goal. The IEP goals were set to be achieved in a year and reviewed after six months. In this section, only three IEP goals will be discussed in depth. Fae worked with the EIPIC team to achieve these goals. It is important to note that, in this Singaporean EIPIC context, occupational therapists do not have separate OT goals but work toward the IEP goals of the team. Regarding PEO, the goals for Teddy centered around occupations, while also considering personal and environmental factors.

The three IEP goals discussed in this section are:

Goal 1: Teddy will participate in worktime by completing simple worksheets. We will know that he can do this when he uses lines and circles to match or indicate the answer (e.g., matching mama cat to baby kitten, circling the dog, etc.) when asked by adults at home and in school, all the time, across two weeks.

Goal 2: Teddy will participate in playtime by engaging in pretend play. We will know that he can do this when he enacts play themes related to familiar home routines, carries out three to four play action sequences for each theme, and uses similar-looking objects as needed objects (e.g., yarn strands as noodles) at home and in school, three times a week, across two weeks.

Goal 3: Teddy will participate in mealtimes by feeding himself and accepting a variety of food textures. We will know that he can do this when he brings the spoon into his mouth (after it is filled) and bites and chews shredded meat or vegetables using a munching pattern for three types of new food across two weeks.

Intervention related to feeding

Considering that Teddy's occupational performance in eating was compromised, Fae started by gathering knowledge about what his mother had attempted, what worked, what her expectations were, and the environment where his meals took place by using the PEO model and a coaching approach. To understand what was happening at home, she asked Teddy's mother to complete a three-day food diary (see Table 10.5) and take a video of his real performance at mealtime. It was clearly observed that Teddy was attending to the digital device and did not attend to the food given to him. He would open his mouth when the teaspoon reached his lips, and without much chewing, he would swallow the food.

Table 10.5 A three-day food diary for Teddy

	Saturday	Sunday	Monday (today)
Breakfast	■ Rice and sweet potato porridge (fed, ate sweet potato only) ■ Snow beans and minced pork (fed, did not finish)	■ 1 banana ■ Sandwich (toast 2 pieces, 1 egg, 1 sliced cheese) ■ Milk 150 ml ■ Some dragon fruit	■ 2 chicken nuggets (self-fed, vomited out) After that, ■ Package drinking yogurt 90 ml ■ Packet chocolate brownie ■ Family-cooked soup noodles (did not eat)
Lunch	■ Fries (self-fed) ■ Packet chocolate brownie (self-fed) ■ Packet chocolate milk 125 ml (self-fed) ■ Half red dragon fruit (fed)	■ Rice half a bowl (fed) ■ Fish and pumpkin (fed) ■ Fresh milk 250 ml (self-fed)	■ Millet porridge half a bowl (fed) ■ Fish and broccoli (fed)
Dinner	■ Fish rice porridge (fed, did not finish) ■ Homemade juice 200 ml ■ Family-cooked noodles (did not eat)	■ Porridge full bowl (fed) ■ Fish, chopped broccoli, and chopped carrot (fed and finished)	■ Small rice ball with minced chicken (self-fed, tried to remove chicken pieces)
Snacks	■ Chocolate cookie – 10:15 am ■ Fresh milk 3 cups total 300 ml – 11:30 am ■ Half red dragon fruit – 4:30 pm ■ Fresh milk, another 2 cups 200 ml – 5:30 pm ■ 1 banana – 10:20 pm before sleep	■ Brownie – 11:30 am ■ Chocolate cookie – 4 pm	■ Chocolate cookie – 11 am ■ Homemade fresh juice 300 ml – 2 pm ■ Brownie – 4 pm ■ Fresh milk 2 cups 200 ml – 5 pm

Fae did a home visit to observe Teddy's mealtime performance and his home environment. Using the principles from Occupational Performance Coaching (OPC) (Graham et al., 2021), she coached Teddy's mother on how to improve Teddy's feeding by finding feasible solutions at home. OPC is a shared process that uses collaborative performance analysis, observations in natural environments (in person or via digital recording), reflective listening, guidance, and encouragement. With feedback, Fae used OPC to help Teddy's mother develop the understanding and necessary skills that allowed her to create her own solutions to meet Teddy's feeding needs. For example, using the food diary and tapping into his mother's memory of the occasions where mealtime seemed easier, they first explored what might have worked in the past. Teddy's mother commented that on days when they were out in the afternoon and missed his afternoon milk, Teddy seemed hungrier, more interested in the food, and could eat more. With this knowledge, they explored removing the 5 pm milk time and served dinner slightly earlier to when Teddy was hungry.

After trying this method for two weeks, Teddy's mother reported to Fae that Teddy's performance in feeding had improved. He was able to eat more during dinner and seemed more interested in the food presented to him when he was hungrier. From there, Fae continued to work with his mother, as the environmental enabler, by introducing child-friendly cutlery, particularly spoons with larger handles that Teddy could grasp easily. She also recommended a bowl with a suction pad so that the bowl would not move around when Teddy attempted to feed himself some porridge. At dinner, Teddy's mother would present him with the food that he liked when he was hungry, and encouraged him to self-feed. Learning about the concept of the family meal, Teddy started having dinner alongside other family members. His mother would only start feeding him if he became distracted or tired from feeding himself.

Fae coached Teddy's mother in making conversation about the food, such as the texture, color, and smell during their meals. She also taught the mother to demonstrate to Teddy the way she chewed using her molars, encouraging Teddy to do the same with shredded meat. Teddy's mother stopped starting the meals with the digital device, but when frustrated, she would still turn it on toward the end of a meal to get him to eat more or finish up. Fae and Teddy's mother agreed to work on weaning him off the digital device as the next goal.

Intervention on pretend play

In the EIPIC class, Fae sat in the class to work with Teddy during playtime. She paired him with another child with better play skills. Fae started off by introducing a kitchen set and got the two children to imitate a few play actions. She demonstrated the following sequence: cutting the toy vegetables, putting them in a pot, stirring them in the pot, and dishing out the vegetables. Positive reinforcement is important for peer modeling to take place (Rodger et al., 2015). When the other child successfully imitated the steps, Fae praised the other child and encouraged Teddy to do the same. Teddy and his friend imitated the steps and repeated them with various dishes, such as toy sausages and fish. Fae succeeded in getting Teddy to increase the sequence of actions during cooking and their play session lasted for six minutes. Over the next four sessions, Fae introduced various play actions, such as the kitchen set, making a hot drink, having a meal, and washing up the dishes. Her intention was to introduce various play ideas to Teddy and his friend. To improve object substitution in pretend play, she also introduced similar-looking objects for play, such as an ice cream stick as a spoon, yarn strands as noodles, etc. After two weeks, they were able to perform five to six related play actions with the kitchen set and their play session lasted around ten minutes.

Next, Fae wanted to work on the goal of extending play themes beyond the events that took place at home (e.g., cooking). Being family-centered, she checked with Teddy's mother on what they frequently did on the weekend or in their free time. Teddy's mother shared that the family did grocery shopping together every Saturday. They would also frequent either a park or playground in the neighborhood. From this information, Fae picked the supermarket as the play theme to work on next. When the supermarket toys were first introduced to Teddy, he could only press the button on the toy cashier machine to make a "ding" sound. In the classroom, Fae partnered with a speech therapist in this play scene, with Teddy playing the role of a cashier. The speech therapist would push a toy trolley with some toy drink bottles to Teddy. Fae gave Teddy a four-step play sequence: scan the price tags, ask for money, collect the money, and put the toy drink bottles in a shopping bag. Along with this play theme, the speech therapist worked on the IEP goal of getting Teddy to use short greetings such as saying to his customer, "Hello, how is your day?" or "Good bye, hope to see you soon". Within three months, Teddy was observed to show improvements in both the pretend play and his language skills.

Intervention to participate in worktime

In Singapore preschools, it is common for children to be tasked with table-top work such as coloring pictures or completing simple worksheets. In addition to pretend play, Fae sat with Teddy in his EIPIC class to improve his pencil skills at table-top tasks. Fae chose pictures that he was interested in, such as cars and baby sharks. She scaffolded by getting him to imitate a line to connect two dots near to each other and then slowly increasing the distance between the dots. She then introduced the idea of matching and joining two baby sharks together. Fae demonstrated samples of good work versus scribbles and made it explicit by giving lots of stickers to a piece of work with neat lines versus none for the one that was scribbled over. Thicker crayons or color pencils were provided to Teddy. Fae highlighted the importance of keeping the non-dominant hand on the table, and would pull his paper away when his non-dominant hand was not there to stabilize or "protect" the paper. Based on his current pencil skills, she recommended to the teachers the types of worksheets that Teddy was ready for.

In class, Fae also worked on other fine motor activities to improve Teddy's bilateral coordination. By threading beads, she got Teddy's non-dominant hand to hold a bead, while the dominant hand did the threading. Through numerous practices of fine motor activities using both hands, Teddy reduced the frequency of switching hands and was able to engage longer in table-top activities. Teddy's attention span for table-top tasks improved with the use of a visual schedule in his class. He was able to complete the tasks on the schedule before leaving his seat. With improved fine motor skills, he also got less frustrated when attempting fine motor activities such as puzzles.

By the first six-month review, Teddy had made good progress with his IEP goals. Fae evaluated the effectiveness of her OT intervention. She was pleased with the outcome of coaching the mother in addressing mealtime concerns (self-care), working with the speech therapist to jointly improve pretend play and language (leisure/play), and working within the classroom and with Teddy's teachers to improve his participation in table-top tasks (productivity).

Reflections on the similarities and differences of occupational therapy across the three regions

The case study in this chapter highlights several cultural similarities and differences in the provision of pediatric OT services across Taiwan, Hong Kong, and Singapore. First, pediatric occupational therapists in all three regions collaborate with other professionals to develop individualized treatment plans that address children's needs, help them achieve developmental milestones, and maximize their independence in ADL.

However, differences in laws and regulations have resulted in various service settings for pediatric occupational therapists in each region. For example, in Taiwan, where there is a National Health Insurance system, most pediatric occupational therapists work in hospitals or clinics. In Hong Kong, pediatric occupational therapists work mostly in non-governmental organizations (NGOs), subvented by the Social Welfare Department. In Singapore, pediatric occupational therapists work in diverse settings such as hospitals, clinics, and community-based centers, which provide EI services supported by the government.

Second, the PEO model was used to analyze Teddy's problems and guide assessment in all three regions, but the selection of the assessments and approaches varied depending on cultural considerations. For instance, the therapists in Taiwan and Hong Kong conducted sensory-related and fine motor-related assessments with Teddy, but different tools were used due to the availability of culturally adapted tools in each region. The therapists in Singapore might be more inclined to use a top-down approach to assessment by obtaining information about Teddy's play, the way he ate his meals, and his food choices. In contrast, the therapists in Taiwan and Hong Kong focused more on a bottom-up assessment approach related to Teddy's sensory processing and fine motor skills. These differences might be related to the service settings in which the therapists worked, such as hospitals in Taiwan versus EIPIC centers in Singapore.

Third, the differences in service settings have resulted in varying foci for the interventions given to Teddy. For instance, more intervention goals on his performance component skills appeared to be targeted in Taiwanese hospital settings, whereas no specific OT goals were formulated in Singaporean EIPIC settings. Instead, shared functional goals were set for the transdisciplinary EI team to work toward. However, despite these slight variations, the overarching goals for OT services across the three regions were similar, which were to enhance Teddy's performance in certain meaningful occupations. The focus on these occupations in the intervention plan could vary across regions due to the cultural influences that shaped different customs, beliefs, activity patterns, behavioral standards, and expectations. For instance, Teddy's dressing issue was not addressed in the Taiwanese context as his parents helped him directly, and it was not a major concern at that moment. In contrast, Teddy's performance in table tasks was formulated as the first goal in the Hong Kong context. This corresponds to Hong Kong parents' emerging concern for children's academic performance since kindergarten. As a pediatric occupational therapist, it is important to be aware of how culture can influence the focus of OT service provision.

Important considerations for provision of occupational therapy services with pediatric cases

Culture can influence OT service provision, but there are four common considerations that OT students should keep in mind when working with pediatric cases in the future, regardless of the cultural context. Importantly, these considerations vary from those related to the OT service provision for adults with DD, and this also requires students' special attention. The four considerations are a family-centered approach, children's developmental milestones at various stages, the crucial role of caregivers, and play as a means and end in therapy toward school readiness.

Family-centered approach

A family-centered approach is often used in pediatric OT practice, particularly for therapists working in EI services or the school system. Under this approach, caregivers/parents are acknowledged as experts who know their children best and have ultimate responsibility for their care (Rosenbaum et al., 1998). Each family is considered unique and has various needs and strengths. Unlike working with adult clients, as presented in other chapters, occupational therapists must partner with the child's caregivers/parents to ensure the active involvement of the family in decision-making in all stages of the child's care. For example, Teddy's mother was involved in all three regions to set goals that were currently meaningful to the entire family and to define intervention priorities in collaboration with the therapists. Additionally, the family routine in the Singaporean context or family members other than parents in the Taiwanese context were considered as part of the intervention strategies. These examples highlight the importance of occupational therapists not only serving as information providers to enable caregivers/parents to make informed decisions, but also working with the entire family to implement treatment for children with DD.

Children's developmental milestones at various stages

One consideration when providing pediatric OT services is recognizing children's potential for development over time. This consideration has been demonstrated in our case study across the three regions. For example, the developmental milestones of Teddy's fine motor and play skills were assessed using several norm-referenced standardized tests (e.g., the PDMS-2-FM and the HK-PFMDA). These assessments allowed occupational therapists to determine if Teddy's performance component skills were delayed compared to his same-age peers. Weaker areas, such as grasping (percentile rank of 1 in the PDMS-2-FM) and fine motor skills (standard deviation of −1.12 in the HK-PFMDA), were targeted for further intervention in the Taiwanese and Hong Kong contexts, respectively. In the Singaporean context, therapists focused on promoting Teddy's pretend play skills based on the SIPDC results, which indicated a significant lag in his pretend play level. Challenging activities that are just the right level of difficulty must be designed to facilitate skill development and help Teddy progress to higher levels.

Additionally, occupational therapists have to possess a solid understanding of diagnostic criteria and related symptoms, drawing upon neurological knowledge. This is crucial as DD encompasses various neurodevelopmental disorders, as previously mentioned. With diagnostic knowledge, occupational therapists can efficiently identify key areas to be included in the initial assessment, enabling them to understand the impact of neurodevelopmental disorders on children's development. For example, in the case of Teddy, who received a diagnosis of ASD, it is widely recognized that impairment in social interaction, communication difficulties, sensory processing dysfunction, and restricted interests are common characteristics. Consequently, the therapists in both the Taiwanese and Hong Kong contexts conducted sensory-related assessments to evaluate the typicality of Teddy's sensory performance. The consideration of developmental milestones in children with DD holds significant importance for therapists when devising assessment and subsequent intervention plans.

Crucial role of caregivers

Caregivers play a crucial role in the care of children with DD and in extending therapy to the home environment. This is especially important considering that each child typically receives only one 30-minute or 60-minute OT session per week. To maximize the effectiveness of treatment, occupational therapists must actively involve caregivers/parents as participants and facilitators in implementing home training during the remaining time. It is also necessary for therapists to explore what strategies the caregivers/parents are already trying outside of the therapy context and whether they are working (Lim et al., 2021). The development of suitable home programs, along with the provision of parental education and training, is a significant aspect of pediatric OT services. Teddy's case illustrates the implementation of several home programs focusing on eating or upper limb coordination in the Taiwanese and Hong Kong contexts. This highlights the importance of equipping caregivers/parents with the necessary knowledge and skills to support their children's therapy at home.

Parent-focused interventions have become the practice-of-choice in pediatric rehabilitation and EI services. One such intervention, OPC (Graham et al., 2021), exemplified in the Singaporean context, can effectively enhance Teddy's occupational performance and participation through coaching his mother. Occupational therapists, by using goal-specific, open-ended questions, are able to coach caregivers/parents in identifying practical strategies to improve their children's participation in daily activities within the natural environment (Chien et al., 2020). This approach can help to improve parents' confidence and ultimately serve to benefit the children's development of motor, cognitive, and social skills.

Play as a means and end in therapy toward school readiness

Play is a primary occupation of children and serves as a cornerstone for their development across various skill areas. Occupational therapists make use of play as both a therapeutic means and end to capture children's attention, facilitate skill practice, promote overall development, and foster enjoyment. For example, children with DD may have limited opportunities to interact with toys, which puts them at a higher risk of fine motor delay compared to typically developing peers, potentially dampening their interest in play. Occupational therapists can attempt to understand play stages (such as sensorimotor, constructive, or pretend play), the child's play repertoires, and his/her preferences to create engaging play environments for therapy. Suitable play materials and activities can thus be selected to encourage the child's participation in manipulative play, enhance his/her fine motor skills, and cultivate a sense of enjoyment.

Unlike adult clients, therapeutic play in pediatric OT services also aims to foster school readiness in areas such as prewriting, self-care, and social skills before children's transition to primary education. This aspect is crucial considering that the first six years of a child's life are pivotal for development, and many EI services may conclude around this age. OT goals for preschool-aged children often involve self-care, prewriting, socialization, and self-regulation. Through play, which provides a relaxing and fun context, children can practice and master various skills and abilities that are vital for their school lives. Play serves as a central occupation within OT intervention and as a means to develop skills while simultaneously providing children with a sense of pleasure and intrinsic motivation as the end.

Summary

This chapter provides an illustration of the diverse OT assessments and interventions used for a four-year-old boy with ASD in Taiwan, Hong Kong, and Singapore, employing the PEO model. Notably, OT services in Taiwan are more likely to be hospital-based, whereas the services in the other two regions are primarily center-based or school-based. The choice of assessment varies across the three regions, influenced by therapists' clinical reasoning based on the PEO model, intervention focus, and the availability of locally relevant assessment tools. In Taiwan and Hong Kong, the OT interventions appear to target fine motor skills and sensory processing, while in Singapore, the focus seems to be on functional areas such as eating meals and play. These differences may stem from the goals set by caregivers/parents within their unique cultural contexts.

However, there are also notable similarities. The PEO model is utilized in all three regions, and occupational therapists collaborate closely with other professionals and teachers.

Clinical observations are employed to assess children's occupational performance in activities of interest. Self-care activities (e.g., eating) and school participation (including peer interaction and table-related activities) are the primary areas of focus in intervention services across the three regions. Occupational therapists provide direct interventions to the children and act as consultants/coaches, working with caregivers/parents and teachers to enhance the children's performance at home and school.

Based on the case illustrations from the three Oriental regions, there are four principles that OT students should consider when learning about pediatric OT. First, they must adopt a family-centered approach and view pediatric cases and their families as a whole. Second, an understanding of children's developmental milestones is crucial for selecting appropriate assessments and designing effective interventions. Third, active involvement of the children's caregivers/parents in implementing rehabilitation training outside of therapeutic settings is essential. Fourth, recognizing that play is a primary occupation for children, students should learn about play and utilize it as a means and end to promote the development, skills, participation, and enjoyment of children with DD, ultimately preparing them for school. Last but not least, gaining proficiency in using the PEO model is also essential for aspiring pediatric OT practitioners.

References

Bornstein, M. H., & Hendricks, C. (2013). Screening for developmental disabilities in developing countries. *Social Science & Medicine, 97*, 307–315. https://doi.org/10.1016/j.socscimed.2012.09.049

Bruininks, R. H., & Bruininks, B. D. (2005). *BOT-2: Bruininks-Oseretsky test of motor proficiency* (2nd ed.). AGS Publishing.

Case-Smith, J. (2015). *Occupational therapy for children and adolescents* (7th ed.). Elsevier Mosby.

Case-Smith, J., Weaver, L. L., & Fristad, M. A. (2015). A systematic review of sensory processing interventions for children with autism spectrum disorders. *Autism, 19*(2), 133–148. https://doi.org/10.1177/1362361313517762

Chapin, S., McNaughton, D., Boyle, S., & Babb, S. (2018). Effects of peer support interventions on the communication of preschoolers with autism spectrum disorder: A systematic review. *Seminars in Speech and Language, 39*(5), 443–457. https://doi.org/10.1055/s-0038-1670670

Chien, C. W., Lai, Y. Y. C., Lin, C. Y., & Graham, F. (2020). Occupational performance coaching with parents to promote community participation and quality of life of young children with developmental disabilities: A feasibility evaluation in Hong Kong. *International Journal of Environmental Research and Public Health*, 17(21), 7993. https://doi.org/10.3390/ijerph17217993

Chien, C. W., & Lo, J. L. (2009). Pediatric occupational therapy in Taiwan: Education, service provision, and ongoing development. *Journal of Occupational Therapy, Schools, & Early Intervention*, 2(3–4), 238–245.

Folio, M. R., & Fewell, R. R. (2000). *Peabody Developmental Motor Scales: Examiner's manual* (2nd ed.). PRO-ED.

Graham, F., Kennedy-Behr, A., & Ziviani, J. (2021). *Occupational performance coaching: A manual for practitioners and researchers*. Routledge.

Kaplan, M. (2010). A frame of reference for motor skill acquisition. In P. Kramer, & J. Hinojosa (Eds.), *Frames of reference for pediatric occupational therapy* (3rd ed., pp. 390–424). Lippincott Williams & Wilkins.

Lai, C. Y. Y., Yung, T. W. K., Gomez, I. N. B., & Siu, A. M. H. (2019). Psychometric properties of Sensory Processing and Self-Regulation Checklist (SPSRC). *Occupational Therapy International*, 2019(1), 8796042. https://doi.org/10.1155/2019/8796042

Lane, A. E., Molloy, C. A., & Bishop, S. L. (2014). Classification of children with autism spectrum disorder by sensory subtype: A case for sensory-based phenotypes. *Autism Research*, 7(3), 322–333. https://doi.org/10.1002/aur.1368

Law, M., Cooper, B., Strong, S., Stewart, D., Rigby, P., & Letts, L. (1996). The Person-Environment-Occupation Model: A transactive approach to occupational performance. *Canadian Journal of Occupational Therapy*, 63(1), 9–23. https://doi.org/10.1177/000841749606300103

Lim, S. M., & Jones, F. (2017). Occupational transitions for children and young people. In S. Rodger, & A. Kennedy-Behr (Eds.), *Occupation-centred practice with children: A practical guide for occupational therapists* (2nd ed., pp. 111–132). Wiley-Blackwell.

Lim, S. M., Nyoman, L., Tan, Y. J., & Yin, Y. Y. (2021). Transition practice before entering primary school: A longitudinal study of children with and without special needs across a year. *Hong Kong Journal of Occupational Therapy*, 34(2), 63–72. https://doi.org/10.1177/15691861211013427

Luebben, A. J., & Royeen, C. B. (2010). An acquisitional frame of reference. In P. Kramer, & J. Hinojosa (Eds.), *Frames of reference for pediatric occupational therapy* (3rd ed., pp. 461–488). Lippincott Williams & Wilkins.

McWilliam, R. A., Boavida, T., Bull, K., Cañadas, M., Hwang, A.-W., Józefacka, N., Lim, H. H., Pedernera, M., Sergnese, T., & Woodward, J. (2020). The routines-based model internationally implemented. *International Journal of Environmental Research and Public Health*, 17(22), 8308. https://doi.org/10.3390/ijerph17228308

McWilliam, R. A., Casey, A. M., & Sims, J. L. (2009). The routines-based interview: A method for gathering information and assessing needs. *Infants & Young Children*, 22(3), 224–233.

Ministry of Social and Family Development. (2021). *Professional practice guidelines: Developmental and psycho-educational assessments and provisions for preschool-aged children*. Ministry of Education, Ministry of Social and Family Development and Early Childhood Development Agency. https://www.ecda.gov.sg/docs/default-source/default-document-library/parents/guidelines-(for-professionals)-2021.pdf

Planck, Z., & Bisognin, S. (2016). *Oral defensiveness*. Bright Start Therapy. https://brightstart-therapy.com.au/for-parents/parent-resources/

Rodger, S., Ziviani, J., & Lim, S. M. (2015). Occupations of childhood and adolescence. In C. H. Christiansen, C. M. Baum, & J. D. Bass (Eds.), *Occupational therapy: Performance, participation, and well-being* (4th ed., pp. 129–155). Slack Incorporated.

Rosenbaum, P., King, S., Law, M., King, G., & Evans, J. (1998). Family-centred service: A conceptual framework and research review. *Physical & Occupational Therapy in Pediatrics*, 18(1), 1–20. https://doi.org/10.1080/J006v18n01_01

Siu, A. M. H., Lai, C. Y. Y., Chiu, A. S. M., & Yip, C. C. K. (2011). Development and validation of a fine-motor assessment tool for use with young children in a Chinese population. *Research in Developmental Disabilities*, 32(1), 107–114. https://doi.org/10.1016/j.ridd.2010.09.003

Stagnitti, K. (1998). *Learn to play: A practical program to develop a child's imaginative play skills*. Co-ordinates Publications.

Tang, K. M. L., Chen, T. Y. K., Lau, V. W. Y., & Wu, M. M. F. (2008). Clinical profile of young children with mental retardation and developmental delay in Hong Kong. *Hong Kong Medical Journal, 14*(2), 97–102. https://www.hkmj.org/abstracts/v14n2/97.htm

Tsang, M. H., & Chen, K. L. (2012). *Chinese version of Pediatric Evaluation of Disability Inventory: Instructor manual.* Psychological Publishing Co., Ltd.

Tseng, M. H. (1998). *Development of the Screening Instrument for Sensory Processing Functions.* National Science Council.

Wu, J.-C., Chiang, C.-H., Hou, Y.-M., Liu, J.-H., Chu, C.-L., & Sung, W.-C. (2014). The validity of Childhood Autism Rating Scale in diagnosing autism spectrum disorders in young children. *Educational and Psychological Research, 37*, 37–58.

CHAPTER 11

Schizophrenia

Shu-Mei Wang, Kino Chiu Kim Lam, Vera Wai Man Lam,
Soo Fung Ho, Kamaldin Bin Ibrahim, and Yogeswary Maniam

Case background

Jeff is a 22-year-old man living in Hong Kong who has been diagnosed with schizophrenia. His father died in an accident when Jeff was a child. He currently lives with his mother, who is 49 years old. His 27-year-old sister got married and lives with her husband. When Jeff was 21 years old, he was first hospitalized in a Hospital Authority public hospital due to delusions, hallucinations, social withdrawal, and several difficulties in occupational performance.

At both primary and secondary school, Jeff was an introvert and a diligent student with good academic performance. He believed that he was able to gain good results through hard work. He also felt confident in studying. He had a high expectation for his future because he wanted to take good care of the family after the death of his father. He did not have many friends because he mainly focused on studying and did not know how to establish friendships. His only close friend was Neal, a classmate who proactively got close to him. Jeff treasured this friendship. They usually played basketball together at break time to relieve stress. In the last year of secondary school, Jeff prepared for the Hong Kong Diploma of Secondary Education Examination and was under an overwhelming amount of stress. He started to complain about hearing noises at night and thus did not sleep well. His family did not take his complaint seriously and thought that his sensitivity to sounds resulted from his high stress. In that year, Jeff also found it difficult to concentrate on reading. Despite these challenges, he still tried hard to get through the examination and was admitted to a university program in accounting. However, he felt unsatisfied with his performance. He also felt sad that Neal and he did not study at the same university.

According to Jeff, he did not have a happy university life. Although he wanted to make new friends, he turned out to have none during these years. He felt that he was unable to get along with his classmates and that his classmates usually grouped together, made fun of him, and said he was nerdy. Jeff thought that they were jealous

DOI: 10.4324/9781032721170-15

of his intelligence. Sometimes Jeff lost his temper and shouted at them directly. Jeff did not join any clubs at university because he had no interest in them. He also had no specific hobbies. Sometimes he played basketball with Neal on the weekend when Neal called him. Most of the time after classes, Jeff did not know what to do. When Jeff was a sophomore, he began working part-time in various fast-food restaurants to get away from his classmates. He also wanted to earn money to reduce the financial burden on his family. However, Jeff was unable to maintain each job for more than half a year because he thought that he always had bad fellow workers and bosses. Jeff felt that his fellow employees and bosses slandered him saying that he was goofing around and doing nothing during work hours. Jeff either quit or was fired due to bitter quarrels with his colleagues or bosses.

The situation worsened in Jeff's fourth year at university. He kept hearing voices that scolded him and asked him to rebel against the bullying by his classmates. He believed that his teachers and bosses were drugging him to make him study or work harder. He also regularly saw someone spying on him, although no one else saw this person, and so he felt terrified. He had trouble concentrating and memorizing anything in daily life. He also lost the motivation to study and work. He stayed at home and was socially isolated. He even did not want to hang out with Neal. Jeff isolated himself in his room, talking to and shouting at the voices he heard. He was angry, nervous, terrified, and could not sleep at night or sleep regularly. His self-care became poor, and his mother and sister needed to take leave from work to accompany him at home. Jeff conversed with the family in sentences that were disorganized and not understandable. His movements were slow and rigid. Since Jeff did not attend classes in school and skipped work, he failed all his subjects and was laid off again.

Jeff's mother had worked hard to take care of her two children after the death of her husband. She had high expectations for her children's academic performance, and they had also never disappointed her. Since Jeff's mother usually worked long hours, Jeff spent much time with his elder sister at home after school during his primary and secondary school years. He was close to his sister and would seek advice from her if needed. Jeff always wanted to reciprocate the efforts of his family when he grew up. He aimed to be more independent and able to manage his own affairs after becoming an undergraduate. As such, even though he had difficult relationships with his classmates and fellow workers, he chose not to talk about it with his family. In the third year of university, Jeff experienced a drastic life change and was under stress because his sister got married and moved into her new home. Jeff did not know how to deal with his mixed emotions, so he suppressed them. Afterward, in his fourth year of university, he showed an obvious deterioration in his self-care, studies, and work, along with worsening illness symptoms. Jeff's mother did not understand Jeff's changes and felt very disappointed, which, in turn, put a lot of stress on Jeff.

After searching for information online, Jeff's sister contacted various Early Assessment Service for Young People with Early Psychosis (E.A.S.Y.) centers via their hotlines and discussed Jeff's conditions with them. Shortly thereafter, Jeff was admitted to a hospital for a month to receive professional medical treatment. However, eight months after his discharge, Jeff was admitted to the hospital again because he stopped taking his antipsychotics and had a relapse. Upon leaving the acute ward this time, Jeff continued receiving occupational therapy (OT) in a day hospital.

Occupational therapy assessments in Hong Kong

The acute stage

This was Jeff's second admission to the acute ward because he stopped taking his antipsychotics and had a relapse. The occupational therapists adopted the stress-vulnerability model (Zubin & Spring, 1977) in interviews and encouraged Jeff to explore his *stressors* related to this relapse, as well as his *protective factors* (including illness management skills), which helped him resist the influence of stress in the recovery journey.

Interviews

During the interview, Jeff expressed the following details about the stressors he faced over the past year.

Therapist: What have you found most stressful in the past year?

Jeff: I found that there were many stressors in my life. It seemed that I could not mix well with my classmates. I always had arguments with them.

Therapist: What else?

Jeff: When I had my part-time job, I also had conflicts with my co-workers. Later, I heard voices that were scolding me and asking me to rebel against the bullying by my classmates. I was so mad at that time! The voices existed again this time and I don't know why!

Therapist: Do you experience any stress which is related to your family?

Jeff: My mother always put high expectations on my academic and career performance. It made me feel stressful at times. I used to talk to my sister when I encountered problems. Also, I felt very anxious when my sister got married because afterwards it was difficult to seek her support immediately when I encountered problems.

Jeff identified three major stressors that appeared in the past year: tense relationships with his classmates and co-workers, high expectations from his mother, and reduced support from his sister after her marriage.

During the interview, the occupational therapists worked with Jeff to support him in recognizing his existing protective factors as his strengths to withstand the ramifications of his illness. Jeff also identified challenges in his recovery journey. The following interview extract provides insights into how Jeff managed stress and what social support he had.

Therapist: In general, how did you manage your stress and negative emotions?

Jeff: I tended to bottle up my feelings. The only way I used to reduce my stress was to play basketball with Neal, my old friend.

Therapist: When you face difficulties in your life, who can help you handle stress and give you support?

Jeff: I only talk with Neal. Otherwise, I cannot think of any other people.

Therapist: In terms of your family, who could give you support?

Jeff: My sister used to. However, after she got married and moved out, we could not chat as frequently as before.

Through the interview, the therapists discovered that Jeff managed stress through a particular sport. Potential social support for Jeff came from his good friend, Neal. Based on these existing protective factors, Jeff recognized the challenges and wanted to expand his stress management skills and social circle.

In one of the interview sessions, Jeff expressed his limited understanding of schizophrenia. Jeff told the therapists that he stopped taking antipsychotics in the past when he felt better in terms of his mood. He did not know how long he should maintain pharmacotherapy. About one month prior to his second admission to the acute ward, he started hearing noises and voices when he was alone. He was not sure if it meant a risk of a relapse. Since he was admitted to the acute ward again, he expressed to the therapists that he understood the necessity for a proper understanding of psychiatric intervention so as to retain the treatment effects and avert future relapses.

Interview results and goals of occupational therapy

Based on the stress-vulnerability model, the occupational therapists used several interview sessions to discuss with Jeff about the stressors and challenges he perceived, the existing protective factors as his strengths, and the therapeutic goals during the acute ward period. Throughout the interviews, Jeff recognized illness management as a challenge. In addition, he identified that peer relationships, his mother's expectations, and reduced support from his sister following her marriage were his major stressors.

After discussing with the therapists, Jeff recognized that he had built up some protective factors. For example, he was able to rely on sports and Neal's company to cope with stress. Nevertheless, he realized that he still encountered difficulties in stress management. After discussion and collaboration, Jeff and the occupational therapists worked out the first short-term therapeutic goal to target during the acute ward period, which was to perform illness management once per week in illness management group sessions in a month. Illness management included recognizing symptom fluctuations and signs of relapse, accessing healthcare services, interpreting medication instructions and taking medications regularly, coping with emotions and stress, etc. Another short-term goal was to complete a role play in ward group sessions in a month, where Jeff needed to finish a group project despite having tense relationships with his groupmates. Table 11.1 summarizes all the abovementioned information.

The day hospital stage

The occupational therapists used the Model of Human Occupation (MOHO; see Chapter 1) (Kielhofner, 2008) and the stress-vulnerability model (Zubin & Spring, 1977) to collaborate with Jeff to explore his strengths and challenges. Interviews and assessments were used to collect information on the three subsystems (volition, habituation, and performance), as well as opportunities and demands from environments in MOHO. In addition, interviews were also conducted to collect information on stressors and protective factors in the stress-vulnerability model. Detailed results are shown below.

Interviews

The occupational therapists used individual interviews to obtain information on the volition subsystem and environments of MOHO. The volition subsystem includes personal causation (related to a sense of personal capacity and self-efficacy), values (related

Table 11.1 Summary of Jeff's interview results and corresponding short-term OT goals in the acute stage

Model	Interview results	Short-term goals
SVM – Stressors and challenges	■ Facing challenges of illness management.	■ Jeff can perform illness management once per week in illness management group sessions in a month.
		(This goal is also related to stress management mentioned in the next point because illness management includes stress management.)

	■ Feeling stressful because of:
	  ■ Tense relationships with classmates and co-workers;
	  ■ High expectations from his mother; and
	  ■ Reduced support from his sister after her marriage.
	■ Still facing difficulties in stress management despite existing coping strategies mentioned in protective factors.
		■ Jeff can complete a role play in ward group sessions in a month, where he needs to finish a group project despite having tense relationships with his groupmates.

SVM – Protective factors	■ Able to rely on sports and Neal's company to cope with stress.	

Abbreviation: SVM = Stress-vulnerability model.

to importance and meaningfulness of activities), and interests. Below is an extract of the interview regarding Jeff's personal causation and values.

Therapist: What are your important goals in life?

Jeff: I want to take good care of my mother, you know, since I'm the only son and the only male member in my family after my father's death. I want to get good academic grades at university and find a stable accounting job after graduation to apply what I have learned at university and to earn money.

Therapist: How do you achieve these desired outcomes?

Jeff: I think I need to study hard and get good results, then I may get a good job. I used to get satisfactory academic results because I worked hard in both primary and secondary school.

Therapist: What are your current performances when you study and work part-time?

Jeff: Since I had abnormal experiences, I have found a deterioration in my academic performance. Now I am not so confident that I could study as well as before. I worry that I will not get good grades even though I study hard. I am anxious and distressed. I need to complete my bachelor's degree by this year. I have not yet achieved my goals!

Therapist: What else do you want to achieve?

Jeff: I think I have poor social skills so that I only have one friend. I may want to know how to make friends in the future.

For personal causation, Jeff found it difficult to understand his own studying abilities, indicating a limited sense of personal capacity. He did not believe that he could use his ability to achieve the desired academic outcomes, showing limited self-efficacy. For values, Jeff thought that having good academic performance, then getting a stable job, and ultimately taking care of his family were important for him. In addition, Jeff also thought that friendship and making friends were important.

Social environments might provide opportunities or place demands on Jeff. The occupational therapists asked questions during the interviews to collect related information and observed that opportunities from Jeff's social environments included support from his sister and his friend, Neal. Although Jeff's sister had gotten married and reduced the number of long talks with Jeff, she was still able to provide support when Jeff proactively contacted her. Also, although Neal and Jeff studied at different universities, Neal regularly played basketball with Jeff and provided support to him. On the other hand, demands from Jeff's social environments were related to the high expectations of his mother, who had a limited understanding of mental illness. Jeff felt stressful and guilty because he could not maintain good academic grades and meet his mother's expectations after the onset of schizophrenia. His mother did not know about the psychotic symptoms that Jeff experienced, so Jeff rarely talked to her about the disease and his distress.

Based on the stress-vulnerability model, the occupational therapists also collaborated with Jeff in the interviews to explore his stressors and protective factors. Moving from the acute stage to the day hospital stage, Jeff faced similar stressors but had already performed illness management and completed a role play related to stress management. He could recall some key knowledge about schizophrenia, psychotic symptoms, medications, signs of relapse, and strategies for stress management.

Assessments

The occupational therapists not only relied on interviews but also adopted various checklists, questionnaires, assessment batteries, and work samples to collect information on the three subsystems of MOHO. As mentioned above, the volition subsystem includes personal causation, values, and interests. The habituation subsystem includes the concepts of habits/routines and roles. The performance subsystem includes capacities and skills that support performance in various occupational areas. Below are the assessment results in detail.

For Jeff's interests in the volition subsystem, the occupational therapists used interviews to learn that Jeff played basketball. The therapists further used the Modified Interest Checklist (MOHO-IRM Web, 2023) for in-depth exploration. The Modified Interest Checklist consists of several leisure activities that respondents may feel interested in. For each leisure activity, respondents need to indicate past and current interests, as well as the interests that they would like to develop in the future. Jeff's Modified Interest Checklist results showed that, in the past, he had very limited interests and, in the future, he would like to have a dog and maintain his current hobby of playing basketball.

To obtain information on the roles Jeff would like to perform, the occupational therapists adopted the Role Checklist (Oakley et al., 1986), which lists several life roles and requires respondents to indicate whether they played each role in the past, are playing it now, or will play it in the future. Respondents also need to indicate how valuable each role is. The Role Checklist can be used to collect information on roles in the habituation subsystem and values in the volition subsystem. Jeff's Role Checklist results showed that the valuable roles he performed at present were student, worker, friend, and family member, and the valuable roles he would perform in the future were worker, caregiver, friend, and family member.

The performance subsystem is related to various human capacities and skills. After the interviews and discussions, the occupational therapists and Jeff wanted to obtain further information about his work performance, social cognition, and neurocognition. For work performance, because Jeff wanted to look for a job related to accounting or a clerical job in the future, the occupational therapists adopted the VALPAR Component Work Sample #5 (VCWS-5) – Clerical Comprehension and Aptitude (Christopherson & Hayes, 2006) to evaluate a wide range of clerical work skills, such as mail sorting, filing, phone answering, computer use, and bookkeeping (Figure 11.1). The VCWS-5 provides work rate standards to check if examinees demonstrate successful work performance. Although Jeff showed satisfactory working speed (i.e., the rate of work was greater than 100%), he showed poor accuracy in all tasks (Table 11.2). He did not meet the requirements of most tasks, and his performance was far below competitive levels, as indicated by the result of "Did not meet (B)" in Table 11.2. Jeff only achieved the work standard of mail sorting. He was not well prepared for working in open employment as a clerk and required further training.

Social cognition covers cognitive processes regarding social interactions. These cognitive processes include how people perceive and explain social messages from environments (Marcopulos & Kurtz, 2012). The occupational therapists adopted the Chinese Facial Emotion Identification Test (Lo & Siu, 2018) and the social cognition test of the

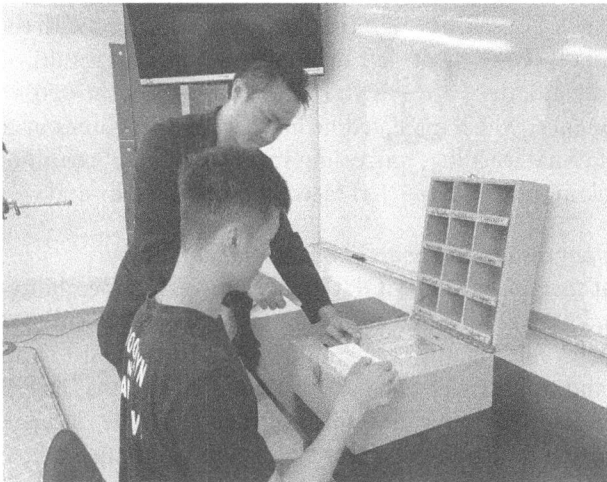

Figure 11.1 An occupational therapist using the VALPAR Component Work Sample #5 – Clerical Comprehension and Aptitude to evaluate the clerical work skills of a client

Table 11.2 Jeff's VCWS-5 – Clerical Comprehension and Aptitude assessment results

Task	Time spent[a]	Errors made	Rate of work	Whether the work standard was met
General clerical section				
Mail sorting	20 m 23 s	2	110%	Met
Alphabetical filing	14 m 52 s	4	145%	Did not meet (B)
Telephone answering	12 m	1	NA[b]	Did not meet (B)
Bookkeeping section				
Disbursement	5 m 10 s	4	140%	Did not meet (B)
Daily log	7 m 51 s	3	140%	Did not meet (B)
Payroll	11 m 12 s	2	140%	Did not meet (B)
Total	24 m 13 s	9	140%	Did not meet (B)

Notes:

[a] Time units: m = minutes; s = seconds.
[b] Not applicable because the time period required to complete this task is fixed.

Abbreviation: VCWS = VALPAR Component Work Sample.

MATRICS Consensus Cognitive Battery (August et al., 2012) to assess Jeff's social cognition. The Chinese Facial Emotion Identification Test is designed to assess facial emotional perception in examinees. It comprises 21 photos showing human faces displaying basic emotions and neutral emotions that examinees must correctly identify. Jeff's assessment results showed that he had limited ability in perceiving other people's emotions, particularly negative emotions.

To assess Jeff's neurocognition, the occupational therapists adopted the MATRICS Consensus Cognitive Battery, which is a standardized assessment battery for assessing attention, memory, problem-solving, learning, and processing speed (Figure 11.2). Although the MATRICS Consensus Cognitive Battery mainly involves neurocognitive tests, it also includes one test concerning social cognition. The obtained score in each test of the MATRICS Consensus Cognitive Battery is compared with the norm to reflect the performance level of the client. Jeff's complete assessment results of the MATRICS Consensus Cognitive Battery are shown in Table 11.3. Jeff showed a borderline level of overall performance, which indicated he had certain difficulties in cognition. Major problems were in visual learning, processing speed, and social cognition. These factors might largely explain the challenges Jeff faced in both his study and work performance.

Interview/assessment results and goals of occupational therapy

The occupational therapists used MOHO and the stress-vulnerability model to guide the interviews and assessments and to collaborate with Jeff to collect his information on the three MOHO subsystems, opportunities and demands from the social environment, stressors, and protective factors. Data gathered from the interviews and assessments were integrated into a meaningful profile of Jeff. The occupational therapists used the client-centered approach to work with Jeff to jointly determine therapeutic goals in the day hospital stage.

Throughout the interviews, assessments, and discussions, Jeff and the occupational therapists identified some long-term therapeutic goals in the day hospital stage, which

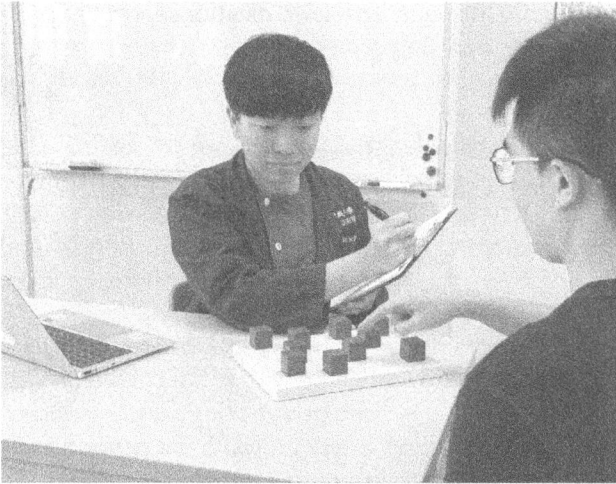

Figure 11.2 An occupational therapist using the MATRICS Consensus Cognitive Battery to evaluate neurocognition in a client. (Photo credit: Department of Occupational Therapy, Pamela Youde Nethersole Eastern Hospital, Hong Kong)

are listed below. In terms of adopting MOHO, because the three MOHO subsystems and environment were interwoven to contribute to Jeff's occupational participation, each goal setting related to MOHO entailed consideration of the interview and assessment results across the MOHO subsystems and environment.

- Jeff will perform a student role on a routine basis with a better sense of personal capacity, self-efficacy, academic performance, social skills, and cognitive skills.
- Jeff will perform a worker role on a routine basis with a better sense of personal capacity, self-efficacy, work performance, social skills, and cognitive skills.
- Jeff will engage in more social activities with more friends and family members.
- Jeff will engage in more leisure activities.
- Jeff will perform better illness management and stress management.

Table 11.3 Jeff's MATRICS Consensus Cognitive Battery assessment results

Test	Performance level
Attention	Average
Working memory	Above average
Problem-solving	Below average
Verbal learning	Average
Visual learning	Very poor
Processing speed	Very poor
Social cognition	Very poor
Overall composite	Borderline

According to MOHO, through the aforementioned occupational participation, occupational performance, and skill demonstration, Jeff will construct a positive occupational identity and accomplish occupational competence, which form Jeff's occupational adaptation.

Based on the long-term goals, Jeff and the therapists discussed the short-term goals. Similarly, Jeff and the therapists collaborated in setting each goal after considering Jeff's information across all MOHO subsystems and his environment, as well as the information on the protective factors and stressors of the stress-vulnerability model. For performing a student role, which Jeff valued, the relevant occupational performances included engaging in class activities, doing assignments, and engaging in social activities with classmates. These occupational performances were associated with Jeff's information in the performance subsystem (having difficulty with social cognition, visual learning, and processing speed) and the MOHO environment (having social support from Neal and his sister, and demands from his mother). These occupational performances were also associated with the difficulties in managing stress analyzed in the stress-vulnerability model. Therefore, the corresponding short-term goals were identified as follows:

- Jeff can attend classes at university twice per week (two sessions per week were required for the subject Jeff took this semester) in a month.
- Jeff can attend social activities (such as having lunch together) with other clients in the day hospital or his classmates at university once per week in a month.
- Jeff can complete an assignment in the subject he took this semester at university in two months.

For performing a worker role, which Jeff also valued, the relevant occupational performances included performing accounting work, working with co-workers, and engaging in social activities with co-workers in vocational training workshops at the day hospital. These occupational performances also involved analyses across the MOHO subsystems and stress-vulnerability model. Jeff and the therapists agreed on the following short-term goals:

- Jeff can perform accounting work two days per week in vocational training workshops in the day hospital in a month.
- Jeff can attend social activities (such as having lunch together) with other clients/co-workers in the day hospital or his classmates at university once per week in a month.
- Jeff can work with co-workers to complete accounting tasks once per week in vocational training workshops in the day hospital in a month.

More short-term goals in the day hospital stage are summarized in Table 11.4. It is important to note that each short-term goal in Table 11.4 was set after Jeff and the therapists considered all assessment results across subsystems, the environment, and models. Therefore, each goal was related to all assessment results. Follow-up interviews and assessments, as well as the setting of new short-term goals, continued with Jeff's changes in occupational participation, occupational performances, and skill demonstration in the day hospital.

Table 11.4 Summary of Jeff's interview and assessment results and short-term OT goals in the day hospital stage. It is important to note that although each assessment result is followed by no, one, or two short-term goals for simplified presentation, each short-term goal is related to all assessment results across subsystems, the environment, and models

Model	Assessment results	Short-term goals

MOHO – Volition	■ Personal causation:
	  ■ Having a limited sense of personal capacity.
	  ■ Having limited self-efficacy.
	■ Values:
	  ■ Achieving good academic performance, getting a stable job, taking care of the family, and making friends were important.
	■ Interests:
	  ■ Playing basketball in the past.
	  ■ A possible new interest in the future: having a dog.
		■ Jeff can perform accounting work two days per week in vocational training workshops in the day hospital in a month.
		
		■ Jeff can engage in one new leisure activity in addition to playing basketball twice per week in a month.

MOHO – Habituation	■ Roles:
	  ■ Present: student, worker, friend, and family member.
	  ■ Future: worker, caregiver, friend, and family member.
		■ Jeff can attend classes at university twice per week (two sessions per week were required for the subject Jeff took this semester) in a month.
		■ Jeff can perform accounting work two days per week in vocational training workshops in the day hospital in a month.

MOHO – Performance	■ Work performances:
	  ■ Facing difficulties in working in jobs related to accounting or clerical jobs.
	  ■ Facing challenges in social cognition (social cognitive skills).
	  ■ Having limited visual learning and processing speed.
		■ Jeff can perform accounting work two days per week in vocational training workshops in the day hospital in a month.
		■ Jeff can attend social activities (such as having lunch together) with other clients in the day hospital or his classmates at university once per week in a month.
		■ Jeff can complete an assignment of the subject he took this semester at university in two months.

Table 11.4 Summary of Jeff's interview and assessment results and short-term OT goals in the day hospital stage. It is important to note that although each assessment result is followed by no, one, or two short-term goals for simplified presentation, each short-term goal is related to all assessment results across subsystems, the environment, and models (*continued*)

Model	Assessment results	Short-term goals
MOHO – Environments	■ Opportunities from social environments: 　■ Having partial support from his sister and his friend, Neal. ■ Demands from social environments: 　■ Facing high expectations from his mother.	■ Jeff's mother and sister can attend caregiver groups once per week in the day hospital in a month. (This goal targets Jeff's social environment [i.e., his mother and sister], not Jeff himself, to create more environmental support and reduce environmental demands. Attaining this goal supports activity engagement in other short-term goals targeting Jeff.)
SVM – Stressors and challenges	■ Facing challenges of illness management.	■ Jeff can perform illness management once per week in illness management group sessions in a month. (This goal is also related to stress management mentioned in the next point because illness management includes stress management.)
	■ Feeling stressful because of: 　■ Tense relationships with classmates and co-workers. 　■ High expectations from his mother. 　■ Reduced support from his sister after her marriage. ■ Still facing difficulties in stress management despite existing coping strategies mentioned in protective factors.	■ Jeff can work with co-workers to complete accounting tasks once per week in vocational training workshops in the day hospital in a month.
SVM – Protective factors	■ Being able to rely on sports and Neal's company to cope with stress.	

Abbreviations: MOHO = Model of Human Occupation; SVM = Stress-vulnerability model.

Occupational therapy intervention in Hong Kong

The acute stage

The first short-term goal for Jeff was to be able to perform illness management once per week in illness management group sessions in a month. For the corresponding intervention, the occupational therapists invited Jeff to join psychoeducational groups about illness management skills, such as the Transforming Relapse and Instilling Prosperity group (Chan, 2009). Such groups aim to educate Jeff about schizophrenia and psychotic symptoms, antipsychotic medications, stress management skills, ways to prevent relapses, etc. Generally, these sessions last less than an hour, with multiple sessions per week across two to four weeks because of the short period of hospitalization in the acute ward. Relapse is a severe issue for clients suffering from schizophrenia because clients' function dramatically decreases with each occurrence of relapse. Research has shown that the illness management groups led by occupational therapists effectively increase illness insights and health in schizophrenia clients, as well as reduce re-hospitalization after discharge from the acute ward (Chan, 2009).

The second short-term goal was that Jeff could complete a role play in ward group sessions in a month, where he needed to finish a group project despite having tense relationships with groupmates. Jeff faced numerous stressors, such as reduced support from his sister, difficulty in meeting his mother's expectations, and getting along with his classmates and co-workers. Although some stress was related to Jeff's psychotic symptoms (e.g., his delusions might result in a hostile reaction toward his classmates and co-workers) and could lessen during remission, numerous stressors still existed for Jeff after his discharge from the acute ward, and these continued to interfere with his work performance. Therefore, enhancing Jeff's coping skills or stress management skills was crucial. The occupational therapists in Hong Kong not only invited Jeff to join illness management groups that covered topics on stress management but also conducted individual therapy, adopting several counseling skills, such as motivational interviewing and solution-focused brief therapy, to help Jeff cope with stressors in his occupational participation. Motivational interviewing aims to increase clients' motivation for change and focuses on collaborative relationships with clients, evoking clients' own reasons for change and their autonomy to decide what to do. Solution-focused brief therapy focuses on clients' resources and strengths that could be used to solve problems instead of focusing on why there are problems. Both motivational interviewing and solution-focused brief therapy emphasize clients' abilities/strengths and changes/solutions (Lewis & Osborn, 2004). Previously, when Jeff faced stressors, he chose to keep the problems to himself and bottle up his negative feelings. During individual therapy, the occupational therapists guided Jeff to think about his desires (what he wanted or wished), his abilities to change (what he could do), the reasons for making the change, and his needs (what he was obliged to do). Through the motivational interviewing process, the therapists elicited Jeff's motivations for changing his behaviors from bottling up negative feelings to other effective coping strategies. The therapists also used solution-focused brief therapy techniques in individual therapy. For example, Jeff was guided to envision a future without his negative feelings and further think about what helped him cope with stressors. This process increased Jeff's awareness of his available resources and strengths and shifted his focus to solutions. The therapists arranged small groups involving two to four clients with similar difficulties in stress management and provided opportunities of role playing for Jeff to practice related skills during activity engagement.

The day hospital stage

The OT intervention targeting each short-term goal in the day hospital stage is described below. It is worth noting that the OT intervention described in a particular paragraph may also contribute to the goals indicated in other paragraphs.

Goal 1: Jeff can attend classes at university twice per week (two sessions per week were required for the subject Jeff took this semester) in a month.

In terms of values and roles in MOHO, Jeff thought that performing the roles of student, worker, friend, and family member was important. The occupational therapists and Jeff decided to target the first three roles in rehabilitation in the day hospital considering the role of family member was not lost. To maintain the student role, after discussing with the occupational therapists, Jeff would keep studying at university. However, the therapists discussed the assessment results with Jeff, particularly those regarding his limitations in neurocognition and stress management, to help him make a feasible study plan. With the academic and therapeutic support from his academic advisor at university and the occupational therapists in the day hospital, Jeff planned to take one subject in the upcoming semester and finish his year-four subjects in two years. The routine of taking classes every week enabled Jeff to maintain a student role, which was important to him.

Goal 2: Jeff can perform accounting work two days per week in vocational training workshops in the day hospital in a month.

Every week, Jeff received OT in the day hospital when he had no class at university. According to MOHO, participation in occupations helps people develop occupational identities, competence, and adaptation. To provide opportunities for Jeff to experience performing the role of worker, and to support him in improving his work performance in jobs related to accounting and clerical duties, the occupational therapists invited Jeff to regularly attend vocational training workshops in the day hospital. The vocational training workshops provide vocational training for clients in the recovery process of mental illnesses in specially designed work environments. Occupational therapists design a variety of simulated work tasks, including accounting and clerical tasks, and assign the tasks to clients according to their levels of performance capacity and their choices. The workshops usually operate at similar hours as an actual workplace. In such vocational training workshops, occupational therapists and their assistants provide constant supervision and assistance in work performance and work-related social skills for clients. By receiving feedback on their work performance from therapists and gaining successful work experience, clients gradually understand their own abilities (a sense of personal capacity) and come to believe that they can apply their abilities in achieving goals (self-efficacy).

Jeff performed accounting work two days per week in vocational training workshops to improve his skills in accounting and clerical jobs and to develop his work endurance and work habits. Because the work environment provided abundant opportunities for Jeff to interact with his colleagues, Jeff was also able to practice the social cognitive skills he learned from the therapeutic groups (described in the next paragraph) and, if necessary, receive mediation from the therapists when he had arguments with co-workers. In addition, after receiving feedback on his work performance from the therapists and his colleagues, Jeff gained a better understanding of his own work abilities (i.e., improved sense of personal capacity). Multiple successful experiences in completing work tasks allowed him to believe that he could use his ability to complete tasks (i.e., improvement in self-efficacy).

Goal 3: Jeff can attend social activities (such as having lunch together) with other clients/co-workers in the day hospital or his classmates at university once per week in a month.

To achieve this goal, Jeff gained support from occupational therapists to improve his social cognitive skills. The therapists provided Jeff with the Social Cognition and Interaction Training program (Lo et al., 2018; Roberts et al., 2015). This is a group-based therapy for improving social cognition in people with schizophrenia, particularly the ability to recognize other people's emotions (i.e., emotion perception), understand other people's intentions/viewpoints (i.e., the theory of mind), and explain causes of positive/negative results in social interactions (i.e., social attributions). It comprises 19–24 weekly sessions that last 45–60 minutes per session for chronic clients and around 10 weekly sessions of the same duration for early psychosis clients. Across the training period, the earlier sessions focus on emotion perception, the middle sessions focus on the theory of mind and social attributions, and the later sessions focus on practice and application to daily life. Research has shown that the Social Cognition and Interaction Training program is effective in improving emotion perception and the theory of mind in clients with schizophrenia (Lo et al., 2018).

The occupational therapists not only used the Social Cognition and Interaction Training program to support Jeff to improve his social cognitive skills, but also allowed program venues become environments where Jeff could make friends with other clients. Jeff could thus increase his experience in performing the role of friend, which was important for him. Jeff attended the complete program of the Social Cognition and Interaction Training. In the earlier sessions, he learned how to distinguish various negative emotions. In the middle sessions, he learned how to be flexible in thinking about social situations and to differentiate his own thoughts about social situations from social facts. In the later sessions, Jeff put the skills and strategies he learned into practice. He was encouraged to bring up troubling interpersonal situations he had faced in workplaces or schools so that he could work with occupational therapists and his groupmates to apply what he learned in the program to solving real-life social problems. During the program, Jeff made a new friend, Tom, who usually paired up with Jeff in the practices and had frequent social interactions with him.

Goal 4: Jeff can complete an assignment of the subject he took this semester at university in two months.

To achieve this goal, Jeff gained support from occupational therapists to enhance his neurocognition, particularly his visual learning and processing speed. The therapists adopted the cognitive remediation approach, which emphasizes neural plasticity and improving neurocognition in clients after their learning (Medalia

& Saperstein, 2013). The occupational therapists provided Jeff with individualized computerized cognitive training programs, the effectiveness of which for clients with schizophrenia has been supported in a recent meta-analysis publication (Prikken et al., 2019). These individualized computerized cognitive training programs, such as CogniPlus, comprise various training modules that target separate neurocognitive skills. The programs use realistic designs and daily tasks in the training modules to motivate clients and increase the generalization of improved neurocognitive skills to real-life contexts. The programs also automatically adjust the training difficulty according to the clients' ability, which simulates how occupational therapists grade intervention to provide a challenge of just the right level for clients. With the aid of the computerized training programs, the occupational therapists worked with Jeff to develop a tailor-made individual neurocognitive training plan for him. Training modules regarding visual memory/learning and processing speed in the computerized programs were adopted. Jeff received this neurocognitive training in three sessions per week with one hour per session. At the end of each week's training, the therapists provided Jeff with feedback on his performance, discussed his changes, and, more importantly, discussed the application to real-life situations, such as doing an assignment at university.

As Jeff was young and had experienced the first episode of schizophrenia less than one year ago, he had great potential for improvement in neurocognition after the intervention. Therefore, the therapists adopted remediation intervention, i.e., the neurocognitive training described above, and worked with Jeff to plan the training. In other scenarios, particularly for chronic schizophrenia clients with persistent neurocognitive limitations, occupational therapists may consider simultaneously adopting the compensation approach to support clients so that they will still be able to engage in activities when they need to live with residual symptoms. The compensation approach focuses on adaptive strategies and environmental modifications. One example of compensatory therapy for neurocognition provided in Hong Kong is the Compensatory Cognitive Training for People with Severe Mental Illnesses. This training protocol is a translated version (in Chinese) of the Cognitive Symptom Management and Rehabilitation Therapy program (Twamley et al., 2014), which targets each neurocognitive ability and teaches clients corresponding daily compensatory strategies.

Goal 5: Jeff can engage in one new leisure activity in addition to playing basketball twice per week in a month.

To support Jeff in exploring new leisure activities, the occupational therapists invited him to join various leisure groups in the day hospital, particularly a sports group and a group involving information and hands-on experience in taking care of animals. When Jeff participated in these groups, the therapists also encouraged him to initiate conversations with groupmates by talking about common interests in sports and pets. Jeff could practice making friends in these leisure groups, which improved his experience in performing the role of friend.

Goal 6: Jeff's mother and sister can attend caregiver groups once per week in the day hospital in a month.

Jeff's mother's knowledge of schizophrenia was limited, including the symptoms, prognosis, and relapse signs, which led to her unrealistic expectations for Jeff and the stress it caused him. It was expected that by enhancing the family's under-standing of schizophrenia, family interactions and family support for Jeff would improve, which, in turn, helped Jeff perform the roles he wanted. The occupational therapists held psychoeducational talks and caregiver groups, and invited Jeff's mother and sister to join to provide family intervention for Jeff's family members. Family intervention involves psychoeducation regarding schizophrenia, antipsychotic medications, early signs of relapse, and the ways to assist clients in symptom management. Family intervention may also include training of problem-solving skills, communication skills, and emotion management to support caregivers in handling caregiving challenges and alleviating stress. It has been shown that family intervention is beneficial to benign family interactions, decision-making regarding taking medications, and reducing the risk of relapses in clients with schizophrenia (Caqueo-Urízar et al., 2017).

Goal 7: Jeff can perform illness management once per week in illness management group sessions in a month.

Although short-term illness management groups were provided when Jeff was in the acute ward, long-term and continuous training in the day hospital stage was needed to consolidate Jeff's illness management skills. In the day hospital setting, in which clients receive relatively longer rehabilitation, occupational therapists provide three-month to nine-month illness management groups on a weekly basis, such as the Illness Management and Recovery program (Mueser et al., 2006). Topics cover personal recovery goals, knowledge of schizophrenia, relevant symptoms, antipsychotic medications, the stress-vulnerability model, ways to increase social support, coping strategies for stress and persistent symptoms, mental health resources, and ways to prevent relapses. Research has provided initial evidence regarding the effectiveness of the Illness Management and Recovery program in clients with schizophrenia in outpatient settings (Färdig et al., 2011). In Hong Kong, an abridged Chinese version of the Illness Management and Recovery program has been used in day hospitals.

Goal 8: Jeff can work with co-workers to complete accounting tasks once per week in vocational training workshops in the day hospital in a month.

Jeff faced difficulties in stress management when he argued with his co-workers. Even though coping strategies for stress are included in the aforementioned illness management training, given the Chinese cultural background, occupational therapists in Hong Kong also adopt health *qigong* as supplementary therapy for stress management. Health *qigong* (Wang et al., 2014) is a type of mind-body practice that emphasizes concentration to guide inner *qi* (energy) in the human body, coordination between bodily movements and breathing regulation, and relaxation (see Chapter 1). The Hong Kong Occupational Therapy Association (HKOTA) provides local therapists with regular training courses of *Baduanjin*, one of the popular forms of health *qigong*, and recommends therapists apply *Baduanjin* to clinical practice to reduce stress and enhance health in clients. Preliminary evidence (Zhu et al., 2021) has shown the effects of *Baduanjin* on reducing stress. For Jeff, the occupational therapists invited him to attend daily *Baduanjin* sessions (around 30 minutes per session). Afterward, Jeff practiced *Baduanjin* regularly and applied this coping skill when he felt stressed working with co-workers to complete accounting tasks in vocational training workshops.

After the day hospital stage

During the day hospital stage, the occupational therapists conducted assessments regularly to identify changes in Jeff and worked with him to adjust the intervention plans if necessary. Depending on Jeff's status of functional recovery and employment, after discharge from the day hospital, Jeff might be advised to receive further supported employment services, which adopt the Individual Placement and Support model found in non-governmental organizations. Supported employment services adopting the Individual Placement and Support model aim to help clients directly obtain a competitive job instead of providing long pre-employment training, focus on clients' job choices, and give continuous support to help clients maintain the job (Bond, 2004; Wong et al., 2008).

Occupational therapy assessments and intervention in Singapore

The previous section outlined OT assessments and interventions used in Hong Kong. This section explores assessments and interventions of the early psychosis intervention program (EPIP) in Singapore, which would be applicable to occupational therapists in a case like Jeff's.

The Institute of Mental Health in Singapore began EPIP in 2001 to cater to first-episode psychosis clients. They are managed by the same treatment team throughout the first three years of their inpatient/outpatient journey. This team includes occupational therapists, case managers, peer support specialists (people with similar experiences), psychologists, medical social workers, pharmacists, doctors, and nurses. Clients are transferred to other psychiatric services within the Institute of Mental Health at the end of their third year at EPIP. The Institute of Mental Health runs two outpatient psychosocial rehabilitation programs. The first program, Club EPIP, is managed within the early psychosis program. The second program, Occupational Therapy: Activities, Vocation and Empowerment (OCTAVE), is for outpatients from general psychiatry wards and outpatient clinics. Clients in EPIP attend Club EPIP and may be referred to OCTAVE for work rehabilitation and supported employment when deemed suitable. Job support is provided by occupational therapists from OCTAVE.

Assessments in the acute stage

Jeff was admitted to the EPIP ward where, as part of the ward program, he was invited to attend group activities such as cooking, yoga, creative expression, medication management, and group art therapy sessions. The activities lasted between one and one-and-a-half hours, run by various members of the multidisciplinary team. He also attended individual sessions with a peer support specialist, primarily to hear the specialist's experiences and gain some insights into his own recovery journey.

During the third week of admission, the team felt that Jeff was ready to see the occupational therapist for an initial assessment. He was referred primarily for cognitive assessment and to explore vocational opportunities. The following information was gathered during the initial assessment: educational history, employment history, social support, hobbies, perceived strengths, long-term goals, and areas of concern. The occupational therapist elicited Jeff's thoughts on his illness, his understanding of his recovery journey, and his treatment plans. In addition to administering the Montreal Cognitive Assessment (Nasreddine et al., 2005) and Allen's Cognitive Level Screen, the occupational therapist collated reports from other team members who had seen Jeff in their groups. From all the assessments and feedback obtained, the following was formulated.

Social history

Jeff lives with his mother. His father passed away when Jeff was a child. Jeff has a caring elder sister who is married and lives in her own home. He has one close male friend, Neal. They particularly enjoyed playing basketball together in the past. Jeff is currently distant from both his sister and Neal. He did not have any friends at university and had awkward social relationships with his workmates. He appeared to have limited social support and has struggled to make friends since he was young.

Educational and employment history

Jeff passed secondary school with good grades. He is now in year five, studying accountancy at a university. Although he passed earlier university exams satisfactorily, he was struggling with his studies. He worked part-time jobs at fast-food restaurants in the past few years but could not sustain these jobs for longer than six months, possibly due to interpersonal and cognitive difficulties.

Challenges, strengths, and goals

Jeff had significant cognitive challenges, especially in terms of attention and processing speed. Although he was not able to identify the strengths within himself, the occupational therapist recognized that he had a strong sense of filial duty. Jeff wanted to quickly graduate and find work to help support his mother. He expressed that he wanted to continue part-time employment while attending classes at university to lighten the family burden. The occupational therapist also noted that Jeff struggled to develop friendships.

Cognitive assessment findings

Jeff scored 25 points in the Montreal Cognitive Assessment, which indicated mild cognitive impairments. His score in Allen's Cognitive Level Screen was at Level 4. This suggested that his global cognition was moderately impaired, and increased assistance in all cognitive skills might be required. Level 4 indicates that clients have difficulty solving new problems, are unable to learn new information independently, and require much repetition to learn and retain new information (Allen, 1991). The occupational therapist observed that Jeff persevered in the tasks of Allen's Cognitive Level Screen and had not given up but constantly sought reassurance that he was doing the tasks correctly. Considering that Jeff was about to be discharged and that he said he was tired of being subjected to assessments, the occupational therapist recommended administering the Brief Assessment of Cognition in Schizophrenia (Keefe et al., 2004) to Jeff when he continued as an outpatient.

Assessments in the outpatient stage

Jeff attended outpatient sessions with the occupational therapist at Club EPIP. The occupational therapist used MOHO to guide the interviews and assessments and observed Jeff's behaviors in ward activities. During the outpatient sessions, the Brief Assessment of Cognition in Schizophrenia, Role Checklist, and Interest Checklist were administered. The Brief Assessment of Cognition in Schizophrenia was used to assess Jeff's cognitive functioning and impairments. This includes brief assessments of executive functions, verbal fluency, attention, verbal memory, working memory, and motor speed. The final composite score is the sum of z-scores based on comparisons with a normative sample of 400 healthy controls. Its reliability and validity have been established empirically (Keefe et al., 2004). The relevant results of Jeff's interviews and assessments are shown below.

Volition subsystem

Jeff's interests were initially limited to only playing basketball, but during the outpatient sessions, he was more willing to try other sports. He also mentioned an interest in having a pet dog. His valued goals were graduating from university, sustaining a job, contributing to the family's well-being, and making friends. However, he had decreased confidence in himself.

Habituation subsystem

The Role Checklist showed that Jeff considered the roles of being a family member, student, worker, and friend to be important. His habits were keeping things to himself and brooding over situations without asking for help when required. He would habitually quit jobs when feeling stressed or unhappy at work.

Performance subsystem

Although Jeff had good physical skills, his activity endurance was poor. He had difficulty sustaining employment and struggled in school (he did not pass some subjects). During group activities, he was observed to have poor communication skills, limited social awareness, and poor presentation skills. He expressed that he had difficulty making friends. The results of the Brief Assessment of Cognition in Schizophrenia (Table 11.5) showed that Jeff's overall cognitive performance was borderline. This could account for his difficulties in school and poor ability to complete work tasks.

Environment

Jeff had limited social support, which came only from his sister and his friend Neal.

Intervention in the acute stage

During the acute stage, intervention was limited to ward group activities. These served both as general clinical assessments and intervention opportunities for the team. The

Table 11.5 Jeff's Brief Assessment of Cognition in Schizophrenia results

Type of measure	Z-score	Performance
Verbal memory	0.55	Average
Working memory	1.25	High average
Motor speed	−1.25	Low average
Semantic fluency	−1.45	Borderline difficulty
Attention and processing speed	−2.33	Moderate difficulty
Reasoning and problem-solving	−0.75	Low average
Composite score	−1.45	Borderline difficulty

medication management group was facilitated by the ward pharmacist, who educated Jeff about the importance of medication and its correlation to the prevention of relapses. Jeff's psychiatrist, case manager, and occupational therapist held a family session in the fourth week of the inpatient admission to discuss and establish treatment plans for subsequent outpatient care. Based on the results of cognitive assessments and clinical observations of Jeff's behaviors in the acute ward, the team recommended that Jeff defer university studies for six months and attend Club EPIP. During this period, Jeff could work on his endurance and social skills and continue to see the peer support specialist to better understand the recovery process.

Intervention in the outpatient stage
Jeff attended monthly individual sessions with the occupational therapist and Club EPIP group sessions at least four times per week. The aims of the group sessions were to facilitate social rehabilitation, reinforce work behavior skills, improve cognition, and provide support. Individual sessions with the occupational therapist emphasized the generalization of life skills, the development of effective coping skills, and supportive counseling. The occupational therapist and Jeff jointly evaluated the treatment goals and adjusted the intervention methods when necessary.

Individual sessions provided Jeff with the opportunity to talk about his progress and discuss with the occupational therapist about how intervention helped him in his areas of concern. The case manager and Jeff's mother were sometimes invited to these sessions. Such sessions enabled Jeff's mother to better understand Jeff's recovery process and helped her adjust her expectations.

Jeff was enrolled in a **cognitive remediation training** program to address his cognitive problems. Cognitive remediation training utilizes components from the Neurocognitive Educational Approach to Remediation (NEAR), which has been shown to improve cognition such as attention (Bell et al., 2001), processing speed (McGurk et al., 2007), and memory (Lee et al., 2013). NEAR is a method of cognitive remediation that is highly individualized and administered in a group setting. After discussion with occupational therapists, clients select their cognitive tasks and work on the tasks at their own pace. Examples of goals involved in NEAR include: improve cognition that impacts one's global functioning, and develop competence and confidence in one's ability to acquire skills (Medalia et al., 2009). It is delivered through fun and interactive computer games that provide a positive learning experience (Figure 11.3).

The cognitive remediation training program that Jeff attended had 24 sessions in total and was conducted in a group format with a total of five clients in each session. It was conducted twice per week for three months, with each session lasting one-and-a-half hours. Jeff was given structured neurocognitive exercises concerning attention, memory, speed of apprehension, visual motor, and reaction. The occupational therapist tailored the sessions by increasing or decreasing the difficulty level based on Jeff's performance. The therapist used various methods such as drills, practice, and strategy coaching in the training sessions. Bridging sessions were conducted where Jeff and his group members discussed the strategies they had learned and practiced. The therapist also facilitated discussions on how group members could use these strategies in their various roles in real-life situations. Such discussions enabled Jeff to participate in social

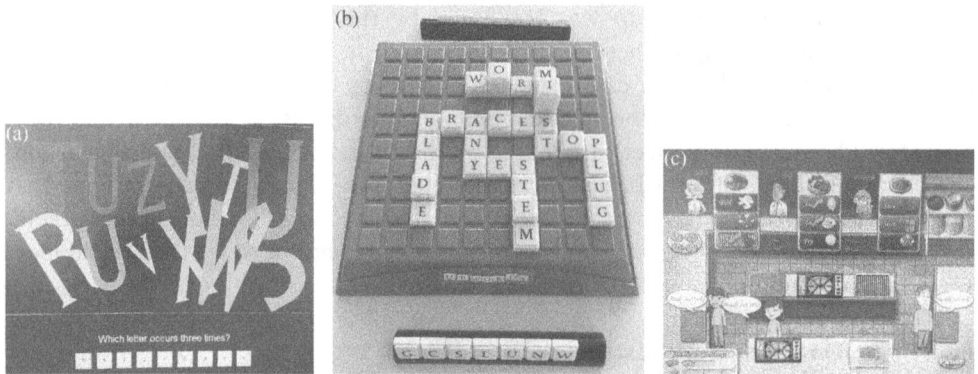

Figure 11.3 The cognitive remediation training program is initially conducted using structured cognitive exercises available in "Cogpack" (a). As the client progresses, other commercially available games (b and c) are used to facilitate training. The exercises are built in a hierarchical manner starting with improving attention and moving on to problem-solving. (Photo credit: Occupational Therapy Department, Institute of Mental Health, Singapore)

interactions, providing opportunities to build his self-confidence and transfer the skills he learned into real-life scenarios.

Jeff also attended **sports and discussion-based groups** run by the occupational therapist. The occupational therapist and Jeff collaboratively agreed to work on two goals: develop Jeff's confidence and improve his interpersonal skills and endurance. The sports and discussion-based groups were two-hour sessions, held once per week, with each group interconnected with the others. Jeff participated in activities such as basketball, captain's ball, dodgeball, Frisbee, and soccer in the **sports group**. The group was divided into two teams, and the teams were asked to create a name and slogan for themselves. Every member had a specific role such as captain, defender, striker, goal-keeper, and scorer. This allowed them to interact and learn negotiation and leadership skills. Work behaviors such as cooperation, teamwork, turn-taking, and social communication were emphasized in such activities. Prior to the start of the game, the teams discussed and decided how many goals they wanted to score. The teams used half-time to reassess their goals, discuss their strategies about how to achieve their goals and, at times, change their goals. At the end of the game, team members gathered together and each member led the team in cool-down exercises. The subsequent discussion examined the strengths demonstrated by each team member, the improvements they noticed, and the areas they wanted to improve in the next session (for example, being assertive and confident or taking leadership roles). They also nominated one member from their team to be given a sportsmanship award. The occupational therapist facilitated group discussions, oversaw the administration of the sports program, and gently encouraged Jeff to try out the leadership position. Jeff used these sessions to practice problem-solving, negotiation, and communication skills.

The **discussion-based group** that Jeff attended mainly focused on current affairs and life skills such as managing money, stress, and jobs. Clients were organized into small groups of about four per group and were given some articles to read. They were also given pertinent questions to explore and subsequently answer. Each member was asked to answer one question. Others were invited to probe and provide feedback. Presenting teams questioned members in the audience to facilitate learning and recall. These sessions helped hone clients' public speaking skills, such as voice projection, maintaining eye contact, and interacting with an audience. They also provided opportunities to practice strategies for overcoming anxiety and learn how to give and receive feedback.

Jeff attended **movie screenings** at Club EPIP once a month. The occupational therapist conducted a discussion at the end of each movie. Discussion topics covered themes that had emerged in the movie, characters whom members identified with, and how members would craft the ending of the movie if they were the director. These discussion-based sessions were helpful in improving cognitive skills such as paying attention to details and memory. At times, the occupational therapist led a **six-word-memoir** activity during discussion-based group sessions. This facilitated abstract and creative thinking. In addition, memoirs were used as personal messages of hope and support for themselves. These sessions enabled Jeff to apply newly learned skills and strategies in his daily life.

Jeff also attended a six-week **recovery program** led by a peer support specialist and his case manager. The program covered topics such as understanding mental illnesses, identifying one's support system, and sustaining hope. Jeff's conversations with the peer support specialist instilled hope and provided Jeff with a sense of not being alone in his struggle.

During **individual sessions** with Jeff, the occupational therapist provided feedback on his progress in the various group sessions in which he had participated. The therapist also role-played scenarios to increase his confidence in public speaking and in the instances when he needed to initiate conversations. The occupational therapist explored **activity scheduling** and gave him homework occasionally, such as requiring him to talk to another group member.

Jeff and the occupational therapist collaboratively identified Jeff's stress triggers and management techniques via the **stress bucket**. Jeff was encouraged to think about the size and shape of his bucket and the various constituent stressors he had in terms of friendships, groups, school, and part-time employment. He was asked how full the bucket was and what were some signs that would inform him that the bucket was reaching its limit. Their discussions also revolved around what could potentially help reduce Jeff's level of stress. The occupational therapist taught him stress management techniques such as deep breathing and relaxation exercises as identified through the stress bucket exercise. Cognitive strategies from cognitive remediation training were reinforced during these sessions. Jeff was encouraged to talk about his goals and what he wanted to achieve in group sessions. Jeff's desire to own a dog was explored during one of these sessions, which resulted in him being tasked to research the steps of owning a pet. As an initial step, the occupational therapist encouraged him to volunteer at a dog shelter and helped him through this process.

During another individual session some weeks later, the occupational therapist introduced a **vocational rehabilitation program** available in OCTAVE. Jeff chose **Food and Beverage training** because he wanted to improve his work skills and learn to manage the stress that he expected to experience in a fast-food restaurant, where he hoped to work in the future. Jeff was referred to OCTAVE and attended Food and Beverage

training. This took place in a café within the Institute of Mental Health. Prior to starting work training in the café, Jeff attended cooking and baking sessions twice a week at
OCTAVE. This activity group was conducted by a therapy assistant, supervised by an
occupational therapist. Jeff learned new skills regarding food handling techniques and
practiced how to work amicably with others. He used strategies of cognitive remediation training that he had learned and applied breathing techniques to manage stress.
After eight weeks of learning to cook and bake, he was placed in the frontline crew of
the café training program. He learned how to take orders from patrons, offer purchas-
ing suggestions, cook simple dishes, and handle the cash register. After three months of
café training, he was selected for an internship, doing part-time work in a fast-food restaurant. The occupational therapist at OCTAVE followed through with workplace visits.

Jeff resumed university classes at about the same time that he started supported
employment. Prior to starting the classes, Jeff and the EPIP occupational therapist
visited the university to identify suitable locations within the campus where he could
retreat when feeling stressed. He adopted suggestions by the occupational therapist
to negotiate for a lighter study load and register for student counseling opportunities
offered by the university. He was more at ease with himself and had started to socialize with two Club EPIP members with whom he had forged satisfying friendships. He
had been volunteering regularly at the dog shelter and had started discussions to adopt
a dog. Jeff continued monthly follow-ups with the EPIP occupational therapist. Their
focus shifted to reintegration and sustenance at the university.

Conclusion

Jeff was diagnosed with schizophrenia and received OT services in the acute stage
and the day hospital/outpatient stage. The clinical practice of OT in Hong Kong and
Singapore has been described in detail, and Jeff and his therapists collaborated on
assessments and discussed intervention plans.

Overall, in the acute stage, the occupational therapists in Hong Kong and Singapore
conducted interviews related to the stress-vulnerability model and assessments using
the Montreal Cognitive Assessment and Allen's Cognitive Level Screen. Because the
stay in the acute ward was short, Jeff and his therapists agreed that interventions should
focus on illness and stress management.

In the day hospital/outpatient stage, the therapists in Hong Kong and Singapore
adopted MOHO and the stress-vulnerability model to conduct interviews, clinical
observations, and assessments, using the Interest Checklist, Role Checklist, VALPAR
Component Work Samples, MATRICS Consensus Cognitive Battery, and Brief
Assessment of Cognition in Schizophrenia. Interventions in the day hospital/outpatient
stage aimed to support Jeff's engagement in activities related to his student and worker
roles, in his social and leisure activities, and in his illness and stress management.
These interventions included individual sessions, involvement of peer support specialists, vocational training, Social Cognition and Interaction Training, cognitive training, leisure groups, caregiver groups, the Illness Management and Recovery program,
health *qigong*, and discussion-based groups.

This chapter presented an example of how occupational therapists in Asian cultures
(primarily Hong Kong and Singapore) collaborated with a client with schizophrenia on

assessments, goal setting, and intervention. The content covers several models, assessment tools, and therapeutic programs. However, there are other frames of reference, tools, and interventions that have not been mentioned. In clinical practice, occupational therapists make clinical decisions on the choice of appropriate theories, assessment tools, and therapeutic activities after discussing with clients about their goals for occupational participation and their preferences.

References

Allen, C. K. (1991). Cognitive disability and reimbursement for rehabilitation and psychiatry. *Journal of Insurance Medicine*, 23(4), 245–247.

August, S. M., Kiwanuka, J. N., McMahon, R. P., & Gold, J. M. (2012). The MATRICS Consensus Cognitive Battery (MCCB): Clinical and cognitive correlates. *Schizophrenia Research*, 134(1), 76–82. https://doi.org/10.1016/j.schres.2011.10.015

Bell, M., Bryson, G., Greig, T., Corcoran, C., & Wexler, B. E. (2001). Neurocognitive enhancement therapy with work therapy: Effects on neuropsychological test performance. *Archives of General Psychiatry*, 58(8), 763–768. https://doi.org/10.1001/archpsyc.58.8.763

Bond, G. R. (2004). Supported employment: Evidence for an evidence-based practice. *Psychiatric Rehabilitation Journal*, 27(4), 345–359. https://doi.org/10.2975/27.2004.345.359

Caqueo-Urízar, A., Rus-Calafell, M., Craig, T. K. J., Irarrazaval, M., Urzúa, A., Boyer, L., & Williams, D. R. (2017). Schizophrenia: Impact on family dynamics. *Current Psychiatry Reports*, 19(1), 2. https://doi.org/10.1007/s11920-017-0756-z

Chan, S. H.-W. (2009). Illness management training: Transforming relapse and instilling prosperity in an acute psychiatric ward. In I. Söderback (Ed.), *International handbook of occupational therapy interventions* (pp. 261–267). Springer. https://link.springer.com/chapter/10.1007/978-0-387-75424-6_25

Christopherson, B. B., & Hayes, P. D. (2006). *Valpar component work samples uses in allied health*. Valpar International Corporation.

Färdig, R., Lewander, T., Melin, L., Folke, F., & Fredriksson, A. (2011). A randomized controlled trial of the illness management and recovery program for persons with schizophrenia. *Psychiatric Services*, 62(6), 606–612. https://doi.org/10.1176/ps.62.6.pss6206_0606

Keefe, R. S. E., Goldberg, T. E., Harvey, P. D., Gold, J. M., Poe, M. P., & Coughenour, L. (2004). The brief assessment of cognition in schizophrenia: Reliability, sensitivity, and comparison with a standard neurocognitive battery. *Schizophrenia Research*, 68(2–3), 283–297. https://doi.org/10.1016/j.schres.2003.09.011

Kielhofner, G. (2008). *Model of human occupation: Theory and application* (4th ed.). Lippincott Williams & Wilkins.

Lee, R. S. C., Redoblado-Hodge, M. A., Naismith, S. L., Hermens, D. F., Porter, M. A., & Hickie, I. B. (2013). Cognitive remediation improves memory and psychosocial functioning in first-episode psychiatric out-patients. *Psychological Medicine*, 43(6), 1161–1173. https://doi.org/10.1017/S0033291712002127

Lewis, T. F., & Osborn, C. J. (2004). Solution-focused counseling and motivational interviewing: A consideration of confluence. *Journal of Counseling & Development*, 82(1), 38–48. https://doi.org/10.1002/j.1556-6678.2004.tb00284.x

Lo, P. M. T., & Siu, A. M. H. (2018). Assessing social cognition of persons with schizophrenia in a Chinese population: A pilot study. *Frontiers in Psychiatry*, 8, 302. https://doi.org/10.3389/fpsyt.2017.00302

Lo, P. M. T., Siu, A. M. H., & Roberts, D. L. (2018). Adaptation of the social cognition and interaction training (SCIT) for promoting functional recovery in Chinese persons with schizophrenia in Hong Kong. In M. Knight, & B. McCoy (Eds.), *Understanding social cognition: Theory, perspectives and cultural differences* (pp. 79–103). Nova Science Publishers.

Marcopulos, B. A., & Kurtz, M. M. (2012). *Clinical neuropsychological foundations of schizophrenia*. Routledge.

McGurk, S. R., Twamley, E. W., Sitzer, D. I., McHugo, G. J., & Mueser, K. T. (2007). A meta-analysis of cognitive remediation in schizophrenia. *American Journal of Psychiatry*, 164(12), 1791–1802. https://doi.org/10.1176/appi.ajp.2007.07060906

Medalia, A., Revheim, N., & Herlands, T. (2009). *Cognitive remediation for psychological disorders: Therapist guide.* Oxford University Press.

Medalia, A., & Saperstein, A. M. (2013). Does cognitive remediation for schizophrenia improve functional outcomes? *Current Opinion in Psychiatry, 26*(2), 151–157. https://doi.org/10.1097/YCO.0b013e32835dcbd4

MOHO-IRM Web. (2023). *Modified Interest Checklist.* Retrieved August 1, 2023, from https://moho-irm.uic.edu/productDetails.aspx?aid=38

Mueser, K. T., Meyer, P. S., Penn, D. L., Clancy, R., Clancy, D. M., & Salyers, M. P. (2006). The illness management and recovery program: Rationale, development, and preliminary findings. *Schizophrenia Bulletin, 32*(S1), S32–S43. https://doi.org/10.1093/schbul/sbl022

Nasreddine, Z. S., Phillips, N. A., Bédirian, V., Charbonneau, S., Whitehead, V., Collin, I., Cummings, J. L., & Chertkow, H. (2005). The Montreal Cognitive Assessment, MoCA: A brief screening tool for mild cognitive impairment. *Journal of the American Geriatrics Society, 53*(4), 695–699. https://doi.org/10.1111/j.1532-5415.2005.53221.x

Oakley, F., Kielhofner, G., Barris, R., & Reichler, R. K. (1986). The Role Checklist: Development and empirical assessment of reliability. *Occupational Therapy Journal of Research, 6*(3), 157–170. https://doi.org/10.1177/153944928600600303

Prikken, M., Konings, M. J., Lei, W. U., Begemann, M. J. H., & Sommer, I. E. C. (2019). The efficacy of computerized cognitive drill and practice training for patients with a schizophrenia-spectrum disorder: A meta-analysis. *Schizophrenia Research, 204*, 368–374. https://doi.org/10.1016/j.schres.2018.07.034

Roberts, D. L., Penn, D. L., & Combs, D. R. (2015). *Social cognition and interaction training (SCIT): Group psychotherapy for schizophrenia and other psychotic disorders. Clinician guide.* Oxford University Press.

Twamley, E. W., Jak, A. J., Delis, D. C., Bondi, M. W., & Lohr, J. B. (2014). Cognitive symptom management and rehabilitation therapy (CogSMART) for veterans with traumatic brain injury: Pilot randomized controlled trial. *Journal of Rehabilitation Research and Development, 51*(1), 59–70. https://doi.org/10.1682/JRRD.2013.01.0020

Wang, C.-W., Chan, C. H. Y., Ho, R. T. H., Chan, J. S. M., Ng, S.-M., & Chan, C. L. W. (2014). Managing stress and anxiety through qigong exercise in healthy adults: A systematic review and meta-analysis of randomized controlled trials. *BMC Complementary and Alternative Medicine, 14*, 8. https://doi.org/10.1186/1472-6882-14-8

Wong, K. K., Chiu, R., Tang, B., Mak, D., Liu, J., & Chiu, S. N. (2008). A randomized controlled trial of a supported employment program for persons with long-term mental illness in Hong Kong. *Psychiatric Services, 59*(1), 84–90. https://doi.org/10.1176/ps.2008.59.1.84

Zhu, X., Chu, T., Yu, Q., Li, J., Zhang, X., Zhang, Y., & Zou, L. (2021). Effectiveness of mind-body exercise on burnout and stress in female undergraduate students. *International Journal of Mental Health Promotion, 23*(3), 353–360. https://doi.org/10.32604/IJMHP.2021.016339

Zubin, J., & Spring, B. (1977). Vulnerability: A new view of schizophrenia. *Journal of Abnormal Psychology, 86*(2), 103–126. https://doi.org/10.1037/0021-843X.86.2.103

Future trends

CHAPTER 12

Evidence-based practice in occupational therapy

Hector Wing Hong Tsang, Benson Wui Man Lau, and Jessie Jingxia Lin

As occupational therapists, we often need to make decisions about which treatment is most effective for the client. Along with considering the needs and preferences of the client, an important component of these decisions should involve an appraisal of the existing research evidence among various available treatment options and interventions. With such critical evaluation included in the clinical decisions, the possibility that the selected treatment will result in beneficial and effective outcomes will certainly be increased. But what constitutes evidence-based practice (EBP)? Where did the term come from? How can it help occupational therapists make evidence-based decisions about the effectiveness of their practice? This chapter attempts to answer these questions with examples for illustration.

Development of evidence-based practice

The term "evidence-based medicine" was coined in the 1980s as a method of problem-based clinical learning and teaching that searched for and evaluated the evidence for clinical practice at McMaster University (Bennett et al., 1987; Shin et al., 1993). John Wennberg, a physician, conducted a series of small area variation studies and found that physicians treated the same medical condition differently, not depending on scientific evidence but largely on their demographic similarity (Wennberg & Gittelsohn, 1973). He concluded that physicians made medical decisions by heavily relying on factors such as traditions and norms, and that they were unsure about treatment for their clients. Wennberg and others suggested a paradigm shift to evidence-based medicine (Tanenbaum, 2006). The work of Archie Cochrane, an epidemiologist, has been key to the development of evidence-based medicine through the championing of randomized controlled trials (RCTs) and systematic reviews to evaluate the effectiveness and efficacy of interventions (Cochrane, 1972).

What exactly is EBP? A tremendous amount of literature has attempted to answer this question. Sackett et al. (1996, p. 71) defined evidence-based medicine as "the

DOI: 10.4324/9781032721170-17

conscientious, explicit and judicious use of current best evidence in making decisions about the care of individual patients". Torrey et al. (2005, p. 91) suggested a simpler and yet specific definition: "Evidence-based practice refers to health services that are bolstered by a strong scientific base, preferably accumulated through a plethora of randomized clinical trials performed by different research teams in multiple research sites and even in different places of the world". The explicit and clearly articulated decision process is the essence of EBP, and decisions can be explained to the client and justified to colleagues. The needs of the client, the demands of the healthcare system, and the up-to-date best evidence are weighted together to provide the best care to the client. EBP should be viewed as critical thinking and one of the tools of clinical practice.

EBP has been explored and discussed in the occupational therapy (OT) discipline for decades. Dubouloz et al. (1999) remarked that research evidence has been slowly integrated into clinical decision-making processes by occupational therapists. To recognize the range of evidence in OT, evidence-based OT was defined as "the client-centred enablement of occupation, based on client information and a critical review of relevant research, expert consensus and past experience" (Law et al., 1998). Holm (2000) highlighted in the 2000 Eleanor Clarke Slagle Lecture that the OT Code of Ethics had confirmed the essence of and need for EBP. Principle 4.E of the Code of Ethics states, "Critically examine evidence so they may perform their duties on the basis of current information" (Cameron et al., 2005). Thus, evidence-based OT is a form of critical appraisal of the research evidence and all aspects of OT interventions within a framework of reflection and clinical reasoning in order to explore the skills and activities that enable us to become evidence-based occupational therapists.

Levels of evidence

Hierarchy of evidence
The evidence in EBP is not created equally. Various strengths of evidence come from sampling and methods in the research. A hierarchy of evidence has been suggested, which provides guidance about the types of research study. This hierarchy classifies evidence based on its strengths at various levels (Evans, 2003) as shown in Figure 12.1.

There are seven levels of evidence depending on the type of clinical question. For intervention/treatment questions, quantitative research (e.g., a systematic review of RCTs) is ranked at the highest level of confidence compared with designs such as qualitative and descriptive studies, which have lower levels of confidence. In the hierarchy model, the higher a study design is ranked, the more likely the study results accurately represent the actual condition and the more confidence in implementing the treatment to clients by health professionals.

A systematic review or meta-analysis provides the highest level of evidence because it combines and analyzes a large number of RCTs with similar designs. This synthesis of data from numerous studies results in the most reliable and least biased evidence for evaluating the effectiveness of a treatment. Such systematic reviews have been regarded as the "heart of EBP" (Stevens, 2001).

The next level consists of RCTs. An RCT recruits a sample of participants and then allocates them to a treatment group or control group using an unbiased randomized procedure. The design controls for numerous confounding factors that might account

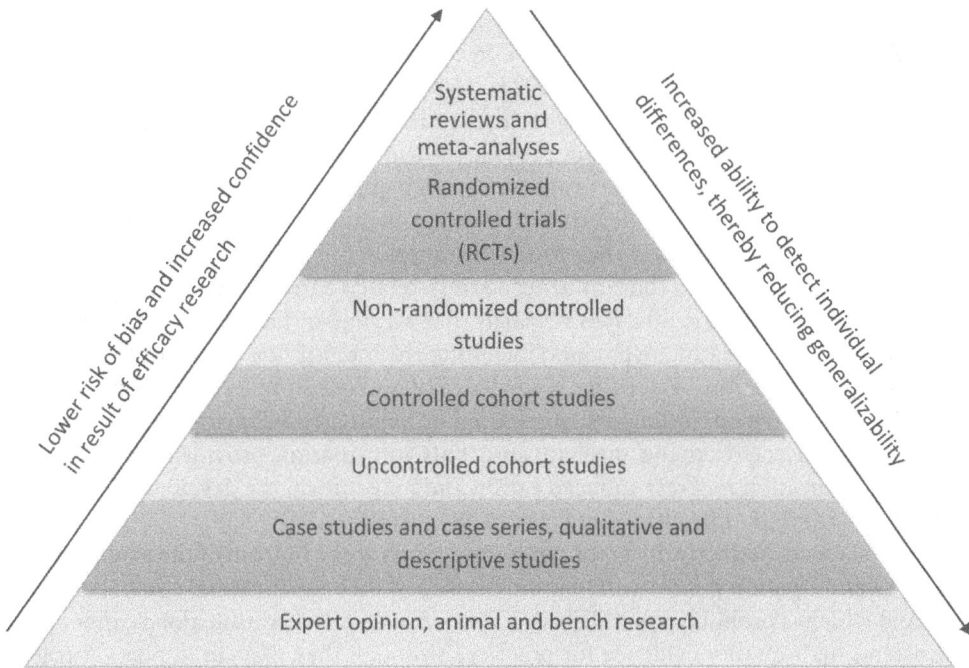

Figure 12.1 Hierarchy of evidence for evaluating studies that examine the efficacy of interventions for groups of people (modified from Evans, 2003)

for a difference among groups and provides the strongest confidence for a single efficacy study. With an RCT design, the results are more likely to be attributable to the intervention itself and not to other factors (e.g., automatic recovery or the placebo effect). In the non-randomized controlled design, a comparison (control) group exists to be compared with the treatment group; however, participants are not randomly allocated to these groups. This non-randomized method could have an impact on the results and affect confidence in the evidence. For example, if initial participants are assigned in the intervention group, then these individuals may have higher motivation and be more eager to change.

Cohort studies, either prospective or retrospective in design, involve the study of groups based on exposure or intervention and are evaluated for differences in the outcome measures. The primary difference between an RCT and a cohort study is that in the RCT participants are randomly allocated to intervention groups, while cohort studies lack random allocation. Retrospective cohort studies identify participants based on exposure or intervention at a certain time point in the past and then follow the groups forward. Thus, random allocation in this method is not possible, and the results of cohort studies can be affected by numerous factors outside the investigators' control.

The next level of evidence is drawn from non-experimental studies such as case studies and case series, and qualitative and descriptive studies. By design, case studies provide no statistical comparison but rather describe the procedures of treatment and the outcomes of the cases. There is a lack of information regarding the outcome for individuals without treatment. For example, Wilcox used a case report to describe OT evaluation and treatment approaches, the plan of care, and the associated outcomes on prolonged symptoms from the novel coronavirus disease 2019 (COVID-19) in the outpatient setting (Wilcox & Frank, 2021). Case studies and case series provide information under certain conditions or when the study focuses on rare diseases. Qualitative studies have no efficacy evidence but provide information that is complementary to the research question and may not be available through quantitative approaches. For example, in a qualitative study of determinants of stress-induced eating in adults, participants were invited to reflect on their food consumption following stressor exposure and to elaborate on the factors that influenced stress-related eating behaviors (Leow et al., 2021). Reflexive thematic analyses revealed that a range of factors significantly influenced stress-induced eating behaviors, including the intensity or nature of the stressor, aspects of prioritization, rewarding, knowledge of and perceptions about food, normative (e.g., family, friend) influences, automated or habituated behaviors, the availability of food, and selected coping mechanisms. This information provided directions for research in variation in stress-induced eating and may inform the development of interventions to alleviate unhealthy dietary responses to stress.

There are two distinctly different types of research at the bottom of the evidence hierarchy. Expert opinion refers to an opinion developed through informal clinical observation and which is probably unpublished. Experience and observation alone cannot yield consistent, high-quality evidence for practice, although they play an important role in decision-making. Animal and bench research, often referred to as laboratory studies, focuses on investigating the physiological and biomechanical mechanisms underlying diseases or treatments. Conclusions drawn from bench and animal research cannot be directly generalized to human beings. However, this work is important in forming the foundation of human clinical trials and advancing healthcare practice.

Comparison with the upstream/downstream research continuum

There is a concept of "upstream" and "downstream" factors in public health, which is related to McKinlay's (1979) river analogy, describing the impacts of pre-existing psychosocial, cultural, financial, and environmental factors on health promotion and outcomes in a profound manner. The analogy goes that a man standing by a fast-flowing river kept jumping in to save people from drowning. The task of saving people exhausted his resources, meaning he was unable to go upstream to prevent them from falling into the river in the first place (Sánchez-Vidaña et al., 2017). This story emphasizes the importance of upstream planning and action in health promotion.

These ideas are now also embedded in OT research and practice. Occupational therapists normally focus on downstream secondary or tertiary health promotion, facilitating individuals to develop personal skills to cope with the symptoms of chronic diseases or disabilities. A significant secondary prevention role in OT, for example, is teaching avoidance skills in fall prevention programs and providing education and lifestyle management training for the elderly. Tertiary prevention strategies in OT include rehabilitation programs using assistive technology for individuals with chronic conditions, such as stroke or neurological diseases.

Upstream thinking targets primary health promotion and aims to prevent illness and disabilities through lifestyle intervention or public policy changes. As Scriven and Atwal (2004) highlighted, upstream primary healthcare focuses on and targets the determinants of health instead of the illness itself (Fung et al., 2021). It develops indicators of health, and involves service users and the general population as equal partners in the development of health to embrace the goal of improving health equality. Furthermore, upstream primary healthcare prioritizes sustainable interventions to build a social system for health. Adopting upstream primary preventative roles in the general population would undoubtedly contribute to a much wider mandate for occupational therapists and enhanced early intervention. Emerging evidence has demonstrated the potential of occupational therapists in primary preventative roles. A systematic review by Elliott and Leland (2018) examined the evidence for the effectiveness of OT fall prevention interventions in improving occupational performance and quality of life for community-dwelling older adults. Synthesized results of 50 articles found mixed evidence for single-component and multifactorial interventions, strong evidence for multicomponent interventions, and moderate evidence for population-based interventions. Tobar et al. (2017) evaluated studies of OT in the prevention of delirium in critically ill clients in an intensive care unit. The findings suggested a significantly lower incidence of delirium, higher level of functional independence, and better cognitive performance in clients receiving OT compared to the control group (Yim et al., 2009).

The important role of occupation in promoting health and wellbeing has been emphasized since the 1980s (Ruan et al., 2014), and echoed through the scientific research in OT. Upstream OT research may add a positive dimension to health prevention and promotion due to the comprehensive understanding of its impact on individuals' self-esteem, as well as their physical and mental health. Further upstream research is needed to support and modernize professional practice, and to facilitate the core functions of OT to accommodate the upstream primary health prevention role in addition to downstream activities. Such a paradigm shift in OT research and practice can help occupational therapists work upstream in the dynamic, multidisciplinary field of public mental healthcare.

Evidence-based practice – Efficacy studies

Randomized controlled trials: Gold standard to test treatment effects

In the EBP community, RCTs are seen as the gold standard for providing evidence of the effectiveness of treatments and interventions. An RCT provides the strongest evidence for a single intervention study due to the design, which controls for numerous confounding factors related to a difference among groups. This means, with an RCT design, the results are more likely induced by the treatment itself and not by other factors. It is important for occupational therapists to be able to understand and critically appraise RCTs in their EBP.

The aim of a clinical trial is to investigate the effectiveness of a treatment, compared with another form of treatment or with no treatment. RCT is the most rigorous form of clinical trial, with other less rigorous forms being controlled clinical trials, pretest–posttest trials, and single-subject trials. An RCT usually consists of three steps: baseline assessment, intervention, and post-intervention assessment, as illustrated in Figure 12.2. A study by Clark et al. (2012) compared the effect of an OT on pain, vitality, social functioning, mental health, and life satisfaction in older people with a no-treatment control condition. Participants were randomly allocated to either the OT group or the control

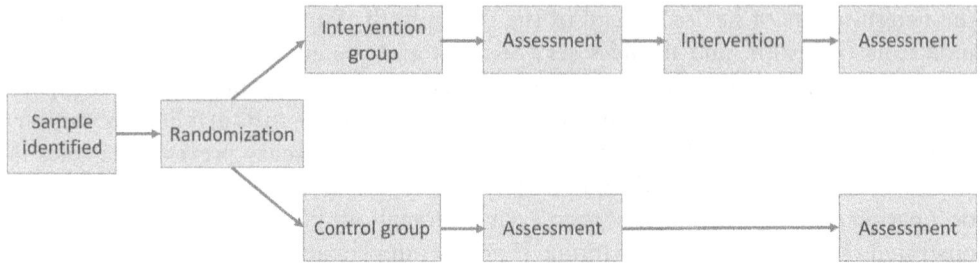

Figure 12.2 RCT steps

group and then assessed using a variety of standardized measures of function and psychosocial health at baseline and six months after the intervention.

Some trials are more complicated in their design. For example, Lee et al. (2021) investigated the effects of robot-assisted therapy (RT) on the sensorimotor and hand function of clients with stroke using a crossover design. Following initial screening, participants were randomized into either the RT or the conventional therapy (CT). Data on hand function and daily living function were collected at baseline and six weeks after intervention. The RT group then received six-week CT, and the CT group received six-week RT. There was a one-month washout period in between the crossover of the interventions. Outcome data were collected from both groups at the end of the 16-week study period.

The process of randomization is the main reason why RCTs are regarded as the gold standard to assess the effectiveness of any treatment. Each participant has an equal opportunity of being allocated to the treatment group or non-treatment (control) group during randomization. This ensures that bias is minimized and that there are no significant differences at baseline among the groups. Another strength of RCTs is the inclusion of the control group. There are several approaches to the use of a control group, including receiving no treatment, receiving standard care, receiving an alternative treatment, or a combination. The use of alternative treatment or standard care reduces the risk of a placebo effect and results in fewer ethical concerns. The control group provides a baseline, and any changes in the treatment group can be compared against it to test the effectiveness of the treatment.

Evidence-based practice – Beyond efficacy studies

Animal and laboratory studies: Exploration of problems, mechanisms, and solutions

From the clinical perspective, evidence generated from various types of research can be classified into levels of evidence, with animal and laboratory studies usually placed at the bottom of the hierarchy. Placement order is determined by the readiness of applying the findings in clinical practice. Animal or laboratory studies, while at the bottom of the hierarchy, can be crucial to clinical applications. In fact, many therapeutic interventions have originated from these fundamental studies. However, the importance of animal and *in vitro* studies cannot be overestimated due to their uniqueness of not involving human subjects and the possibility of testing novel and advanced treatment options.

From the early days of practice in clinical medicine, classic animal model studies have provided a theoretical basis for understanding the physiology of biological systems and the pathology of various diseases, as well as providing a platform for predicting the human response in a range of physiological conditions (El-Nahhas, 2011). The results from animal studies are used to extrapolate and explain the mechanism of human disease conditions, and even to predict the response in human beings in various treatment conditions. Once the principle has been proven in animal models, it would provide a basis and rationale to test if similar responses can be induced in humans. By comparing the basic principles of science generated from animal studies, tests can be conducted to see if existing treatment can be supported by the known principles and the factors which affect the recovery can be defined. The comparison would provide a potential roadmap for future investigation of treatments and recovery for particular diseases (Raymer et al., 2008).

One of the lines of translational study being conducted by the authors' team is to explore the therapeutic mechanisms of essential oils, which provides preliminary scientific evidence to support the application of essential oils and aromatherapy, and delineate the factors which may affect the therapeutic effects of aromatherapy (Fung et al., 2021; Sánchez-Vidaña et al., 2017; 2019; Yim et al., 2009). From our animal studies, it was proven that exposure to lavender essential oil could effectively reduce anxiety-like behaviors (measured by behavioral tests specific for animals, i.e., elevated plus maze and open field tests) in an animal model of experimental anxiety disorder (Tsang et al., 2013), or reduce depression-like behaviors (measured by forced swimming tests) in an animal model of depression (Sánchez-Vidaña et al., 2019). Further analyses of the biochemistry and histology of the brain revealed that, as expected, there was an associated increase in the frontal lobe serotonin level and neurogenesis (Sánchez-Vidaña et al., 2019; Tsang et al., 2013). These findings provided preliminary scientific evidence to support the application of essential oils in two aspects. First, the use of animal models provided unbiased evidence for the anti-depressant and anxiolytic effects of essential oils. Second, biological assays on neurotransmitters and neurogenesis allowed in-depth exploration of related biological or physiological mechanisms. Our group found that the effects of essential oils can be exerted through various routes and mechanisms via both the nervous and respiratory systems (Fung et al., 2021), which implies that future treatment with essential oils may focus on the related mechanisms and routes of delivery (e.g., enhancing intake by the circulatory system and the respiratory system).

In recent years, there have been efforts to translate the knowledge of environmental enrichment obtained from basic scientific research to clinical applications. Environmental enrichment is defined as the provision of an environment with various arrays of sensory, social, and motor stimulation (Musselman et al., 2018). Animal studies have shown that an enriched environment has a powerful and positive impact on neuroplasticity in animals, leading to improvements in cognition and emotion. It has been suggested that with the application of principles derived from animal studies (e.g., provision of multiple stimulations which change with time), there might be a way to bring about both functional and brain structural changes in humans, particularly in those suffering from neurological disorders, including but not limited to traumatic brain injury (Bondi et al., 2015), stroke (McDonald et al., 2018), and neurodegenerative disorders (Menalled & Brunner, 2014). Although the positive effects of an enriched environment have been well established in the laboratory, translational research leading to application is still needed to solve the problems that affect actual clinical application.

For instance, is there a need to standardize the enriched environment in various clinical settings to ensure the reproducibility of effects? Can the observed biological changes in animals be found in human beings (McDonald et al., 2018)? What are the critical and active components to enhance brain plasticity? How to determine the optimal "dosages" of enrichment? Before having a protocol and guideline for introducing an enriched environment in the clinical treatment of neurological disorders, further studies on these issues are needed.

Apart from the abovementioned studies, there are other ongoing studies that explore the translation between basic scientific research and clinical applications, such as the focus on spinal cord injuries (Musselman et al., 2018), cardiovascular diseases (Gevaert et al., 2020), and pulmonary rehabilitation (Jones et al., 2012), etc. Although the findings from animal studies may not be immediately ready for advising clinical practice, their importance in the exploration of mechanisms would shed light on the continuum of biomedical research.

Systematic review and meta-analysis: Toward clinical application

A systematic review or meta-analysis collects possible primary sources of data on a particular topic, summarizes the results of the reports, and provides a conclusion that informs clinical practice. The major difference between a systematic review and a meta-analysis is the presence of collective statistical analyses in the latter. If a pooled estimate is possible (e.g., common assessment tools used across various studies with comparable subjects), a meta-analysis is usually recommended. The pooled estimate would provide convincing results for the research question being asked. In addition, analyses of qualitative data are also involved in a systematic review. As most OT studies adopt quantitative designs, systematic reviews and meta-analyses of quantitative data will be the focus of this section.

To have the highest level of evidence, the key objective of a systematic review and a meta-analysis is to provide valid, objective, and scientific results to a clinical question (Ahn & Kang, 2018). Usually, RCTs are collected via a standardized procedure, and the guidelines for conducting the systematic review or meta-analysis are suggested by the Preferred Reporting Items for Systematic Reviews and Meta-Analyses (PRISMA) statement (Liberati et al., 2009) and the Quality of Reporting of Meta-analyses (QUOROM) statement (Moher et al., 1999). These types of studies have contributed to clinical practice in multiple ways, including informing processes of diagnosis, therapeutic values of treatments, and management of diseases, etc. For example, Arbesman et al. (2013) reported the results of a systematic review of the literature on children's mental health using a public health model consisting of three levels of mental health service. They found strong evidence for the effectiveness of occupation- and activity-based interventions on children's mental wellbeing at the universal level. At the targeted level, strong evidence indicated that social and life skills programs were effective for children who were aggressive or who had intellectual impairments, developmental delays, or learning disabilities. Furthermore, evidence for the effectiveness of the social skills program was strong for children with clinical diagnoses (e.g., autism spectrum disorders) at the intensive level. The study findings shed light on the implementation of various evidence-based OT in a range of target groups at different levels, leading to effective improvements in social behavior and self-management of these individuals.

In the OT field, earlier systematic reviews or meta-analyses often examined the generic effects of OT on different populations, such as individuals with dementia (Kim et al., 2012) or stroke (Steultjens et al., 2003), or community-dwelling elderly (Steultjens et al., 2004), particularly focusing on the functioning of activities of daily living (ADL). Recently, interest has shifted to the effectiveness of particular treatment options, for instance, narrative exposure therapy for clients with post-trauma stress disorder (Correll et al., 2018), telerehabilitation (Hung & Fong, 2019), and virtual reality treatment in upper limb rehabilitation (Mekbib et al., 2020), etc. The changes in topic indicate the higher acceptance and better understanding of OT as an EBP in the management of various disorders in recent years. There is also an increasing interest in the exploration of the therapeutic values of specific treatment options related to OT. Based on this trend, it is expected that systematic reviews or meta-analyses of OT will help to distinguish treatment options of particular importance, and clinical practice may be informed by these reviews.

The quality of a systematic review or meta-analysis can be judged in several aspects: planning of the study, selection of studies, analysis of data (for meta-analysis), and presentation of results.

Planning of the study

At the beginning stage of a systematic review or meta-analysis, a research question should be clearly defined, and it would be desirable to construct the question with population, intervention, comparison, and outcome parameters (i.e., the PICO structure). The research question should be backed up with a good rationale, clearly stating the clinical value of the study. After deciding on the research question, the protocol of the study should be designed with inclusion and exclusion criteria, keywords to be used for the literature search, and databases to be searched. The protocol of the study is recommended to be registered, which ensures the transparency of the study process. The most commonly used registration links include the International Clinical Trials Registry Platform (ICTRP; https://trialsearch.who.int), Cochrane Central Register of Controlled Trials (CENTRAL; https://www.cochranelibrary.com/central/about-central), and ClinicalTrials.gov (https://clinicaltrials.gov).

Selection of studies

The literature search should be done to include as many studies as possible to meet the inclusion criteria. For OT, typically used databases include CINAHL, Cochrane Library, Medline, PubMed, etc. After collecting a literature list, researchers should select appropriate studies based on the abstracts and full texts. Usually, this process should be done by at least two independent researchers. The quality of the included studies should be assessed (e.g., Jadad scale [Qingmei, 2020]), which would have an impact on the quality of the review directly.

Analysis of data

If a pooled estimate is possible after reviewing the studies, clinical effectiveness will be evaluated by a meta-analysis. Often, forest plots will be used to present the odds ratios (ORs), which show the 95% confidence intervals (CIs) of various studies and, more importantly, the combined results from the included studies. The diamond in a forest plot represents every study analyzed in the meta-analysis's overall effect within the 95% CIs. If the diamond does not cross the value of "1" on the plot, it indicates the overall intervention effect is statistically significant. To ensure the quality of the conclusion, an analysis of potential publication bias should be included in the meta-analysis to ensure the conclusion is not due to one or a few studies with a large population size. Publication bias can be assessed by a funnel plot, which is a scatter plot with the effect size on the x-axis and the sample size/precision on the y-axis. If the distribution of the studies shows a mostly symmetrical upside-down funnel shape, it indicates studies with larger samples have less variance and should have ORs similar to the overall effect. This would suggest a low risk of publication bias. If the funnel plot is asymmetric in shape and large studies or many studies fall outside the 95% confidence interval lines, it would suggest a high risk of publication bias.

In addition to the forest and funnel plots, the measure of heterogeneity of the meta-analysis should be considered. To measure the heterogeneity of the meta-analysis, the I^2 value needs to be examined. The I^2 value explains why a proportion of the variation in observed effects is due to variation. If I^2 is closer to 0%, then the results would indicate that much of the meta-analysis calculated effect is due to the true effect of an intervention, and the variance would be minimal. If I^2 is closer to 100%, then most of the observed variance in the meta-analysis would remain. If I^2 is <50%, studies are considered homogenous, and a fixed-effect model of a meta-analysis can be used. If I^2 is >50%, heterogeneity is considered high, and a random-effects model should be used for the meta-analysis (Borenstein et al., 2017).

Presentation of results

The results section of a systematic review or meta-analysis should consist of a flowchart of the literature selection process according to the inclusion and exclusion criteria. A table that summarizes the characteristics of included studies should be present, including the assessment of the quality of studies. Forest plots should also be presented in the results section of a meta-analysis.

Tsang and his team recently conducted a systematic review and meta-analysis to examine the impacts of acupressure on depression in various populations (Lin et al., 2022). A systematic literature search was performed on six databases in both English and Chinese. Data were synthesized using a random-effects model or a fixed-effect model. Subgroup comparisons and meta-regression analyses were performed to explore the factors relevant to the greater or lesser effects of treating symptoms. A total of 14 RCTs were identified, with 1,439 participants. An analysis of the between-group showed that acupressure was significantly effective in reducing depression ($P < 0.0001$) and anxiety ($P < 0.0001$) in participants with mild-to-moderate primary and secondary depression. Subgroup analyses suggested that acupressure significantly reduced depressive symptoms compared with various controlled conditions and in participants of various ages, clinical conditions, and durations of intervention. The main results of the risk of bias evaluation and meta-analysis are presented in Figures 12.3 and 12.4.

To conclude, systematic reviews and meta-analyses inform clinical practice with the highest level of evidence. In the OT field, the focus of systematic reviews or meta-analyses has shifted from the overall effectiveness of OT for various diseases to the effectiveness of particular treatments. To consider adopting the suggestions from systematic reviews or meta-analyses, the quality of the reviews should be assessed from various aspects.

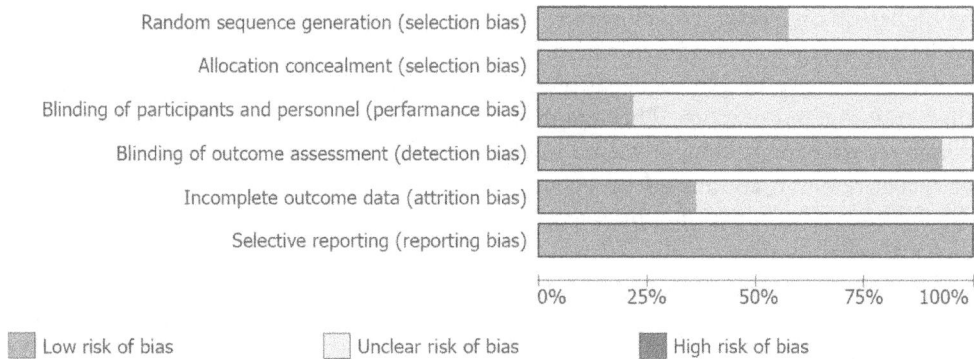

Figure 12.3 Risk of bias evaluation for the included studies

Evidence-based interventions in occupational therapy

Examples of randomized controlled trials of occupational therapy research

Cusick and McClusky (2000) advised occupational therapists to incorporate EBP into their professional role to remain competent, relevant, and clinically effective. This has happened in all subfields of OT research, including mental health, pediatrics, geriatrics, and physical rehabilitation. The scientific publications show that active research has been conducted across various populations by occupational therapists. The emphasis on EBP and an increase in occupational therapists with a doctoral degree are leading

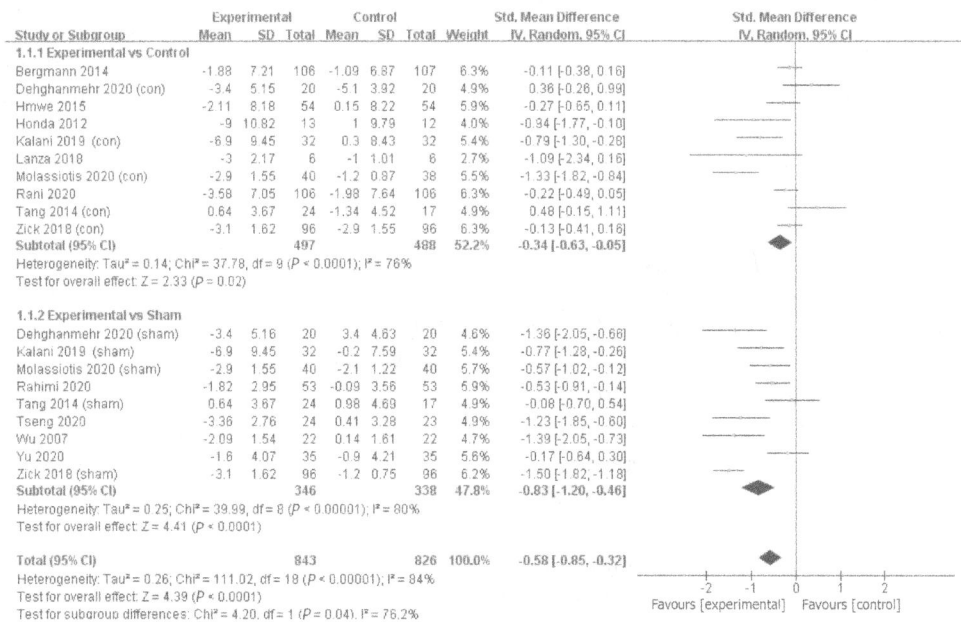

Figure 12.4 Effects of acupressure on depression. 1.1.1: Subgroup meta-analyses of studies used treat-as-usual (TAU) as controls. 1.1.2: Subgroup meta-analyses of studies used sham controls

to higher-quality research. However, there is still space for further development of RCTs and meta-analyses in this field. Tse et al. (2004) urged the importance of EBP and the necessity to arm occupational therapists with evidence-based knowledge in their training and practice. They emphasized the significance of practitioners and academic researchers in being involved in clinical research. Table 12.1 provides a sample of recent research conducted by occupational therapists in various populations, and the evidence of occupational interventions in mental health, pediatrics, geriatrics, and physical rehabilitation.

Occupational therapists have been active in conducting research and contributing to EBP to facilitate the mediating, enabling, and advocating roles in improving the mental and physical health of their clients. It is necessary to develop OT research to improve the status of OT as a health profession for individuals with various disabilities. OT research provides valuable information related to functional and occupational assessments, as well as the development, implementation, and efficacy of interventions. Moreover, increasing RCTs used in efficacy studies and emerging upstream research targeting preventive roles have directed OT to influence public health policy through more strategic activities to promote cost-effective healthcare interventions.

Evidence-based psychosocial interventions

Pharmacological treatment is a standard first-line intervention for people with psychiatric disorders. However, the effectiveness of medication is limited, and psychiatric symptoms and disability are rarely totally relieved. It was reported that approximately 30% of clients with psychotic disorders benefited little from standard antipsychotic treatment and were considered as treatment-resistant (Demjaha et al., 2017). Additionally, medication non-adherence has been identified as one of the major reasons for antipsychotic treatment failure due to the side effects of the medication (Lally & MacCabe, 2015) and internalized stigma (Tsang et al., 2006). Given the limited effects of medication and the growing concerns about long-term antipsychotic prescriptions, psychosocial intervention has been widely accepted for people with psychiatric disabilities.

Psychosocial interventions refer to those treatments that are designed to help clients achieve independence, recovery, employment, meaningful interpersonal relationships, and an enhanced quality of life (Antai-Otong, 2003). These interventions address individual factors (e.g., symptom management, social knowledge and skills, and cognitive functioning), target occupational performances (e.g., work, parenting, and independent living), and consider environmental barriers interfering with successful and satisfying community life. In recent decades, a wide range of psychosocial interventions have been developed and applied in the rehabilitative treatment of people with mental illnesses.

However, not all psychosocial treatments are evidence-based. Established guidelines for best practice are common indicators for identifying EBP. During the development of EBP in mental healthcare, several indicators have been put forward for determining whether a particular psychosocial intervention is considered evidence-based.

Table 12.1 Overview of OT interventions in various areas

Author (year)	Design	Purpose	Results
Mental health			
Employment			
Au et al. (2015)	RCT	Evaluate the effectiveness of Integrated Supported Employment (ISE) plus cognitive remediation training (CRT) for people with schizophrenia and schizoaffective disorders.	Both ISE and ISE+CRT yielded similar improvements across several outcome domains assessed immediately after the interventions and at both 7- and 11-month follow-ups. Significant positive trends over time in vocational, clinical, and cognitive outcomes consistently favored the ISE+CRT condition.
Zhang et al. (2017)	RCT	Evaluate the effectiveness of ISE compared with Individual Placement and Support (IPS) and traditional vocational rehabilitation (TVR) for people with schizophrenia.	Significant higher employment rate and longer job tenure in the ISE group compared with the other two groups.
Noyes et al. (2018)	Systematic review	Review occupational interventions for people with severe mental illness.	Strong evidence for IPS and moderate evidence for supported education interventions.
Leisure			
Esmaili et al. (2019)	RCT	Review the effect of peer-play activities on children with a specific learning disability.	Intervention resulted in moderate to large effects on executive function.
Kim (2020)	RCT	Evaluate the effectiveness of recollection-based OT for mild-stage Alzheimer's disease.	Participants receiving therapy presented improved cognitive functions, reduced depression, and enhanced quality of life.
Health promotion			
Arbesman et al. (2013)	Systematic review	Review the literature on children's mental health at three levels of mental health service.	Identified the effective interventions at each level: occupation- and activity-based interventions at the universal level, and social and life skills programs at the targeted and intensive levels.

Table 12.1 Overview of OT interventions in various areas (*continued*)

Author (year)	Design	Purpose	Results
Schmidt et al. (2021)	Qualitative	Study the context of, barriers to, and recommendations for sex education for people with intellectual and developmental disabilities.	Four barriers to sex education were identified, and participants recommended proactive and formal sex education provided by multiple stakeholders.
Family/caregivers			
DiZazzo-Miller et al. (2017)	RCT	Evaluate the effectiveness of Family Caregiver Training Program for caregivers of people with dementia.	Participants demonstrated an increase in knowledge of daily living activities and improvements in confidence.
Abrahams et al. (2018)	Systematic review and meta-analysis	Evaluate the effects of multicomponent interventions on burden, depression, health, and social support for family caregivers of people with dementia.	Significant effectiveness was found for all four outcomes.
Aqdassi et al. (2021)	Pretest–posttest	Review the efficacy of a family-based telerehabilitation program for children with high-functioning autism.	The program significantly improved motor skills in children with high-functioning autism.
Substance abuse			
Mueser et al. (2013)	RCT	Examine the impact of family intervention on people with substance abuse.	Participants in the family intervention group had significantly less severe psychotic symptoms and tended to improve more in terms of functioning.
Rojo-Mota et al. (2017)	Systematic review	Review OT in the treatment of addiction.	Theoretical and professional role studies, and qualitative and quantitative studies were reviewed; low levels of evidence were found.
Pediatrics			
Romagnoli et al. (2019)	Systematic review	Evaluate the efficacy of OT interventions in pediatric clients with Asperger's syndrome (AS).	OT interventions could help AS children overcome social issues and improve their social skills.
An et al. (2019)	RCT	Determine if a collaborative intervention process between therapists and parents can improve interactions between the two parties.	The intervention improved interactions between parents and therapists, and increased parent participation in the intervention process.

Table 12.1 Overview of OT interventions in various areas (*continued*)

Author (year)	Design	Purpose	Results
Hahn-Markowitz et al. (2020)	RCT	Examine the efficacy of a cognitive-function intervention for children with ADHD.	The intervention resulted in improvements in parent-reported outcomes and self-reported gains. No effect was observed on teachers.
Geriatrics			
Smallfield and Kaldenberg (2020)	Systematic review	Determine the effectiveness of OT interventions in improving reading performance of older adults with low vision.	Electronic magnification, eccentric viewing training, and low vision services could be incorporated in OT practice for older adults with low vision.
Li et al. (2022)	RCT	Investigate the effects of home-based OT telerehabilitation via smartphones on increasing performance and fall efficacy in outpatients after hip fracture surgery.	Significant improvements in fall efficacy and IADL performance were found in the group with the intervention.
Torpil et al. (2021)	RCT	Evaluate the effectiveness of a virtual reality (VR) program in improving cognitive functions in older adults with mild cognitive impairment (MCI).	VR-based rehabilitation enhanced cognitive functions in older adults with MCI.
Physical rehabilitation			
Lee et al. (2019)	Systematic review and meta-analysis	Determine if OT improves ADL and overall physical functioning in clients after hip fracture surgery.	A trend toward improvements in ADL, physical function, and fall occurrence was found. Health perception and client emotions were reported to have significant improvements.
Waliño-Paniagua et al. (2019)	RCT	Analyze if an OT intervention combined with VR can improve manual dexterity of clients with multiple sclerosis.	Precision of movement and execution time, and efficiency of certain functional tasks in the Purdue Pegboard Test and Jebsen-Taylor Hand Function Test were found, although dexterity did not show significant improvements.

The Substance Abuse and Mental Health Services Administration (SAMHSA) has released three foundation guidelines to promote the implementation of EBP (Steenrod, 2009):

- Guideline 1 suggests that the intervention should be formed with a solid and validated theoretical framework.
- Guideline 2 asserts that the effectiveness of the intervention should be supported by empirical evidence.
- Guideline 3 suggests that the intervention should be judged by a group of informed experts to be effective in terms of its underlying theoretical framework, research outcomes, and practice experience.

SAMHSA has established a web-based searchable database, the National Registry of Evidence-based Programs and Practices, to provide information about evidence-based interventions for individuals with co-occurring disorders.

The following subsections introduce several psychosocial interventions that fall within OT's domain and which meet SAMHSA's criteria for EBP. A brief description of the interventions together with supporting research evidence are presented. Further discussion of the details of these interventions is presented in other chapters of the book. The strong research support for these interventions increases the possibility of positive outcomes for clients. Therefore, it is important for occupational therapists to be familiar with these interventions and, when applicable, consider implementing them in practice.

Supported employment

Employment is an important life domain that promotes positive mental health and community participation. Challenges in employment are highly prevalent among people with severe mental illness. For example, according to a study, people with psychotic disorders had poor outcomes related to employment, and as few as 10% of them were employed on a competitive basis (Marwaha et al., 2007). Some studies suggested that around half of clients with schizophrenia had difficulty in sustaining a competitive job (McGurk et al., 2003). Employment challenges span a full range of elements, including obtaining employment and sustaining a job after being employed (Becker & Drake, 2003).

Vocational rehabilitation aims to help people with severe mental illness succeed in employment (Mueser & Bond, 2000) and facilitate their recovery process (Antai-Otong, 2003). The "train and then place" approach was the essential philosophy in traditional vocational rehabilitation. Within this framework, people were expected to develop the necessary skills before seeking employment through sheltered workshops or prevocational training programs. However, unfavorable outcomes associated with this approach were reported (Clark & Samnaliev, 2005). Tsang et al. (2004) reported that only 2.5% of participants who received traditional vocational rehabilitation intervention went on to obtain competitive employment.

In view of the limited effects of traditional vocational rehabilitation, the Individual Placement and Support (IPS) model was developed to improve treatment outcomes for people with severe mental illness (Becker & Drake, 1993; Drake & Becker, 1996). IPS is a specific model of Supported Employment (SE) that aims to facilitate people with psychiatric disabilities to succeed in competitive employment (Drake & Becker, 1996).

According to Bond et al. (2001) and Bond (2004), contrary to the traditional "train and then place" model, IPS adopts a "place and then train" approach. There are seven key principles included in IPS:

- Seeking competitive employment;
- Conducting a rapid job search;
- Integrating mental health services;
- Emphasizing individuals' preferences;
- Implementing continuous and comprehensive assessment;
- Providing time-unlimited support; and
- Conducting benefits counseling.

Empirical evidence indicated that the IPS approach improved short-term employment among people with psychotic disorders (Drake et al., 1999; Lehman et al., 2002). A systematic review by Bond (2004) found that 56% of participants were able to achieve competitive employment after receiving IPS. Moreover, Probyn et al. (2021) reviewed ten RCTs investigating the effectiveness of IPS in people with conditions other than severe mental illness and found significant improvements in competitive employment. Overall, multiple RCTs demonstrated that SE was superior to traditional vocational rehabilitation approaches (e.g., prevocational training, sheltered workshops, etc.) (Bond et al., 2008; Cook et al., 2008). However, nearly half of the participants receiving SE intervention failed to obtain or sustain jobs. The effectiveness of the IPS approach in improving job satisfaction, job tenure, and other nonvocational outcomes has not been fully addressed.

Based on the IPS model proposed by Becker and Drake, researchers have integrated skills training elements into the model to augment its effectiveness (Cook et al., 2005; McGurk et al., 2005). It has been reported that individuals tended to work more hours and have an increased income after taking the IPS program with cognitive training (McGurk et al., 2005). Tsang et al. (2009) incorporated social skills training (SST) in the IPS program and found that the competitive employment rate increased to 78.8% and participants tended to have a longer sustained working period within 15 months of service (Tsang et al., 2010). A wide range of various enhanced SE interventions are being explored.

Social skills training
Social skills are the basis of effective social interaction (Bellack & Mueser, 1993) and enable individuals to succeed in daily functioning (Kopelowicz et al., 2006). SST was developed based on social learning theory (Bandura, 1969) and the principles of operant conditioning (Liberman, 1972). The primary focus of SST is on social functioning improvement and specific skills enhancement in individuals, such as identifying and mending problems in social relationships, daily life, work, and leisure (Lauriello et al., 1999). SST aims to optimize the social functioning of individuals with psychiatric disabilities (Antai-Otong, 2003) and to improve their repertoire of skills for community functioning (Corrigan et al., 1992).

The key components of SST include warm-up activities, behaviorally based instructions, demonstration, corrective feedback, and homework assignments (Lehman et al.,

2003; Wallace et al., 1980). Behavioral techniques such as prompting, shaping, reinforcing, and modeling are used to help individuals acquire and sustain social skills (Glynn, 2003). There are three models of SST: basic, social problem-solving, and cognitive remediation (Bellack & Mueser, 1993). Each model focuses on different components of skills training. The basic model emphasizes corrective learning, in which complex social repertoires are broken down into simple steps for understanding and practice. The social problem-solving model works on the hypothesis that impairments in information processing induce social skill deficits. The model targets the skill deficit of the corresponding daily life function in terms of reception, processing, and transmission. The cognitive remediation model hypothesizes that learning and generalization of social skills can be achieved by lowering the level of cognitive deficits, and thus fundamental cognitive functions are trained using this model.

The effectiveness of SST in enhancing skill acquisition in people with psychiatric disabilities has been widely demonstrated (Bustillo et al., 2001; Heinssen et al., 2000; Lehman et al., 2003). A meta-analysis conducted by Turner et al. (2018) identified 27 RCTs, including 1,437 participants with psychosis, and found significant superiority of SST for symptoms and social outcomes compared to other interventions. In view of the effectiveness of SST in successful employment, Tsang and Pearson (1996) developed a structural work-related social skills training (WSST) program for people with schizophrenia. The WSST program trained participants to learn the social skills necessary for handling general and specific work-related conditions, in addition to practicing basic social communication and survival skills (Tsang & Pearson, 1996). Tsang (2001) conducted an RCT to examine the effectiveness of the WSST program for clients with schizophrenia. The findings suggested that participants had better social competence after the WSST training compared with those receiving standard treatment. The competitive employment rate of the WSST group reached 46.7%. The WSST program is currently being used as a part of psychiatric rehabilitation programs in Hong Kong, Australia, and Germany (Tsang & Cheung, 2005).

According to Becker et al. (1998), skills training programs should be tailored to the required skills of a particular job. In view of the importance of acquiring job-specific social skills for success in the workplace, Cheung et al. (2006) developed a job-specific social skills training (JSST) program based on earlier efforts in this line of study, with a specific focus on the job of a salesperson because this job was found to be popular for people with psychotic disorders (Tsang et al., 2002). Tsang and Cheung (2005) conducted a study of 106 salespeople to identify the required specific social skills and used these elements to develop the JSST program.

A systematic literature review (Tsang & Cheung, 2005) of the effectiveness of SST for people with psychiatric disabilities suggested a consistently strong and positive impact on social skills acquisition among participants. However, inconsistent findings were still reported, including those in symptom elimination, relapse prevention, rehospitalization reduction, and short-term maintenance of skills. In addition, the long-term outcomes of SST, the generalization of behaviors, and the potential neurophysiological mechanism underlying the effectiveness remain unclear.

Cognitive behavioral therapy

Cognitive behavioral therapy (CBT) is a problem-oriented approach that works to improve emotional states and cognitive functioning by changing distorted thinking

(Reinecke et al., 1998). CBT was first developed to treat depression and anxiety (Beck, 1976; Haddock et al., 1998). It has subsequently been used as an add-on treatment to pharmacotherapy for people with schizophrenia and bipolar disorders (Gould et al., 2001) to reduce hallucinations and delusions and lower the level of social disability and risk of relapse (Bustillo et al., 2001; Glynn, 2003).

It is assumed in CBT that the symptom or problematic issue is manifested and maintained by the mediation of cognitive and environmental processes, and modification of these processes can be accomplished by training individuals with more adaptive cognitive and behavioral skills (Haddock et al., 1998). Kingdon and Turkington (1994) proposed a two-pronged approach to CBT: first, test the validity of potential irrational beliefs through logical reasoning, then test various management strategies such as problem-solving and distraction if the targeted concern cannot be eliminated via logical reasoning. Several psychotherapy modalities, such as psychoeducation, cognitive reconstruction, and skills training, are integrated in CBT programs (Kingdon & Turkington, 1994).

CBT was initially developed for individuals with depression, with a focus on changing negative thinking. There is strong evidence for the efficacy of CBT in reducing depressive symptoms, and it has equal effects when compared to medication (Feldman, 2007). A recent systematic review and network meta-analysis compared the effectiveness of various types of therapy, various components and combinations of components, and a range of delivery methods used in CBT interventions for adult depression. The systematic review of 91 studies found strong evidence that CBT interventions yielded a larger short-term decrease in depression scores compared with treat-as-usual (López-López et al., 2019).

There is also evidence that CBT may be more beneficial than antidepressants for preventing relapse in major depressive disorders (Zhang et al., 2018). There is also evidence that CBT is an effective treatment for anxiety, typically leading to reductions in worry, and studies showed that CBT was equal to pharmaceutical treatment and more effective at a six-month follow-up (Borza, 2017). CBT can be conducted in individual or group formats; the effects on depression and anxiety disorder were found to be significantly stronger in individual CBT compared to group CBT (Carpenter et al., 2018).

Several clinical trials demonstrated the effectiveness of CBT in reducing psychotic symptoms such as delusions and hallucinations (Clark & Samnaliev, 2005; Morrison et al., 2018; Pot-Kolder et al., 2018). A meta-analysis conducted by Zimmermann et al. (2005) investigated 14 RCTs of CBT and showed a mean effect size of 0.37 in eliminating positive symptoms. A recent systematic review and meta-analysis of 25 RCTs suggested that CBT interventions offered a large effect size improvement in personal recovery at post-treatment (mean effect size = 2.27), and a large effect size of 2.62 at long-term follow-up (Wang et al., 2019). However, the benefits for relapse prevention, reduction in hospitalization, and promotion of social cognitive functioning for people with psychotic disorders were limited.

Assertive community treatment

Enabling community functioning is a primary aim of mental health services and OT for people with psychiatric disorders (Bustillo et al., 2001). Collaboration and thoughtful allocation of mental health services are facilitated by proper case management systems (Antai-Otong, 2003). Assertive community treatment (ACT) is a community-oriented intensive care management approach that originated in the Mendota Mental Health Institute in Madison in the late 1970s (Stein & Test, 1980). ACT was developed in response to the deinstitutionalization movement of psychiatric rehabilitation (Marshall & Lockwood, 2000).

The key objectives of ACT are to reduce the hospitalization rate among people with the most severe disabilities, develop skills for community life, and promote proper utilization of mental health services (Antai-Otong, 2003). The unique features of ACT allow it to be distinguished from traditional case management models. One of these features is the importance of multidisciplinary teamwork (Bustillo et al., 2001; Lehman et al., 2003). The team draws on the expertise of its members to provide targeted services to clients. The composition of each team may vary, but it typically consists of 10 to 12 mental health professionals, including an occupational therapist, nurse, psychiatrist, social worker, psychologist, employment specialist, substance abuse specialist, peer specialist, or other related experts. All team members are able to serve as case managers (Stein & Santos, 1998). The caseload of staff members is generally low, with approximately one member of staff for every 10 clients. This ensures that staff members can cope with the intensive needs of service recipients (Phillips et al., 2001). The tailor-made service is provided on a 24-hour basis with no arbitrary time limit (Mueser & Glynn, 1998; Phillips et al., 2001). In the design of ACT, clients receive services for as long as needed, and whenever they are needed.

Numerous ACT studies have provided empirical support for its effectiveness in reducing the number of hospitalizations and the total length of stay in psychiatric hospitals, and in improving housing stability among people with psychotic disorders (Nelson et al., 2007; Vanderlip et al., 2017). Studies indicated a range of 10–85% reduction in hospitalization rates among participants who had engaged in ACT programs (Vanderlip et al., 2017). The best outcomes were demonstrated in individuals with serious symptoms and functional deficits (Philips et al., 2001).

However, aside from the reduction in hospitalization rates, the effects of ACT on other clinical and functional outcomes are limited, and there is no consensus regarding its effectiveness in promoting competitive employment, social functioning, and symptom management (Clark & Samnaliev, 2005).

Family therapy

Research has suggested that the family environment is associated with treatment outcomes in people with psychiatric disabilities (Glynn, 2003). Expressed emotion is a concept used to describe the level of family stress due to factors such as criticism, overinvolvement, and hostility (Antai-Otong, 2003). It is important to realize that taking care of mentally ill family members increases both the physical and psychological burden on the family (Tsang et al., 2003). The primary aims of family intervention (FI) are to lower relapse rates, enhance the social adjustment of people with psychotic disorders, and reduce caregivers' stress and burden (Glynn, 2003).

Effective FIs include psychoeducation, problem-solving, crisis management, and crisis intervention (Lehman et al., 2003). FI can be conducted with an individual family or in multiple family groups. Research has suggested that the multiple family groups approach is more effective due to the additional benefit of increased social support among members (Lehman et al., 2003).

The effectiveness of FI in eliminating symptoms, improving functioning, reducing family burden, and promoting family subjective well-being has been well examined by RCTs (Konkolÿ Thege, 2021; McFarlane, 2016; Miklowitz & Chung, 2016). A previous study by Mueser and Glynn (1998) reported that the relapse rate of individuals who had participated in FI was 24%, compared to 64% for those without FI. Moreover, FI was proven to enhance medication compliance and improve the coping skills and knowledge of relatives to take care of and communicate with their mentally ill family members (Pharoah et al., 2010). Empirical evidence supported the durable effect of long-term FI (Mueser & Glynn, 1998), and the beneficial effects of FI were sustained after the termination of services (Jensen et al., 2014).

Motivational interviewing

Motivational interviewing (MI) was originally developed to address problems associated with making behavioral changes for people with substance abuse disorders (Miller et al., 2006); however, it has since been applied to many other behavioral change interventions (e.g., smoking cessation, weight loss, exercise, etc.). One of the primary differences between MI and earlier approaches to substance abuse treatment is the style of interaction. Traditionally, treatment for substance abuse used a confrontational approach, which was based on the theory that people could not change until they "hit rock bottom" or were ready to change. In contrast, MI emphasizes a collaborative approach that seeks to engage and motivate the client to change.

There are four general principles of MI (Miller & Rollnick, 2002):

- Express empathy (let the client know that the change process is difficult);
- Develop discrepancy (identify differences between current behavior and personal goals and values);
- Roll with resistance (avoid confrontation); and
- Support self-efficacy (indicate that you believe the client is capable of making a change).

There is strong evidence supporting the efficacy of MI for substance abuse treatment. A meta-analysis found that MI showed a significant effect on substance use compared with no treatment control at post-intervention, short-term follow-up, and medium-term follow-up (Smedslund et al., 2011). Another systematic review synthesized 16 studies that examined the effectiveness of MI-based compliance therapy to improve psychiatric symptoms in people with severe mental illness. It found that MI-based compliance therapy significantly improved psychiatric symptoms with a moderate effect size of 0.45. Session length and dose effect should be considered when tailoring MI to clients of different ages (Wong-Anuchit et al., 2019). MI is typically offered in a very brief format, sometimes one session. Empirical evidence provided additional support for these short-term approaches (Vasilaki et al., 2006).

Mindfulness-based interventions

The term "mindfulness" refers to two primary concepts: (1) a meta-cognitive exercise involving sustained and intentional attention to experiencing the present moment, while diminishing the emotional and cognitive reactivity generated by the experience, and (2) acceptance of the experience with a non-judgmental attitude. Mindfulness originally came from the Buddhist philosophy and plays a central role within the framework of a conceptual and applied system whose aim is the cessation of suffering (Hanh, 2020).

There are two seminal protocols for mindfulness-based intervention (MBI): mindfulness-based stress reduction (MBSR) (Kabat-Zinn, 1982) and mindfulness-based cognitive therapy (MBCT) (Segal et al., 2018). Both are widely used in mental healthcare and have remarkable empirical support. The popularity of MBIs has increased exponentially over the past 30 years, alongside the volume of research conducted on their effectiveness in treating various psychiatric disorders. Recent reviews of RCTs comparing MBIs with active control conditions indicated that MBIs were effective in treating a wide range of outcomes among diverse populations. These outcomes included depression and anxiety symptoms (Hofmann et al., 2010), stress (Chiesa & Serretti, 2009), quality of life (Godfrin & van Heeringen, 2010), and psychological and emotional distress (Xu et al., 2016).

A recent systematic review and meta-analysis of ten clinical trials on MBCT for bipolar disorder revealed a reduction in symptoms of depression, anxiety, and stress, with small to moderate effect sizes (Xuan et al., 2020). Some studies published in the early 2000s found that the application of therapies, which included mindfulness components, resulted in improvements in clients with schizophrenia (Bach & Hayes, 2002). Chadwick (2006) developed person-based cognitive therapy (PBCT) for distressing psychosis, with the first intervention specifically designed for people with schizophrenia to incorporate mindfulness as a core element, combined with other therapeutic components derived from CBT. A recent systematic review suggested that MBI combined with standard treatments was able to generate significant improvements in a variety of clinical schizophrenia-related parameters, including overall symptomatology, positive and negative symptoms, functioning level, and awareness of illness (Hodann-Caudevilla et al., 2020).

Besides emotional symptoms, it is clear that the empirical evidence of MBIs for other psychosocial outcomes such as cognitive functioning and occupational rehabilitation is scarce. It is therefore necessary to conduct further studies in order to draw sound conclusions on the effectiveness of MBIs in a wide range of psychiatric disabilities, and to examine the underlying neural mechanisms of these effects using imaging techniques.

Recommendations for strengthening evidence-based occupational therapy practice

As a young profession compared to medicine and nursing, the research evidence originating from OT is still limited. The following recommendations are proposed to increase the contribution of OT to clinical research.

(1) The curriculum of both undergraduate and postgraduate entry-level professional education of occupational therapists should include more credits on research, biostatistics, and their application in clinical practice. Joint employment between clinical and academic settings in the institutions should be encouraged for implementation of collaborative translational research on OT interventions.

(2) Occupational therapists globally have developed a wide spectrum of standardized and manualized programs and interventions that are ideal targets for evaluation research. For example, the Integrated Supported Employment (ISE) program conceptualized by Tsang and Pearson (1996), which combined IPS (Bond et al.,

1997) and WSST (Tsang & Pearson, 2001), was found to be significantly effective in improving employment outcomes in individuals with severe mental illness as well as their quality of life in Hong Kong and mainland China using RCTs (Tsang et al., 2009; Zhang et al., 2017). Further evaluation research in different clinical settings and populations is also needed.

(3) Lloyd et al. (2005) reported the benefits of forming a collaborative partnership between OT clinicians and an academic institution in order to conduct research within a clinical setting. The Department of Rehabilitation Sciences at The Hong Kong Polytechnic University (PolyU) has established the Rehabilitation Clinic on campus to facilitate teaching and research, and to provide both physiotherapy and OT rehabilitation services to the public. This setting has demonstrated that collaboration at the service provision level has the potential to overcome the low level of involvement in clinical research. It also outlines the steps involved in developing a collaboration between clinicians and academic researchers. Clinicians can provide access to the population and therapists to carry out the intervention, whereas academic researchers can design the study, select outcome measures, and analyze the data. In terms of research collaboration, the Mental Health Research Centre (MHRC) at PolyU is a good example. MHRC was established in 2021 to function as a collaborative research hub that integrates basic and translational animal models, neuroimaging and neurophysiological techniques, and social and cultural factors to explore the neurobiological underpinnings of mental illnesses and neurocognitive mechanisms, as well as to understand the impact of environmental and social determinants on help-seeking and social functioning in people with mental illnesses. Experts from various professional and scientific disciplines apart from OT have been contributing to MHRC, including neuroscientists, biochemists, computer scientists, psychologists, psychiatrists, sociologists, policy researchers, etc.

(4) Although there are several barriers to the implementation of experimental research, quasi-experimental and observational studies can provide important quantitative evidence, and qualitative research also helps answer "how" and "why" OT interventions work. When experimental studies are not feasible, occupational therapists may consider other research designs.

(5) Case studies in journals and textbooks should attempt to knit theory, practice, and research together by demonstrating how EBP can be implemented within a coherent theoretical framework. Occupational therapists can submit case studies to journals that describe the approach to an individual case in terms of a theoretical perspective, the clinical reasoning and intervention provided, and the outcomes collected.

(6) With the development of digital techniques, occupational therapists should incorporate high-level techniques into clinical practice. Research on digital mental health interventions in OT is still in its infancy, but it offers a promising direction for conducting research in related fields, thereby providing more evidence to clinicians and mental health professionals and facilitating the allocation of resources in the healthcare system.

EBP includes the assimilation of empirical evidence for clinical decisions. Therapists and other experts in the profession should conduct regular reviews to synthesize empirical evidence from OT and other fields to support clinical reasoning. An excellent example is the review conducted by Stoffel and Moyers (2004) on substance abuse treatments. In this review, they identified four EBPs: brief intervention, CBT, MI, and 12-step programs. Of particular help in the review was an analysis of the role of OT in each of these practices.

Summary

This chapter reviews the definition and development of EBP, outlines the evidence-based interventions in OT, and provides recommendations for expanding the scope of research in this field. It addresses the common misconception regarding the interpretation and application of existing research data and findings in clinical practice. It aims to assist readers in consuming and interpreting research data and literature to evaluate the effectiveness of treatments and interventions, thereby facilitating their application in clinical practice. The knowledge obtained from the chapter can be used as a practical guide to EBP.

References

Abrahams, R., Liu, K. P. Y., Bissett, M., Fahey, P., Cheung, K. S. L., Bye, R., Chaudhary, K., & Chu, L.-W. (2018). Effectiveness of interventions for co-residing family caregivers of people with dementia: Systematic review and meta-analysis. *Australian Occupational Therapy Journal*, 65(3), 208–224. https://doi.org/10.1111/1440-1630.12464

Ahn, E., & Kang, H. (2018). Introduction to systematic review and meta-analysis. *Korean Journal of Anesthesiology*, 71(2), 103–112. https://doi.org/10.4097/kjae.2018.71.2.103

An, M., Palisano, R. J., Yi, C.-H., Chiarello, L. A., Dunst, C. J., & Gracely, E. J. (2019). Effects of a collaborative intervention process on parent-therapist interaction: A randomized controlled trial. *Physical & Occupational Therapy in Pediatrics*, 39(3), 259–275. https://doi.org/10.1080/01942638.2018.1496965

Antai-Otong, D. (2003). Psychosocial rehabilitation. *Nursing Clinics of North America*, 38(1), 151–160. https://doi.org/10.1016/S0029-6465(02)00068-3

Aqdassi, L., Sadeghi, S., Pouretemad, H. R., & Fathabadi, J. (2021). A family-based telerehabilitation program for improving gross motor skills in children with high functioning autism spectrum disorder. *Journal of Modern Rehabilitation*, 15(3), 173–182. https://doi.org/10.18502/jmr.v15i3.7738

Arbesman, M., Bazyk, S., & Nochajski, S. M. (2013). Systematic review of occupational therapy and mental health promotion, prevention, and intervention for children and youth. *American Journal of Occupational Therapy*, 67(6), e120–e130.

Au, D. W. H., Tsang, H. W. H., So, W. W. Y., Bell, M. D., Cheung, V., Yiu, M. G. C., Tam, K. L., & Lee, G. T.-H. (2015). Effects of integrated supported employment plus cognitive remediation training for people with schizophrenia and schizoaffective disorders. *Schizophrenia Research*, 166(1–3), 297–303. https://doi.org/10.1016/j.schres.2015.05.013

Bach, P., & Hayes, S. C. (2002). The use of acceptance and commitment therapy to prevent the rehospitalization of psychotic patients: A randomized controlled trial. *Journal of Consulting and Clinical Psychology*, 70(5), 1129–1139. https://doi.org/10.1037/0022-006X.70.5.1129

Bandura, A. (1969). *Principles of behavior modification*. Holt, Rinehart and Winston.

Beck, A. T. (1976). *Cognitive therapy and the emotional disorders*. International Universities Press.

Becker, D. R., & Drake, R. E. (1993). *A working life: The Individual Placement and Support (IPS) Program*. New Hampshire-Dartmouth Psychiatric Research Center.

Becker, D. R., & Drake, R. E. (2003). *A working life for people with severe mental illness*. Oxford University Press.

Becker, D. R., Drake, R. E., Bond, G. R., Xie, H., Dain, B. J., & Harrison, K. (1998). Job terminations among persons with severe mental illness participating in supported employment. *Community Mental Health Journal*, 34(1), 71–82. https://doi.org/10.1023/a:1018716313218

Bellack, A. S., & Mueser, K. T. (1993). Psychosocial treatment for schizophrenia. *Schizophrenia Bulletin, 19*(2), 317–336. https://doi.org/10.1093/schbul/19.2.317

Bennett, K. J., Sackett, D. L., Haynes, R. B., Neufeld, V. R., Tugwell, P., & Roberts, R. (1987). A controlled trial of teaching critical appraisal of the clinical literature to medical students. *Journal of the American Medical Association, 257*(18), 2451–2454. https://doi.org/10.1001/jama.1987.03390180069025

Bond, G. R. (2004). Supported employment: Evidence for an evidence-based practice. *Psychiatric Rehabilitation Journal, 27*(4), 345–359. https://doi.org/10.2975/27.2004.345.359

Bond, G. R., Becker, D. R., Drake, R. E., Rapp, C. A., Meisler, N., Lehman, A. F., Bell, M. D., & Blyler, C. R. (2001). Implementing supported employment as an evidence-based practice. *Psychiatric Services, 52*(3), 313–322. https://doi.org/10.1176/appi.ps.52.3.313

Bond, G. R., Becker, D. R., Drake, R. E., & Vogler, K. M. (1997). A fidelity scale for the Individual Placement and Support model of supported employment. *Rehabilitation Counseling Bulletin, 40*(4), 265–284.

Bond, G. R., Drake, R. E., & Becker, D. R. (2008). An update on randomized controlled trials of evidence-based supported employment. *Psychiatric Rehabilitation Journal, 31*(4), 280–290. https://doi.org/10.2975/31.4.2008.280.290

Bondi, C. O., Semple, B. D., Noble-Haeusslein, L. J., Osier, N. D., Carlson, S. W., Dixon, C. E., Giza, C. C., & Kline, A. E. (2015). Found in translation: Understanding the biology and behavior of experimental traumatic brain injury, *Neuroscience and Biobehavioral Reviews, 58*, 123–146. https://doi.org/10.1016/j.neubiorev.2014.12.004

Borenstein, M., Higgins, J. P. T., Hedges, L. V., & Rothstein, H. R. (2017). Basics of meta-analysis: I^2 is not an absolute measure of heterogeneity. *Research Synthesis Methods, 8*(1), 5–18. https://onlinelibrary.wiley.com/doi/epdf/10.1002/jrsm.1230

Borza, L. (2017). Cognitive-behavioral therapy for generalized anxiety. *Dialogues in Clinical Neuroscience, 19*(2), 203–208. https://doi.org/10.31887/DCNS.2017.19.2/lborza

Bustillo, J. R., Lauriello, J., Horan, W. P., & Keith, S. J. (2001). The psychosocial treatment of schizophrenia: An update. *The American Journal of Psychiatry, 158*(2), 163–175. https://doi.org/10.1176/appi.ajp.158.2.163

Cameron, K. A. V., Ballantyne, S., Kulbitsky, A., Margolis-Gal, M., Daugherty, T., & Ludwig, F. (2005). Utilization of evidence-based practice by registered occupational therapists. *Occupational Therapy International, 12*(3), 123–136. https://doi.org/10.1002/oti.1

Carpenter, J. K., Andrews, L. A., Witcraft, S. M., Powers, M. B., Smits, J. A. J., & Hofmann, S. G. (2018). Cognitive behavioral therapy for anxiety and related disorders: A meta-analysis of randomized placebo-controlled trials. *Depression and Anxiety, 35*(6), 502–514. https://doi.org/10.1002/da.22728

Chadwick, P. (2006). *Person-based cognitive therapy for distressing psychosis*. John Wiley & Sons Ltd.

Cheung, L. C. C., Tsui, C. U., & Tsang, H. W. H. (2006). Job-specific Social Skills Training (JSST) for people with severe mental illness in Hong Kong. *Journal of Rehabilitation, 72*(4), 14–23.

Chiesa, A., & Serretti, A. (2009). Mindfulness-based stress reduction for stress management in healthy people: A review and meta-analysis. *The Journal of Alternative and Complementary Medicine, 15*(5), 593–600. https://doi.org/10.1089/acm.2008.0495

Clark, F., Jackson, J., Carlson, M., Chou, C.-P., Cherry, B. J., Jordan-Marsh, M., Knight, B. G., Mandel, D., Blanchard, J., Granger, D. A., Wilcox, R. R., Lai, M. Y., White, B., Hay, J., Lam, C., Marterella, A., & Azen, S. P. (2012). Effectiveness of a lifestyle intervention in promoting the well-being of independently living older people: Results of the Well Elderly 2 Randomised Controlled Trial. *Journal of Epidemiology and Community Health, 66*(9), 782–790. https://doi.org/10.1136/jech.2009.099754

Clark, R. E., & Samnaliev, M. (2005). Psychosocial treatment in the 21st century. *International Journal of Law and Psychiatry, 28*(5), 532–544. https://doi.org/10.1016/j.ijlp.2005.08.002

Cochrane, A. (1972). *Effectiveness and efficiency: Random reflections on health services*. Nuffield Provincial Hospitals Trust. https://www.nuffieldtrust.org.uk/research/effectiveness-and-efficiency-random-reflections-on-health-services

Cook, J. A., Blyler, C. R., Leff, H. S., McFarlane, W. R., Goldberg, R. W., Gold, P. B., Mueser, K. T., Shafer, M. S., Onken, S. J., Donegan, K., Carey, M. A., Kaufmann, C., & Razzano,

L. A. (2008). The Employment Intervention Demonstration Program: Major findings and policy implications. *Psychiatric Rehabilitation Journal, 31*(4), 291–295. https://doi.org/10.2975/31.4.2008.291.295

Cook, J. A., Lehman, A. F., Drake, R., McFarlane, W. R., Gold, P. B., Leff, H. S., Blyler, C., Toprac, M. G., Razzano, L. A., Burke-Miller, J. K., Blankertz, L., Shafer, M., Pickett-Schenk, S. A., & Grey, D. D. (2005). Integration of psychiatric and vocational services: A multisite randomized, controlled trial of supported employment. *The American Journal of Psychiatry, 162*(10), 1948–1956. https://doi.org/10.1176/appi.ajp.162.10.1948

Correll, C. U., Galling, B., Pawar, A., Krivko, A., Bonetto, C., Ruggeri, M., Craig, T. J., Nordentoft, M., Srihari, V. H., Guloksuz, S., Hui, C. L. M., Chen, E. Y. H., Valencia, M., Juarez, F., Robinson, D. G., Schooler, N. R., Brunette, M. F., Mueser, K. T., Rosenheck, R. A., & Kane, J. M. (2018). Comparison of early intervention services vs treatment as usual for early-phase psychosis: A systematic review, meta-analysis, and meta-regression. *JAMA Psychiatry, 75*(6), 555–565. http://doi.org/10.1001/jamapsychiatry.2018.0623

Corrigan, P. W., Schade, M. L., & Liberman, R. P. (1992). Social skills training. In R. P. Liberman (Ed.), *Handbook of psychiatric rehabilitation* (pp. 95–126). Macmillan.

Cusick, A., & McCluskey, A. (2000). Becoming an evidence-based practitioner through professional development. *Australian Occupational Therapy Journal, 47*, 159–170. https://doi.org/10.1046/j.1440-1630.2000.00241.x

Demjaha, A., Lappin, J. M., Stahl, D., Patel, M. X., MacCabe, J. H., Howes, O. D., Heslin, M., Reininghaus, U. A., Donoghue, K., Lomas, B., Charalambides, M., Onyejiaka, A., Fearon, P., Jones, P., Doody, G., Morgan, C., Dazzan, P., & Murray, R. M. (2017). Antipsychotic treatment resistance in first-episode psychosis: Prevalence, subtypes and predictors. *Psychological Medicine, 47*, 1981–1989. https://doi.org/10.1017/S0033291717000435

DiZazzo-Miller, R., Winston, K., Winkler, S. L., & Donovan, M. L. (2017). Family Caregiver Training Program (FCTP): A randomized controlled trial. *American Journal of Occupational Therapy, 71*(5), 7105190010p1–7105190010p10.

Drake, R. E., & Becker, D. R. (1996). The individual placement and support model of supported employment. *Psychiatric Services, 47*(5), 473–475.

Drake, R. E., McHugo, G. J., Bebout, R. R., Becker, D. R., Harris, M., Bond, G. R., & Quimby, E. (1999). A randomized clinical trial of supported employment for inner-city patients with severe mental disorders. *Archives of General Psychiatry, 56*(7), 627–633. https://doi.org/10.1001/archpsyc.56.7.627

Dubouloz, C.-J., Egan, M., Vallerand, J., & von Zweck, C. (1999). Occupational therapists' perceptions of evidence-based practice. *American Journal of Occupational Therapy, 53*(5), 445–453. https://www.academia.edu/69219749/Occupational_Therapists_Perceptions_of_Evidence_Based_Practice?uc-g-sw=47947104

Elliott, S., & Leland, N. E. (2018). Occupational therapy fall prevention interventions for community-dwelling older adults: A systematic review. *American Journal of Occupational Therapy, 72*(4), 7204190040p1–7204190040p11.

El-Nahhas, A. M. E.-S. (2011). *Modulation of muscle tightness by manual stretching in children with spastic cerebral palsy (A systematic review)* [Unpublished master's thesis]. Cairo University. https://scholar.cu.edu.eg/sites/default/files/a_elnahhas/files/modulation_of_muscle_tightness_by_manual_stretching_in_children_with_spastic_cerebral_palsy_a_systematic_review_0.pdf

Esmaili, S. K., Mehraban, A. H., Shafaroodi, N., Yazdani, F., Masoumi, T., & Zarei, M. (2019). Participation in peer-play activities among children with specific learning disability: A randomized controlled trial. *American Journal of Occupational Therapy, 73*(2), 7302205110p1–7302205110p9.

Evans, D. (2003). Hierarchy of evidence: A framework for ranking evidence evaluating healthcare interventions. *Journal of Clinical Nursing, 12*(1), 77–84. https://doi.org/10.1046/j.1365-2702.2003.00662.x

Feldman, G. (2007). Cognitive and behavioral therapies for depression: Overview, new directions, and practical recommendations for dissemination. *Psychiatric Clinics of North America, 30*(1), 39–50. https://doi.org/10.1016/j.psc.2006.12.001

Fung, T. K. H., Lau, B. W. M., Ngai, S. P. C., & Tsang, H. W. H. (2021). Therapeutic effect and mechanisms of essential oils in mood disorders: Interaction between the nervous and respiratory systems. *International Journal of Molecular Sciences*, 22(9), 4844. https://doi.org/10.3390/ijms22094844

Gevaert, A. B., Adams, V., Bahls, M., Bowen, T. S., Cornelissen, V., Dörr, M., Hansen, D., Kemps, H. M. C., Leeson, P., Craenenbroeck, E. M. V., & Krankel, N. (2020). Towards a personalised approach in exercise-based cardiovascular rehabilitation: How can translational research help? A 'call to action' from the Section on Secondary Prevention and Cardiac Rehabilitation of the European Association of Preventive Cardiology. *European Journal of Preventive Cardiology*, 27(13), 1369–1385. https://doi.org/10.1177/2047487319877716

Glynn, S. M. (2003). Psychiatric rehabilitation in schizophrenia: Advances and challenges. *Clinical Neuroscience Research*, 3(1–2), 23–33. https://doi.org/10.1016/S1566-2772(03)00016-1

Godfrin, K. A., & van Heeringen, C. (2010). The effects of mindfulness-based cognitive therapy on recurrence of depressive episodes, mental health and quality of life: A randomized controlled study. *Behaviour Research and Therapy*, 48(8), 738–746. https://doi.org/10.1016/j.brat.2010.04.006

Gould, R. A., Mueser, K. T., Bolton, E., Mays, V., & Goff, D. (2001). Cognitive therapy for psychosis in schizophrenia: An effect size analysis. *Schizophrenia Research*, 48(2–3), 335–342. https://doi.org/10.1016/S0920-9964(00)00145-6

Haddock, G., Tarrier, N., Spaulding, W., Yusupoff, L., Kinney, C., & McCarthy, E. (1998). Individual cognitive-behavior therapy in the treatment of hallucinations and delusions: A review. *Clinical Psychology Review*, 18(7), 821–838. https://doi.org/10.1016/S0272-7358(98)00007-5

Hahn-Markowitz, J., Berger, I., Manor, I., & Maeir, A. (2020). Efficacy of Cognitive-Functional (Cog-Fun) occupational therapy intervention among children with ADHD: An RCT. *Journal of Attention Disorders*, 24(5), 655–666. https://doi.org/10.1177/1087054716666955

Hanh, T. N. (2020). *Being peace*. Parallax Press.

Heinssen, R. K., Liberman, R. P., & Kopelowicz, A. (2000). Psychosocial skills training for schizophrenia: Lessons from the laboratory. *Schizophrenia Bulletin*, 26(1), 21–46. https://doi.org/10.1093/oxfordjournals.schbul.a033441

Hodann-Caudevilla, R. M., Díaz-Silveira, C., Burgos-Julián, F. A., & Santed, M. A. (2020). Mindfulness-based interventions for people with schizophrenia: A systematic review and meta-analysis. *International Journal of Environmental Research and Public Health*, 17(13), 4690. https://doi.org/10.3390/ijerph17134690

Hofmann, S. G., Sawyer, A. T., Witt, A. A., & Oh, D. (2010). The effect of mindfulness-based therapy on anxiety and depression: A meta-analytic review. *Journal of Consulting and Clinical Psychology*, 78(2), 169–183. https://doi.org/10.1037/a0018555

Holm, M. B. (2000). Our mandate for the new millennium: Evidence-based practice, 2000 Eleanor Clarke Slagle lecture. *American Journal of Occupational Therapy*, 54(6), 575–585. https://www.academia.edu/77615070/Our_Mandate_for_the_New_Millennium_Evidence_Based_Practice

Hung, G. K. N., & Fong, K. N. K. (2019). Effects of telerehabilitation in occupational therapy practice: A systematic review. *Hong Kong Journal of Occupational Therapy*, 32(1), 3–21. https://doi.org/10.1177/1569186119849119

Jensen, M. R., Wong, J. J., Gonzales, N. A., Dumka, L. E., Millsap, R., & Coxe, S. (2014). Long-term effects of a universal family intervention: Mediation through parent-adolescent conflict. *Journal of Clinical Child and Adolescent Psychology*, 43(3), 415–427. https://doi.org/10.1080/15374416.2014.891228

Jones, S. E., Green, S. A., Clark, A. L., Dickson, M. J., Nolan, A.-M., Moloney, C., Kon, S. S. C., Godden, J., Howe, C., Haselden, B. M., Fleming, S., & Man, W. D.-C. (2012). P102 Post-hospitalisation outpatient pulmonary rehabilitation: A translational gap?. *Thorax*, 67(Suppl. 2), A107–A107. https://doi.org/10.1136/thoraxjnl-2012-202678.385

Kabat-Zinn, J. (1982). An outpatient program in behavioral medicine for chronic pain patients based on the practice of mindfulness meditation: Theoretical considerations and preliminary results. *General Hospital Psychiatry*, 4(1), 33–47. https://doi.org/10.1016/0163-8343(82)90026-3

Kim, D. (2020). The effects of a recollection-based occupational therapy program of Alzheimer's disease: A randomized controlled trial. *Occupational Therapy International*, 2020, 6305727. https://doi.org/10.1155/2020/6305727

Kim, S. Y., Yoo, E. Y., Jung, M. Y., Park, S. H., & Park, J. H. (2012). A systematic review of the effects of occupational therapy for persons with dementia: A meta-analysis of randomized controlled trials. *NeuroRehabilitation*, *31*(2), 107–115. https://www.ncbi.nlm.nih.gov/books/NBK109856/

Kingdon, D. G., & Turkington, D. (1994). *Cognitive-behavioral therapy of schizophrenia*. Guilford Press.

Konkolÿ Thege, B., Petroll, C., Rivas, C., & Scholtens, S. (2021). The effectiveness of family constellation therapy in improving mental health: A systematic review. *Family Process*, *60*(2), 409–423. https://doi.org/10.1111/famp.12636

Kopelowicz, A., Liberman, R. P., & Zarate, R. (2006). Recent advances in social skills training for schizophrenia. *Schizophrenia Bulletin*, *32*(Suppl. 1), S12–S23. https://doi.org/10.1093/schbul/sbl023

Lally, J., & MacCabe, J. H. (2015). Antipsychotic medication in schizophrenia: A review. *British Medical Bulletin*, *114*(1), 169–179. https://doi.org/10.1093/bmb/ldv017

Lauriello, J., Bustillo, J., & Keith, S. J. (1999). A critical review of research on psychosocial treatment of schizophrenia. *Biological Psychiatry*, *46*(10), 1409–1417. https://doi.org/10.1016/S0006-3223(99)00100-6

Law, M. C., Baptiste, S., Carswell, A., McColl, M. A., Polatajko, H. J., & Pollock, N. (1998). *Canadian occupational performance measure*. Canadian Association of Occupational Therapists.

Lee, H.-C., Kuo, F.-L., Lin, Y.-N., Liou, T.-H., Lin, J.-C., & Huang, S.-W. (2021). Effects of robot-assisted rehabilitation on hand function of people with stroke: A randomized, crossover-controlled, assessor-blinded study. *American Journal of Occupational Therapy*, *75*(1), 7501205020p1–7501205020p11.

Lee, S. Y., Jung, S. H., Lee, S.-U., Ha, Y.-C., & Lim, J.-Y. (2019). Is occupational therapy after hip fracture surgery effective in improving function?: A systematic review and meta-analysis of randomized controlled studies. *American Journal of Physical Medicine & Rehabilitation*, *98*(4), 292–298. https://doi.org/10.1097/PHM.0000000000001069

Lehman, A. F., Buchanan, R. W., Dickerson, F. B., Dixon, L. B., Goldberg, R., Green-Paden, L., & Kreyenbuhl, J. (2003). Evidence-based treatment for schizophrenia. *Psychiatric Clinics of North America*, *26*(4), 939–954. https://doi.org/10.1016/S0193-953X(03)00070-4

Lehman, A. F., Goldberg, R., Dixon, L. B., McNary, S., Postrado, L., Hackman, A., & McDonnell, K. (2002). Improving employment outcomes for persons with severe mental illnesses. *Archives of General Psychiatry*, *59*(2), 165–172. https://doi.org/10.1001/archpsyc.59.2.165

Leow, S., Dimmock, J. A., Guelfi, K. J., Alderson, J. A., & Jackson, B. (2021). Understanding the determinants of stress-induced eating – A qualitative study. *Appetite*, *165*, 105318. https://doi.org/10.1016/j.appet.2021.105318

Li, C. T. L., Hung, G. K. N., Fong, K. N. K., Gonzalez, P. C., Wah, S.-H., & Tsang, H. W. H. (2022). Effects of home-based occupational therapy telerehabilitation via smartphone for outpatients after hip fracture surgery: A feasibility randomised controlled study. *Journal of Telemedicine and Telecare*, *28*(4), 239–247. https://doi.org/10.1177/1357633X20932434

Liberati, A., Altman, D. G., Tetzlaff, J., Mulrow, C., Gøtzsche, P. C., Ioannidis, J. P. A., Clarke, M., Devereaux, P. J., Kleijnen, J., & Moher, D. (2009). The PRISMA statement for reporting systematic reviews and meta-analyses of studies that evaluate health care interventions: Explanation and elaboration. *Journal of Clinical Epidemiology*, *62*(10), e1–e34. https://doi.org/10.1016/j.jclinepi.2009.06.006

Liberman, R. P. (1972). *A guide to behavioral treatment for borderline personality disorder*. Guilford Press.

Lin, J., Chen, T., He, J., Chung, R. C. K., Ma, H., & Tsang, H. W. H. (2022). Impacts of acupressure treatment on depression: A systematic review and meta-analysis. *World Journal of Psychiatry*, *12*(1), 169–186. https://doi.org/10.5498/wjp.v12.i1.169

Lloyd, C., King, R., & Bassett, H. (2005). Occupational therapy and clinical research in mental health rehabilitation. *British Journal of Occupational Therapy*, *68*(4), 172–176. https://doi.org/10.1177/030802260506800405

López-López, J. A., Davies, S. R., Caldwell, D. M., Churchill, R., Peters, T. J., Tallon, D., Dawson, S., Wu, Q., Li, J., Taylor, A., Lewis, G., Kessler, D. S., Wiles, N., & Welton, N. J.

(2019). The process and delivery of CBT for depression in adults: A systematic review and network meta-analysis. *Psychological Medicine*, 49(12), 1937–1947. https://doi.org/10.1017/S003329171900120X

Marshall, M., & Lockwood, A. (2000). Assertive community treatment for people with severe mental disorders. *Cochrane Database of Systematic Reviews*, (2), CD001089. https://doi.org/10.1002/14651858.CD001089

Marwaha, S., Johnson, S., Bebbington, P., Stafford, M., Angermeyer, M. C., Brugha, T., Azorin, J.-M., Kilian, R., Hansen, K., & Toumi, M. (2007). Rates and correlates of employment in people with schizophrenia in the UK, France and Germany. *British Journal of Psychiatry*, 191(1), 30–37. https://doi.org/10.1192/bjp.bp.105.020982

McDonald, M. W., Hayward, K. S., Rosbergen, I. C. M., Jeffers, M. S., & Corbett, D. (2018). Is environmental enrichment ready for clinical application in human post-stroke rehabilitation? *Frontiers in Behavioral Neuroscience*, 12, 135. https://doi.org/10.3389/fnbeh.2018.00135

McFarlane, W. R. (2016). Family interventions for schizophrenia and the psychoses: A review. *Family Process*, 55(3), 460–482. https://doi.org/10.1111/famp.12235

McGurk, S. R., Mueser, K. T., Harvey, P. D., LaPuglia, R., & Marder, J. (2003). Cognitive and symptom predictors of work outcomes for clients with schizophrenia in supported employment. *Psychiatric Services*, 54(8), 1129–1135. https://doi.org/10.1176/appi.ps.54.8.1129

McGurk, S. R., Mueser, K. T., & Pascaris, A. (2005). Cognitive training and supported employment for persons with severe mental illness: One-year results from a randomized controlled trial. *Schizophrenia Bulletin*, 31(4), 898–909. https://doi.org/10.1093/schbul/sbi037

McKinlay, J. B. (1979). Epidemiological and political determinants of social policies regarding the public health. *Social Science & Medicine*, 13A(5), 541–558.

Mekbib, D. B., Han, J., Zhang, L., Fang, S., Jiang, H., Zhu, J., Roe, A. W., & Xu, D. (2020). Virtual reality therapy for upper limb rehabilitation in patients with stroke: A meta-analysis of randomized clinical trials. *Brain Injury*, 34(4), 456–465. https://doi.org/10.1080/02699052.2020.1725126

Menalled, L., & Brunner, D. (2014). Animal models of Huntington's disease for translation to the clinic: Best practices. *Movement Disorders*, 29(11), 1375–1390. https://doi.org/10.1002/mds.26006

Miklowitz, D. J., & Chung, B. (2016). Family-focused therapy for bipolar disorder: Reflections on 30 years of research. *Family Process*, 55(3), 483–499. https://doi.org/10.1111/famp.12237

Miller, W. R., Baca, C., Compton, W. M., Ernst, D., Manuel, J. K., Pringle, B., Schermer, C. R., Weiss, R. D., Willenbring, M. L., & Zweben, A. (2006). Addressing substance abuse in health care settings. *Alcoholism: Clinical and Experimental Research*, 30(2), 292–302. https://doi.org/10.1111/j.1530-0277.2006.00027.x

Miller, W. R., & Rollnick, S. (2002). *Motivational interviewing: Preparing people for change* (2nd ed.). Guilford Press.

Moher, D., Cook, D. J., Eastwood, S., Olkin, I., Rennie, D., & Stroup, D. F., Quorom Group. (1999). Improving the quality of reports of meta-analyses of randomised controlled trials: The QUOROM statement. *The Lancet*, 354(9193), 1896–1900. https://doi.org/10.1016/S0140-6736(99)04149-5

Morrison, A. P., Law, H., Carter, L., Sellers, R., Emsley, R., Pyle, M., French, P., Shiers, D., Yung, A. R., Murphy, E. K., Holden, N., Steele, A., Bowe, S. E., Palmier-Claus, J., Brooks, V., Byrne, R., Davies, L., & Haddad, P. M. (2018). Antipsychotic drugs versus cognitive behavioural therapy versus a combination of both in people with psychosis: A randomised controlled pilot and feasibility study. *The Lancet Psychiatry*, 5(5), 411–423. https://doi.org/10.1016/S2215-0366(18)30096-8

Mueser, K. T., & Bond, G. R. (2000). Psychosocial treatment approaches for schizophrenia. *Current Opinion in Psychiatry*, 13(1), 27–35.

Mueser, K. T., & Glynn, S. M. (1998). Family intervention for schizophrenia. In K. S. Dobson, & K. D. Craig (Eds.), *Best practice: Developing and promoting empirically supported interventions* (pp. 157–186). Sage Publications.

Mueser, K. T., Glynn, S. M., Cather, C., Xie, H., Zarate, R., Smith, L. F., Clark, R. E., Gottlieb, J. D., Wolfe, R., & Feldman, J. (2013). A randomized controlled trial of family intervention for co-occurring substance use and severe psychiatric disorders. *Schizophrenia Bulletin*, 39(3), 658–672. https://doi.org/10.1093/schbul/sbr203

Musselman, K. E., Shah, M., & Zariffa, J. (2018). Rehabilitation technologies and interventions for individuals with spinal cord injury: Translational potential of current trends. *Journal of NeuroEngineering and Rehabilitation*, 15(1), 40. https://doi.org/10.1186/s12984-018-0386-7

Nelson, G., Aubry, T., & Lafrance, A. (2007). A review of the literature on the effectiveness of housing and support, assertive community treatment, and intensive case management interventions for persons with mental illness who have been homeless. *American Journal of Orthopsychiatry*, 77(3), 350–361. https://doi.org/10.1037/0002-9432.77.3.350

Noyes, S., Sokolow, H., & Arbesman, M. (2018). Evidence for occupational therapy intervention with employment and education for adults with serious mental illness: A systematic review. *American Journal of Occupational Therapy*, 72(5), 7205190010p1–7205190010p10.

Pharoah, F., Mari, J., Rathbone, J., & Wong, W. (2010). Family intervention for schizophrenia. *Cochrane Database of Systematic Reviews*, (12), CD000088.

Phillips, S. D., Burns, B. J., Edgar, E. R., Mueser, K. T., Linkins, K. W., Rosenheck, R. A., Drake, R. E., & McDonel Herr, E. C. (2001). Moving assertive community treatment into standard practice. *Psychiatric Services*, 52(6), 771–779. https://doi.org/10.1176/appi.ps.52.6.771

Pot-Kolder, R. M. C. A., Geraets, C. N. W., Veling, W., van Beilen, M., Staring, A. B. P., Gijsman, H. J., Delespaul, P. A. E. G., & van der Gaag, M. (2018). Virtual-reality-based cognitive behavioural therapy versus waiting list control for paranoid ideation and social avoidance in patients with psychotic disorders: A single-blind randomised controlled trial. *Lancet Psychiatry*, 5(3), 217–226. https://doi.org/10.1016/S2215-0366(18)30053-1

Probyn, K., Engedahl, M. S., Rajendran, D., Pincus, T., Naeem, K., Mistry, D., Underwood, M., & Froud, R. (2021). The effects of supported employment interventions in populations of people with conditions other than severe mental health: A systematic review. *Primary Health Care Research & Development*, 22, e79. https://doi.org/10.1017/S1463423621000827

Raymer, A. M., Beeson, P., Holland, A., Kendall, D., Maher, L. M., Martin, N., Murray, L., Rose, M., Thompson, C. K., Turkstra, L., Altmann, L., Boyle, M., Conway, T., Hula, W., Kearns, K., Rapp, B., Simmons-Mackie, N., & Rothi, L. J. G. (2008). Translational research in aphasia: From neuroscience to neurorehabilitation. *Journal of Speech, Language, and Hearing Research*, 51(1), S259–275.

Reinecke, M. A., Ryan, N. E., & DuBois, D. L. (1998). Cognitive-behavioral therapy of depression and depressive symptoms during adolescence: A review and meta-analysis. *Journal of the American Academy of Child and Adolescent Psychiatry*, 37(1), 26–34. https://doi.org/10.1097/00004583-199801000-00013

Rojo-Mota, G., Pedrero-Pérez, E. J., & Huertas-Hoyas, E. (2017). Systematic review of occupational therapy in the treatment of addiction: Models, practice, and qualitative and quantitative research. *American Journal of Occupational Therapy*, 71(5), 7105100030p1–7105100030p11.

Romagnoli, G., Leone, A., Sansoni, J., Tofani, M., De Santis, R., Valente, D., & Galeoto, G. (2019). Occupational therapy's efficacy in children with Asperger's syndrome: A systematic review of randomized controlled trials. *La Clinica Terapeutica*, 170(5), e382–e387.

Ruan, L., Lau, B. W.-M., Wang, J., Huang, L., ZhuGe, Q., Wang, B., Jin, K., & So, K.-F. (2014). Neurogenesis in neurological and psychiatric diseases and brain injury: From bench to bedside. *Progress in Neurobiology*, 115, 116–137. https://doi.org/10.1016/j.pneurobio.2013.12.006

Sackett, D. L., Rosenberg, W. M. C., Gray, J. A. M., Haynes, R. B., & Richardson, W. S. (1996). Evidence based medicine: What it is and what it isn't. *British Medical Journal*, 312(7023), 71–72. https://doi.org/10.1136/bmj.312.7023.71

Sánchez-Vidaña, D. I., Ngai, S. P.-C., He, W., Chow, J. K.-W., Lau, B. W.-M., & Tsang, H. W.-H. (2017). The effectiveness of aromatherapy for depressive symptoms: A systematic review. *Evidence-based Complementary and Alternative Medicine*, 2017(1), 5869315. https://doi.org/10.1155/2017/5869315

Sánchez-Vidaña, D. I., Po, K. K.-T., Fung, T. K.-H., Chow, J. K.-W., Lau, W. K.-W., So, P.-K., Lau, B. W.-M., & Tsang, H. W.-H. (2019). Lavender essential oil ameliorates depression-like behavior and increases neurogenesis and dendritic complexity in rats. *Neuroscience Letters*, 701, 180–192. https://doi.org/10.1016/j.neulet.2019.02.042

Schmidt, E. K., Hand, B. N., Havercamp, S., Sommerich, C., Weaver, L., & Darragh, A. (2021). Sex education practices for people with intellectual and developmental disabilities: A qualitative study. *American Journal of Occupational Therapy*, 75(3), 7503180060.

Scriven, A., & Atwal, A. (2004). Occupational therapists as primary health promoters: Opportunities and barriers. *British Journal of Occupational Therapy*, 67(10), 424–429. https://doi.org/10.1177/030802260406701002

Segal, Z., Williams, M., & Teasdale, J. (2018). *Mindfulness-based cognitive therapy for depression.* Guilford Press.

Shin, J. H., Haynes, R. B., & Johnston, M. E. (1993). Effect of problem-based, self-directed undergraduate education on life-long learning. *Canadian Medical Association Journal*, 148(6), 969–976.

Smallfield, S., & Kaldenberg, J. (2020). Occupational therapy interventions to improve reading performance of older adults with low vision: A systematic review. *American Journal of Occupational Therapy*, 74(1), 7401185030p1–7401185030p18. https://pmc.ncbi.nlm.nih.gov/articles/PMC7018456/

Smedslund, G., Berg, R. C., Hammerstrøm, K. T., Steiro, A., Leiknes, K. A., Dahl, H. M., & Karlsen, K. (2011). Motivational interviewing for substance abuse. *Cochrane Database of Systematic Reviews*, 2011(5), CD008063. https://doi.org/10.1002/14651858.CD008063.pub2

Steenrod, S. (2009). A functional guide to the evidence-based practice movement in the substance abuse treatment field. *Journal of Social Work Practice in the Addictions*, 9(4), 353–365. https://doi.org/10.1080/15332560903195808

Stein, L. I., & Santos, A. B. (1998). *Assertive community treatment of persons with severe mental illness.* W. W. Norton & Company.

Stein, L. I., & Test, M. A. (1980). Alternative to mental hospital treatment. I. Conceptual model, treatment program, and clinical evaluation. *Archives of General Psychiatry*, 37(4), 392–397. https://doi.org/10.1001/archpsyc.1980.01780170034003

Steultjens, E. M. J., Dekker, J., Bouter, L. M., Jellema, S., Bakker, E. B., & Van Den Ende, C. H. M. (2004). Occupational therapy for community dwelling elderly people: A systematic review. *Age and Ageing*, 33(5), 453–460. https://doi.org/10.1093/ageing/afh174

Steultjens, E. M. J., Dekker, J., Bouter, L. M., van de Nes, J. C. M., Cup, E. H. C., & van den Ende, C. H. M. (2003). Occupational therapy for stroke patients: A systematic review. *Stroke*, 34(3), 676–687. https://doi.org/10.1161/01.STR.0000057576.77308.30

Stevens, K. R. (2001). Systematic reviews: The heart of evidence-based practice. *AACN Clinical Issues*, 12(4), 529–538.

Stoffel, V. C., & Moyers, P. A. (2004). An evidence-based and occupational perspective of interventions for persons with substance-use disorders. *American Journal of Occupational Therapy*, 58(5), 570–586.

Tanenbaum, S. J. (2006). The role of "evidence" in recovery from mental illness. *Health Care Analysis*, 14, 195–201.

Tobar, E., Alvarez, E., & Garrido, M. (2017). Cognitive stimulation and occupational therapy for delirium prevention. *Revista Brasileira de Terapia Intensiva*, 29(2), 248–252. https://doi.org/10.5935/0103-507X.20170034

Torpil, B., Şahin, S., Pekçetin, S., & Uyanık, M. (2021). The effectiveness of a virtual reality-based intervention on cognitive functions in older adults with mild cognitive impairment: A single-blind, randomized controlled trial. *Games for Health Journal*, 10(2), 109–114.

Torrey, W. C., Rapp, C. A., van Tosh, L., McNabb, C. R. A., & Ralph, R. O. (2005). Recovery principles and evidence-based practice: Essential ingredients of service improvement. *Community Mental Health Journal*, 41(1), 91–100. https://doi.org/10.1007/s10597-005-2608-2

Tsang, H. W.-H. (2001). Applying social skills training in the context of vocational rehabilitation for people with schizophrenia. *The Journal of Nervous and Mental Disease*, 189(2), 90–98. https://doi.org/10.1097/00005053-200102000-00004

Tsang, H. W. H., Chan, A., Wong, A., & Liberman, R. P. (2009). Vocational outcomes of an integrated supported employment program for individuals with persistent and severe mental illness. *Journal of Behavior Therapy and Experimental Psychiatry*, 40(2), 292–305. https://doi.org/10.1016/j.jbtep.2008.12.007

Tsang, H. W. H., Chan, F., & Bond, G. R. (2004). Cultural considerations for adapting psychiatric rehabilitation models in Hong Kong. *American Journal of Psychiatric Rehabilitation*, 7(1), 35–51. https://doi.org/10.1080/15487760490464988

Tsang, H. W. H., & Cheung, L. C. C. (2005). Social skills training for people with schizophrenia: Theory, practice and evidence. In J. E. Pletson (Ed.), *Progress in schizophrenia research* (pp. 181–207). Nova Science Publishers.

Tsang, H. W. H., Fung, K. M. T., & Corrigan, P. W. (2006). Psychosocial treatment compliance scale for people with psychotic disorders. *Australian and New Zealand Journal of Psychiatry*, 40(6–7), 561–569. https://doi.org/10.1080/j.1440-1614.2006.01839.x

Tsang, H. W. H., Fung, K. M. T., Leung, A. Y., Li, S. M. Y., & Cheung, W. M. (2010). Three year follow-up study of an integrated supported employment for individuals with severe mental illness. *Australian and New Zealand Journal of Psychiatry*, 44(1), 49–58. https://doi.org/10.3109/00048670903393613

Tsang, H. W. H., Lo, S. C. L., Chan, C. C. H., Ho, T. Y. C., Fung, K. M. T., Chan, A. H. L., & Au, D. W. H. (2013). Neurophysiological and behavioural effects of lavender oil in rats with experimentally induced anxiety. *Flavour and Fragrance Journal*, 28(3), 168–173. https://doi.org/10.1002/ffj.3148

Tsang, H. W. H., Ng, B. F. L., & Chiu, F. P. F. (2002). Job profiles of people with severe mental illness: Implications for rehabilitation. *International Journal of Rehabilitation Research*, 25(3), 189–196. https://journals.lww.com/intjrehabilres/fulltext/2002/09000/job_profiles_of_people_with_severe_mental_illness_.4.aspx

Tsang, H. W.-H., & Pearson, V. (2001). Work-related social skills training for people with schizophrenia in Hong Kong. *Schizophrenia Bulletin*, 27(1), 139–148. https://doi.org/10.1093/oxfordjournals.schbul.a006852

Tsang, H. W. H., Tam, P. K. C., Chan, F., & Chang, W. M. (2003). Sources of burdens on families of individuals with mental illness. *International Journal of Rehabilitation Research*, 26(2), 123–130. https://doi.org/10.1097/00004356-200306000-00007

Tsang, W.-H. H., & Pearson, V. (1996). A conceptual framework for work-related social skills in psychiatric rehabilitation. *Journal of Rehabilitation*, 62(3), 61–67. https://www.proquest.com/docview/236227043?pq-origsite=gscholar&fromopenview=true&sourcetype=Scholarly%20Journals

Tse, S., Lloyd, C., Penman, M., King, R., & Bassett, H. (2004). Evidence-based practice and rehabilitation: Occupational therapy in Australia and New Zealand experiences. *International Journal of Rehabilitation Research*, 27(4), 269–274. https://doi.org/10.1097/00004356-200412000-00003

Turner, D. T., McGlanaghy, E., Cuijpers, P., van der Gaag, M., Karyotaki, E., & MacBeth, A. (2018). A meta-analysis of social skills training and related interventions for psychosis. *Schizophrenia Bulletin*, 44(3), 475–491. https://doi.org/10.1093/schbul/sbx146

Vanderlip, E. R., Henwood, B. F., Hrouda, D. R., Meyer, P. S., Monroe-DeVita, M., Studer, L. M., Schweikhard, A. J., & Moser, L. L. (2017). Systematic literature review of general health care interventions within programs of assertive community treatment. *Psychiatric Services*, 68(3), 218–224. https://doi.org/10.1176/appi.ps.201600100

Vasilaki, E. I., Hosier, S. G., & Cox, W. M. (2006). The efficacy of motivational interviewing as a brief intervention for excessive drinking: A meta-analytic review. *Alcohol and Alcoholism*, 41(3), 328–335. https://doi.org/10.1093/alcalc/agl016

Waliño-Paniagua, C. N., Gomez-Calero, C., Jiménez-Trujillo, M. I., Aguirre-Tejedor, L., Bermejo-Franco, A., Ortiz-Gutiérrez, R. M., & Cano-de-la-Cuerda, R. (2019). Effects of a game-based virtual reality video capture training program plus occupational therapy on manual dexterity in patients with multiple sclerosis: A randomized controlled trial. *Journal of Healthcare Engineering*, 2019, 9780587. https://doi.org/10.1155/2019/9780587

Wallace, C. J., Nelson, C. J., Liberman, R. P., Aitchison, R. A., Lukoff, D., Elder, J. P., & Ferris, C. (1980). A review and critique of social skills training with schizophrenic patients. *Schizophrenia Bulletin*, 6(1), 42–63. https://doi.org/10.1093/schbul/6.1.42

Wang, W., Zhou, Y., Chai, N., & Liu, D. (2019). Cognitive-behavioural therapy for personal recovery of patients with schizophrenia: A systematic review and meta-analysis. *General Psychiatry*, 32(4), e100040. https://doi.org/10.1136/gpsych-2018-100040

Wennberg, J., & Gittelsohn, A. (1973). Small area variations in health care delivery: A population-based health information system can guide planning and regulatory decision-making. *Science*, 182(4117), 1102–1108. https://doi.org/10.1126/science.182.4117.1102

Wilcox, J., & Frank, E. (2021). Occupational therapy for the long haul of post-COVID syndrome: A case report. *American Journal of Occupational Therapy, 75*(Suppl. 1), 7511210060. https://doi.org/10.5014/ajot.2021.049223

Wong-Anuchit, C., Chantamit-o-pas, C., Schneider, J. K., & Mills, A. C. (2019). Motivational interviewing-based compliance/adherence therapy interventions to improve psychiatric symptoms of people with severe mental illness: Meta-analysis. *Journal of the American Psychiatric Nurses Association, 25*(2), 122–133. https://doi.org/10.1177/1078390318761790

Xu, W., Jia, K., Liu, X., & Hofmann, S. G. (2016). The effects of mindfulness training on emotional health in Chinese long-term male prison inmates. *Mindfulness, 7*(5), 1044–1051. https://doi.org/10.1007/s12671-016-0540-x

Xuan, R., Li, X., Qiao, Y., Guo, Q., Liu, X., Deng, W., Hu, Q., Wang, K., & Zhang, L. (2020). Mindfulness-based cognitive therapy for bipolar disorder: A systematic review and meta-analysis. *Psychiatry Research, 290*, 113116. https://doi.org/10.1016/j.psychres.2020.113116

Yim, V. W. C., Ng, A. K. Y., Tsang, H. W. H., & Leung, A. Y. (2009). A review on the effects of aromatherapy for patients with depressive symptoms. *The Journal of Alternative and Complementary Medicine, 15*(2), 187–195. https://doi.org/10.1089/acm.2008.0333

Zhang, G. F., Tsui, C. M., Lu, A. J. B., Yu, L. B., Tsang, H. W. H., & Li, D. (2017). Integrated supported employment for people with schizophrenia in mainland China: A randomized controlled trial. *American Journal of Occupational Therapy, 71*(6), 7106165020p1–7106165020p8.

Zhang, Z., Zhang, L., Zhang, G., Jin, J., & Zheng, Z. (2018). The effect of CBT and its modifications for relapse prevention in major depressive disorder: A systematic review and meta-analysis. *BMC Psychiatry, 18*(1), 50. https://doi.org/10.1186/s12888-018-1610-5

Zimmermann, G., Favrod, J., Trieu, V. H., & Pomini, V. (2005). The effect of cognitive behavioral treatment on the positive symptoms of schizophrenia spectrum disorders: A meta-analysis. *Schizophrenia Research, 77*(1), 1–9. https://doi.org/10.1016/j.schres.2005.02.018

Zou, Q. (2020). Addition of modified Jadad method to evaluate the rationality of over-explanatory drug use: Taking naloxone as an example. *Pharmaceutical Science and Technology, 4*(2), 40–44. https://doi.org/10.11648/j.pst.20200402.13

Use of advanced technologies in occupational therapy

Kenneth Nai-Kuen Fong, Eddie Yip Kuen Hai,
Jack Jiaqi Zhang, and Winnie Wing Tung Lam

Role of occupational therapy in assistive technology

Assistive technology broadly refers to the use of technology to support individuals with disabilities. It encompasses the application, assessment, and follow-up of systems and services involved in providing assistive products (or assistive technology devices) and related services (World Health Organization, 2024). Assistive devices are aids, tools, or equipment specially designed to facilitate activities of daily living (ADL), and they range from something as simple as an enlarged handled knife to complex environmental control systems (Moy, 1987). With estimates of individuals with disabilities across the world projected to double from one billion in 2021 to two billion by 2050, more than one billion of those people need one or more assistive devices. However, only one in ten has access to assistive technology due to the high costs, lack of awareness, and limited availability of professional consultations (World Health Organization, 2024). Due to rapid aging and longevity in developed countries and regions with an increasing number of older people, as well as people with noncommunicable chronic diseases and children with developmental disorders (owing to advances in medical technology and increased survival rate after birth), the demands for assistive devices will be even greater in the future. Regarding children, according to UNICEF, there are 240 million children with disabilities in the world, and only one in ten children with disabilities have access to assistive devices (Wood & Whittaker, 2022).

Occupational therapists are practitioners in assistive technology who are equipped with a unique set of knowledge and skills in assistive technology. They have the following roles:

- Evaluate the needs of end users (clients and their caregivers) in daily functioning and enhance their participation in self-care, work, and leisure activities;
- Prescribe, design, fabricate, and maintain necessary assistive devices;
- Educate the end users on the use and application of the assistive devices; and
- Make referrals to other experts in manufacturing the assistive devices.

DOI: 10.4324/9781032721170-18

The payers of assistive devices can be clients or their families, as well as third-party payers such as insurance companies, government programs, and charitable organizations. Among the abovementioned roles, educating clients on the use of assistive devices is essential in assistive technology services as many individuals are unfamiliar with advanced technology, and some devices may be too complicated to use or involve too many procedures to operate, making the clients reluctant to try them (Scherer, 2002). As clients' disabilities may change over time or across their lifespan due to aging, and environmental changes may occur due to external factors, continuous follow-up and re-evaluation by occupational therapists is a necessary and ongoing process (Scherer, 2002).

The Human Activity Assistive Technology (HAAT) model (Cook & Hussey, 2001) is a model used in the field of assistive technology. The domains in the model are similar to those in the Person-Environment-Occupation (PEO) model, the professional model used in occupational therapy (OT) (Law et al., 1996) (Figure 13.1). The activity

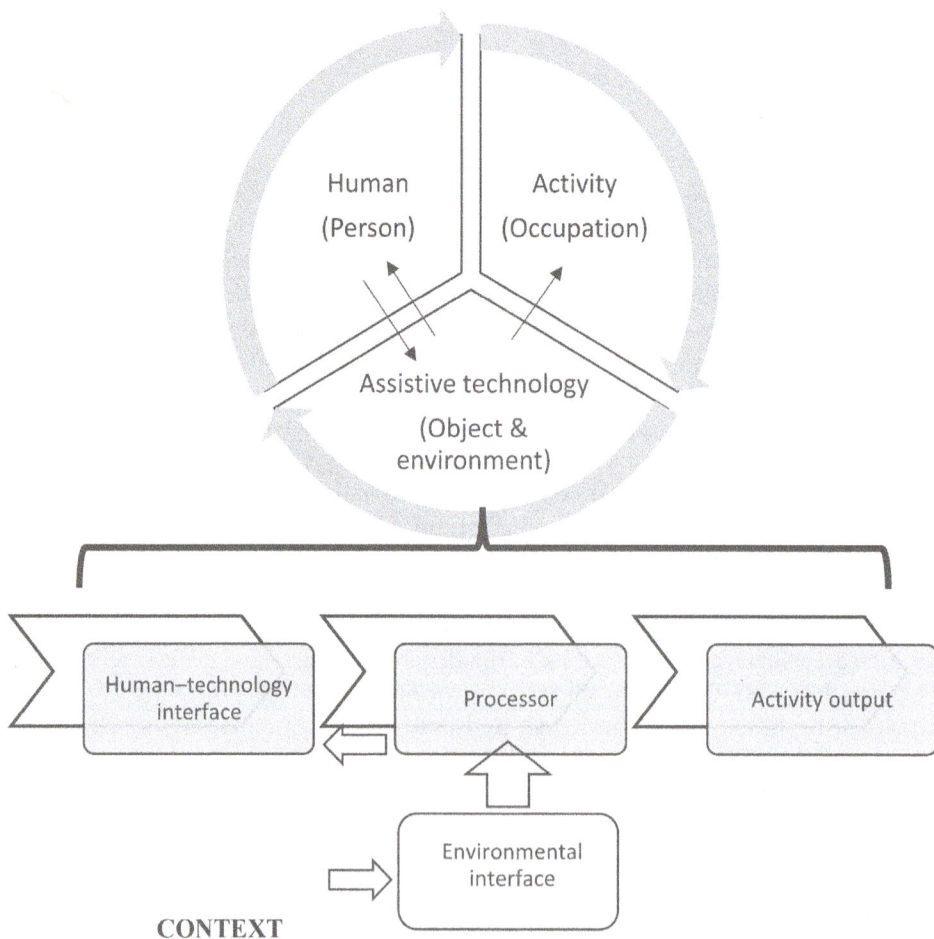

Figure 13.1 Human Occupation and Assistive Technology model (modified from the Human Activity Assistive Technology [HAAT] model [Cook & Hussey, 2001] and the Person-Environment-Occupation [PEO] model [Law et al., 1996])

domain in HAAT resembles human occupation, whereas the context domain refers to the physical, social, and cultural environments. The assistive technology domain in HAAT comprises four components: (1) a human–technology interface that links the hardware or machine with humans, (2) a processor, if any, for interpreting information and data analysis, (3) an environmental interface that interacts with the context, and (4) an activity output system to facilitate or enhance human activity in response to the input from the environment.

For example, to perform the activity of bathing, a person (human) must complete a set of tasks, e.g., taking off/putting on clothing, getting in/out of the bathtub, applying soap, washing, drying, etc. If the person lacks the necessary skills to accomplish the tasks/activity due to, for example, decreased balance to get in/out of the bathtub or difficulty in reaching body parts by the upper extremities, he/she may need assistive devices such as a bath bench with handrails and a long-handle brush in order to be independent for the tasks. The activity of bathing is to be carried out within a context/environment, i.e., the bathtub and bathroom of the client's home.

Assistive products vary from low technology (requiring minimal assistance, e.g., a rod) to high technology (requiring maximal assistance, e.g., robots that involve electronic processing using computers and the Internet). Table 13.1 lists the common assistive devices used by occupational therapists for their clients. Occupational therapists often advise clients to modify the environment or adapt the tasks first before using assistive devices to handle the tasks. Assistive devices range from commercially available non-rehabilitative products that are used by the public to commercially available rehabilitative products or a combination of both technologies. The last option is to fabricate new products or devices if it is impossible to modify commercially available products. The lower the level of functioning the client has, or the more complicated the task, the more likely the occupational therapist will need to consider modifying commercial products to suit the individual needs of the client. Once it has been identified that an assistive device is necessary for the client, the following four aspects need to be considered:

(1) The client's needs, which include the physical needs as well as the psychological and social needs (i.e., whether the device is psychologically and socially acceptable to the client). Continuous monitoring is also essential to ensure that the device still meets the client's needs because his/her condition may change.
(2) The carer's needs, as long as the carer is involved in the use of the device.
(3) The objectives to be achieved in the daily tasks.
(4) Improvisation using available equipment or material as an alternative to commercial products (Moy, 1987). Moy (1987) suggested 14 principles for choosing appropriate assistive devices: design or appearance, method of control, comfort, safety, durability, access, adjustments, weight, dimensions, transportation and storage, cleaning, maintenance and repairs, availability, and price.

We can also explain the HAAT model using the example of high technology. Noninvasive brain-computer interface (BCI) technology is a new training approach designed to achieve motor restoration through a closed-loop system, from brain activity through event-related desynchronization after motor imagery or a movement attempt

Table 13.1 Examples of common assistive devices

Activities of daily living (ADL)

Feeding	Dressing	Grooming	Transfer	Mobility	Toileting	Bathing	Communication	Cognition	Cooking
Universal cuff	Long-handled reacher	Adapted nail cutter	Transfer board	Standard wheelchair	Commode	Long-handled brush	Mouth stick	Notebook	One-handed chopping board
Enlarged/angled spoon	Socking aid	Adapted toothbrush	Monkey pull	Special wheelchair	Raised toilet seat	Non-slip mat	Head pointer	Calendar	Trolley
Manoy plate	Buttonhook	Automatic water tap	Rope ladder	Powered wheelchair	Urinal (male/female)	Shower chair	Writing aid	Memo pad	Bottle opener
Dycem	Adapted shoe horn		Bed height raisers	Quadripod/tripod	Self-inspection mirror	Looped towel	Communication board	Electronic watch/smartphone	Universal opener
Adapted cup with straw	Adapted Velcro opening		Hydraulic hoist	Walking stick/cane	Bed-pan	Bathboard/bathseat/bathbench	Page turner	Medication box	Electric can opener
Nosy cup	Dressing stick		Hydraulic bed	Walking frame/walker			Keyboard guard		Adapted knife
Adapted chopsticks			Nightguard	Rollator			Prism glasses		Rocker knife
Self-feeding device			Pressure-relieving bed mattress	Elbow crutches			Telephone holder		Teapot holder
			Cushion	Portable ramp					
			Geriatric chair						
			Handrail						

to peripheral feedback triggered by an external hepatic device without any real muscle contraction (Bai et al., 2020). In such a case, an electroencephalography (EEG) headset will be the human–technology interface that captures the brain signals; the processor decodes the brain activity signals and then translates them into computerized commands to control external devices such as a virtual game, powered wheelchair, or robot, etc.; the external devices triggered by specific features of brain activity provide the activity output, such as moving the mouse cursor or joystick to play the game, or driving the powered wheelchair, or commanding the robot to give verbal or movement responses. The environmental interface includes factors such as how the headset is worn, its position, and the size, power supply, and other accessories of the BCI equipment.

With the rapid advancement of technology, occupational therapists, both now and in the future, will use advanced equipment to make their treatment or training more effective. A current trend is the use of 3D printing in the design, fabrication, and application of assistive devices. Unlike other major medical users in surgical guide or implant development, occupational therapists are the major rehabilitation professionals utilizing 3D printing to make assistive devices for clients for use in their ADL. 3D printing is a process that transforms shapeless materials (e.g., filaments, liquids, powders) into solid objects with definitive shapes. This is achieved by adding and combining layers to create the final object without using any tools or fixtures. The advantages of 3D printing include improved appearance through the use of various materials, and the ability to easily perform additive and multiple manufacturing in a short period of time. 3D printing is now used in the fabrication of static hand splints, component parts of dynamic splints, prostheses, and assistive devices. There are two categories of advanced technology products: (1) assistive devices that therapists recommend for clients to address their difficulties in daily functioning and enhance participation in self-care, work, and leisure activities, or to facilitate or enhance clients' ability to carry out functional activities independently by helping them master their environment; and (2) training devices used in treatments to enhance the recovery and care of clients, which are utilized under the supervision of therapists.

Emerging technologies

Mobile technology and telerehabilitation

As technology rapidly develops, so too does assistive technology. The use of mobile apps will be a major game changer in the technological world. According to Statista, the number of downloaded mobile apps increased from 140 billion to 230 billion between 2016 and 2021 (Data.ai, 2022), with there being roughly 64% growth in the past five years, and it is only expected to grow in the coming years. The exponential increase in the number of apps being downloaded is due to the rapid growth of the smartphone market. In 2022, there were 4.7 billion smartphone users in the world, and this number is expected to increase to 5.6 billion by 2025 (Statista, 2021).

The advances in mobile technology (i.e., use of mobile phones/smartphones) since 2006 have changed people's habits and ways of connecting to the world. Prior to this, people could only access the Internet at home via a wired connection. However, with the advent of wireless technology, as well as improvements to hardware, people are now able to access the Internet anywhere and anytime, thereby increasing the demand for smartphones.

The rapid increase in the number of smartphone users globally is not just because more people are willing or able to purchase one; it means that more people are able to use smartphones. The concept of digital inclusion began in the early 21st century. As the use of information and communication technology (ICT) rapidly expanded, manufacturers quickly realized that there was a group of people who were unable to access the digital world because the newly developed technology was originally designed for "normal" people. Stakeholders have thought of various ways to lower the threshold for using smartphones so that people with variable functional abilities can make use of them and connect to the world. Thus, the operating systems of smartphones keep evolving and improving. Accessibility settings built into operating systems enable smartphone use by people with various abilities. For example, a high-contrast setting can help people with visual impairments see their screens better. Moreover, the voice-over function can read aloud the contents of screens to users. Developers are also helping people in need. For example, Microsoft has developed Seeing AI, a free app using artificial intelligence (AI) to recognize text, products, people, and colors for the visually impaired. A similar function can be found in OrCam, an assistive device that uses AI to help visually impaired people "see" the world.

Another example of mobile technology is smart home integration (Figure 13.2). In the past, if an individual with a severe physical disability needed to control his/her household appliances, therapists would have to purchase and install a complex and expensive environmental control unit for him/her. However, smart home apps and compatible hardware are now readily available in the market. Together with accessibility settings, such as voice control (e.g., Siri or Google Assistant), users can now control their household appliances with only their voices, maximizing the independence of disabled users. Since both disabled and healthy users can use the same smartphones, stigmatization will be minimized and the extra costs of using specially designed phones can be avoided.

Hardware improvement of mobile technology also plays a key role in assistive technology. One example is the use of LiDAR sensors, a recent technology. LiDAR sensors emit invisible laser beams into the targeted environment and collect reflections that bounce back to the sensor. Using this information, users can calculate the precise distance between objects and the sensor. LiDAR is used for various purposes such as 3D scanning and augmented reality (AR). Recently, it has been used together with WIFI to give electric wheelchairs an automatic driving mode. This is best demonstrated by the Whill Model C2 wheelchair, which uses a pre-learned map for navigation and can avoid obstacles using sensors.

With the rapid development of mobile technology, telerehabilitation (TR) is becoming increasingly common. TR uses ICT to provide rehabilitation services at a distance (Kairy et al., 2009). The World Federation of Occupational Therapists (2014) prefers the term "telehealth" to describe the service delivery model of TR, teletherapy, or telecare, which is the use of ICT to deliver health-related services when the provider and client are in different physical locations and has already acknowledged that TR is an appropriate service delivery model for OT services (World Federation of Occupational Therapists, 2014). The delivery modes of TR can be visualized in terms

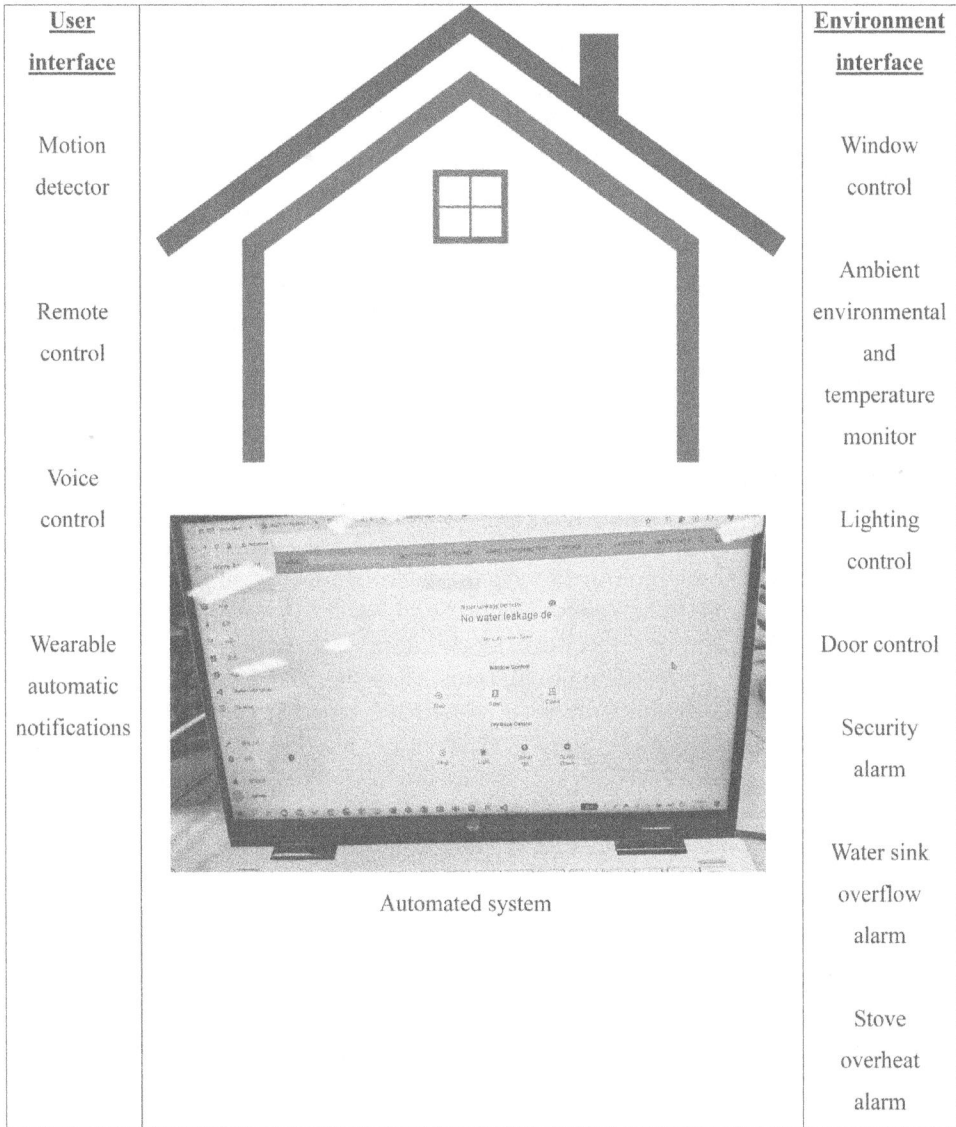

User interface		Environment interface
Motion detector		Window control
Remote control		Ambient environmental and temperature monitor
Voice control		Lighting control
Wearable automatic notifications		Door control
		Security alarm
	Automated system	Water sink overflow alarm
		Stove overheat alarm

Figure 13.2 Conceptual model of a smart house

of: (1) teletherapy, which refers to direct client training, therapeutic services, and treatment, (2) teleconsultation and follow-up services, (3) tele-education, which focuses on preventive client education, and (4) telemonitoring, which refers to remote monitoring of clients (Fong & Kwan, 2020). TR has become increasingly common for the rehabilitation monitoring of clients since the coronavirus (COVID-19) pandemic of 2020, particularly during the restrictions imposed by social distancing. A large number of clients were unable to receive conventional in-person treatment at centers because of the social distancing restrictions and strict infection control measures. TR has been applied to various age populations, including children and the elderly, in the form of a wide range of technologies (Hung & Fong, 2019). One application in the local context was a randomized controlled trial for a group of older adults attending a geriatric day hospital who had undergone hip fracture surgery within 12 weeks of diagnosis (Li et al., 2020). The clients in the experimental group received a three-week TR home program using a smartphone app together with conventional rehabilitation. The comparison group received paper-and-pencil instructions for the home program alongside conventional training on a weekly basis for three weeks. Unlike the comparison group, significant improvements in fall efficacy and instrumental activities of daily living (IADL) performance post-intervention and during follow-up were found in the experimental group (Li et al., 2020). Indeed, mobile technology continues to advance and its use is only growing. It is expected that an increasing number of assistive technologies will use the smart concept with the integration of apps in smartphones.

Wearable technology and functional electrical stimulation

Another recent development has been the use of wearable technologies for home-based rehabilitation. Wearable technologies are electronic hand-free devices such as wristwatches, ear plugs, spectacles, and headset devices worn externally on the body to monitor activities without limiting users' movements (Rodgers et al., 2019). In physical rehabilitation, wearable technologies are commonly used to measure body kinematics, augment posture, and motion correction by providing users with real-time feedback or assistance (passive or active assistance) in terms of cueing, alarms, or reminders (Wang et al., 2017). The most commonly used sensors are pressure sensors, inertial measurement units, and electromyography (EMG) sensors to collect kinematic and muscle activity data (Toh et al., 2023). In one of our recent reviews, we identified that most research on wearable technologies for home-based rehabilitation focused on improving hemiparetic upper limb function, with only a few studies applying wearable technologies in home-based lower limb rehabilitation. Commonly used wearable technologies include virtual reality (VR), stimulation-based training, robotic therapy, and activity trackers. Among them, "strong" evidence was found to support stimulation-based training, "moderate" evidence supported activity trackers, "limited" evidence supported VR, and "inconsistent" evidence supported robotic therapy (Toh et al., 2023). There are two types of stimulation-based training: electrical stimulation of muscles or nerves and the use of vibration to stimulate the skin underneath the device (i.e., the dorsum of the wrist or hand). Unlike electrical stimulation, vibratory stimulation can be applied mechanically with or without the placement of an electrode. They also vary in terms of the mechanism – electrical stimulation targets the tissue responses from the nerves or muscles (Knight & Draper, 2013), while vibratory stimulation targets the cutaneous mechanoreceptors underneath the skin and afferents (Vallbo & Johansson, 1984).

Electrical stimulation is an artificial stimulation of a muscle to provide muscular contractions and functional movements by electrically activating peripheral nerve cells. It is also known as "functional electrical stimulation (FES)" because it aims to restore voluntary motor function, but not lifelong dependence on the FES device. FES can also be used for muscle strengthening and inhibition of antagonist muscles. According to the Canadian Stroke Best Practice Recommendations for Rehabilitation (Teasell et al., 2020), FES targeting wrist and forearm muscles is recommended with level A evidence. FES includes non-voluntary and voluntary control, with non-voluntary control referring to the use of preprogrammed repetitive stimulations, and voluntary control referring to a self-triggered mechanism by the user using either button control, an EMG-triggered positional device, or an accelerometer operated by the non-affected arm. FES can be embedded in a wearable device, with the most common example being the Bioness NESS Handmaster orthosis in the shape of a wrist cock-up (Ring & Rosenthal, 2005). In a controlled study by Ring and Rosenthal (2005), it was found that clients in the neuroprosthesis group after wearing the device had significantly greater improvements in spasticity, active range of motion, and scores in the functional hand test compared to the control group. FES has been used extensively by occupational therapists for promoting upper extremity functions in clients with stroke or spinal cord injury (Dionne & Lenker, 2019; Eraifej et al., 2017; Jolliffe et al., 2019). In a local study, Chan et al. (2009) applied FES to the affected hand of clients with subacute stroke using voluntary control triggered via a positional device on the non-affected hand. After 15 sessions of bilateral arm training with 10 minutes of stretching, 20 minutes of FES, and 60 minutes of conventional OT training every session, the FES group showed significant improvements in arm impairment and functional levels compared to the control group using a placebo simulation and conventional OT training (Chan et al., 2009). FES is user- and state-dependent, meaning that the threshold of electrical current for stimulating the muscle varies from person to person and depends on the distance between the electrodes (anode or positive electrode, and cathode or negative electrode) and the skin condition (such as moisture and conductivity). FES is a safe, noninvasive treatment, but it cannot be used directly in clients with pacemakers or electronic device implants, clients who are pregnant, suffer from epilepsy, or whose skin is allergic to FES. It is suggested that the daily use of FES should not be longer than 30 minutes per session.

Virtual reality

VR is a computer-based technology which allows users to view, navigate, interact, and immerse themselves in a 3D simulated environment and receive augmented feedback on their performance (Rizzo et al., 1997). VR is usually immersive or non-immersive and has various kinds of interactivity according to the various levels of immersion. Regardless of the type of VR, its advantages are that clients can perform activities they cannot do in the real world, and they are motivated by engaging in VR games or treatments (Fong et al., 2010). In addition to immersion, the distinguishing features of VR include a simulated and interactive environment, the use of augmented feedback on performance, and the systematic hierarchical presentation of challenges. VR can be applied to both cognitive and physical training in OT. According to the Canadian Stroke Best Practice Recommendations for Rehabilitation (Teasell et al., 2020), VR is of level A evidence and can be used as an adjunct tool for other rehabilitation therapies following stroke, providing opportunities for engagement, feedback, repetition, intensity, and task-oriented training. Besides VR, AR and mixed reality (MR) are becoming more common in healthcare. AR enables integration of the actual and virtual worlds through the use of a smart device such as a smartphone or tablet (Ovunc et al., 2021). MR is a new technology that fuses the actual world with the virtual world, in which physical entities and digital objects can coexist and interact in real time (Liu et al., 2021). In a systematic review and meta-analysis examining the effectiveness of VR, AR, and MR (VAMR) therapy for upper limb recovery in stroke clients, VAMR therapy was superior to conventional treatment in improving upper limb impairment and daily function outcomes in both subacute and recovery stages, but not in upper limb functional measures (Leong et al., 2022).

One local example of task-specific training using non-immersive VR is a VR automated teller machine (ATM) for clients with brain injuries. In a related study, the intervention group who had received VR ATM training showed a significantly shorter average reaction time in cash withdrawal than the control group who had undergone conventional computer-assisted training (Fong et al., 2010). Another local application is a task-specific VR (TS-VR) program using a leap motion controller device and the Unity3D game engine to promote recovery of the hemiparetic upper extremity in clients with stroke based on a hierarchy of seven functional tasks in the Functional Test for the Hemiplegic Upper Extremity (FTHUE) (Fong et al., 2021).

Artificial intelligence

AI is defined as "a system's ability to correctly interpret external data, to learn from such data, and to use those learnings to achieve specific goals and tasks through flexible adaptation" (Haenlein & Kaplan, 2019). There are two types of machine learning (ML): supervised or unsupervised. In supervised learning, the machine is trained by an expert using the training data set, which is well "labeled", i.e., decision trees of multiple tasks have been created for various correct answers. Unsupervised learning is more complex, allowing the AI model to deal with the unlabeled data and formulate its own correct answers by self-learning.

A supervised learning algorithm learns from labeled training data and helps predict outcomes for unforeseen data. AI could not be used nowadays without the application of the Internet, and cloud-based AI is a million times more powerful than a single system, with the connection of multiple systems as well as access to big electronic databases using the fastest form of transmission, such as 5G. Another new concept named the "Internet of Things (IoT)" is a system that makes use of advanced computer technology to form a network embedded with sensors, software, and other technologies for connecting and exchanging data with other devices and systems over the Internet (Madakam et al., 2015).

AI computes by means of symbolic or subsymbolic AI, such as artificial neural networks (ANNs). Symbolic AI is the classical method which uses mathematical statistics such as logic programming and production rules to direct itself at specific problems with specific goals, and it develops applications mainly using expert systems ("Symbolic Artificial Intelligence," 2022). However, symbolic AI can only solve problems within a framework. As the Internet and mobile technology are commonplace today, and with the hardware developments in graphics processing, ANNs have become more popular and applicable because they primarily capture images for processing. ANN algorithms simulate the human visual neural networks of thinking, including backpropagation, feedforward, and radial basis function networks to investigate the optimal configuration that would give the best classification results (Leonard & Kramer, 1990). One of the ANN techniques is deep learning (DL), which refers to the use of multiple layers in the network powered by algorithms.

The rapid development of computer and AI technology in recent years has meant their potential adoption in the healthcare field. New training devices using VR simulations and sensors in the home that monitor the client's condition are examples of the application of AI and IoT techniques in rehabilitation. The following paragraphs further explore the application of computer technology and AI in OT, which can be categorized into four dimensions: screening, assessment, training, and assisting.

Screening

AI supports feature identification and classification and has been gradually adopted in the medical field in the identification of diseases. Together with motion tracking and analysis methods, AI can act as a developmental monitoring system that screens the symptoms of motor disorders as well as developmental disabilities (e.g., the detection of movement abnormalities in children with cerebral palsy [CP] [Pantzar-Castilla et al., 2018] and the detection of excessive movement in children with hyperactivity disorder [HD] [O'Keefe et al., 2014]). Since the early signs and symptoms of developmental disorders might be difficult for parents to notice, the use of AI in screening would help in the early identification of such diseases. Other types of disease that demonstrate identifiable motor impairments such as bradykinesia, tremors, or rigidity might also be recognized by AI systems. Early screening allows clients to engage in training and rehabilitation at an early stage, which can enhance the rehabilitation prognosis.

Assessment

AI can be used as an accurate measurement of objective assessment items such as range of motion (Schroeder et al., 2020). AI also increases assessment efficacy by reducing the time needed for reading and analyzing the measurement results by the movement analysis algorithm. Besides the use of AI in providing physical assessment, the development of natural language processing (NLP) as a tool has the potential to identify human emotions and mental states (Tanana et al., 2021). The functions of AI that can recognize human emotions can be used as a preliminary assessment for clients with mental health issues (Rajawat et al., 2021). A big database of AI that gathers the signs and symptoms of the disease in the population would make it possible to classify the extent and severity of the symptoms. In the future, it could be a useful tool for therapists to conduct assessments on clients.

Training

Training is a significant area that computer technology and AI contribute to the rehabilitation field. The current use of computer games increases client enjoyment during rehabilitation, and these games could be further expanded to include VR games or training that allow clients to interact with multiple elements in the virtual environment (Afsar et al., 2018). The virtual context can simulate elements in the real world, providing clients with a more realistic training experience. Clients will become more competent in engaging in daily tasks after simulating the tasks in the virtual training. VR training also benefits clients by increasing their training satisfaction, and hence, the motivation and adherence to the rehabilitation program.

Assisting

Together with the IoT system, which gathers information from sensors, AI can analyze clients' conditions and act as a monitoring or supervision system in their daily activities. It can record and remind clients with cognitive impairments of their ADL. It is also reliable in reminding clients of their daily training regime by using wearable devices that detect whether clients have completed their home training. An advanced IoT system is also proposed to assist people with cognitive impairment in navigation and tracking their location if they get lost (Chen et al., 2018). Objects such as personal belongings can also be tracked, which is beneficial to people with weak memory.

Numerous assistive products can now be incorporated into the environment in the form of ambient assistive technology (AAT) to evaluate clients' performance and provide assistance if necessary. This has been made possible over the last decade by the development of new innovative technologies such as sensors, cloud computing, wireless communication technologies, and assistive robots (Ganesan et al., 2019). AAT refers to an array of electronic devices (e.g., sensors and actuators/effectors) that are subtly incorporated into everyday objects (e.g., walls, plugs, doors, stoves, lamps, and screens) in order to monitor the client's status and provide assistance as needed, or to remind the client when he/she forgets the recommended activities (Ganesan et al., 2019). Examples of AAT include the use of markerless motion sensors to detect falls among the elderly, the use of intelligent lighting systems to help regulate the behavioral and psychological symptoms of dementia (BPSD) in clients suffering from the disease, and the use of voice control in an IoT smart home to automate electrical appliances or devices for people with physical disabilities, making operation more convenient. The future development of assistive devices will utilize the "act like a human" characteristic of AI and humanoid robots, further generalizing the use of AI in assistive technology.

Neuromodulation, neurophysiological, and neuroimaging techniques

Neuroplasticity can be broadly described as the ability of the nervous system to adopt a new functional or structural state (Ganguly & Poo, 2013). It occurs spontaneously after the onset of illness or can be induced by OT and rehabilitation (Cassidy & Cramer, 2017). It is important for occupational therapists, particularly those specializing in neurorehabilitation, to understand how therapeutic exercise and activities enhance adaptive neuroplasticity to facilitate functional improvement (Carey, 2010). In this section, we introduce several commonly used neuromodulation, neurophysiological, and neuroimaging technologies that are useful for studying neuroplasticity in association with the efficacy of OT and rehabilitation.

Neuromodulation has been widely applied to drive the brain to a state with enhanced responsiveness to OT and rehabilitation, leading to an optimal rehabilitation outcome (Stoykov & Madhavan, 2015). Neuromodulation technologies also allow researchers and clinicians to understand the neural processes of sensorimotor, cognitive, and affective functions, as well as ascertain the causal relationship between brain regions and human behaviors in healthy and diseased states (Hobot et al., 2021). Neuromodulation technologies include both noninvasive and invasive methods that modify brain activity and function using electrical, electromagnetic, acoustic, optical, or chemical modalities, with the noninvasive form being more commonly used by rehabilitation practitioners. Here, two relatively mature methods, transcranial magnetic stimulation (TMS) and transcranial direct current stimulation (tDCS), are introduced.

According to the current guidelines on repetitive TMS (rTMS) and tDCS, they have been applied to the treatment of various disease conditions, including major depression, stroke (hand motor recovery, visuospatial neglect), Alzheimer's disease (cognitive functions, memory, language), mild cognitive impairment (MCI), addition-related craving (alcohol, drugs, smoking), post-traumatic stress disorder (PTSD), obsessive–compulsive disorder (OCD), etc. (Lefaucheur et al., 2017; 2020). According to the Canadian Stroke Best Practice Recommendations for Rehabilitation (Teasell et al., 2020), rTMS, which is of level A evidence, could be considered as an adjunct to upper limb training following stroke, while tDCS, which is of level B evidence, could be used as an adjunct treatment to improve upper limb function. tDCS is also portable, low cost, and can be applied in home-based rehabilitation.

Transcranial magnetic stimulation

The first TMS machine for human neurophysiological experiments was built in 1985 (Barker et al., 1985). The mechanism of TMS for neuromodulation is based on Faraday's principle of electromagnetic induction (Figure 13.3a). rTMS, using repeated TMS pulses, can induce a measurable modulatory effect on the stimulated cortical areas beyond the duration of stimulation (Hallett, 2000). Typically, high-frequency (≥ 5 Hz) rTMS demonstrates an excitatory after-effect, while low-frequency (0.2–1 Hz) rTMS has an inhibitory after-effect on the stimulated cortical areas (Hallett, 2007). Theta burst stimulation (TBS) is an accelerated and potent form of rTMS. Depending

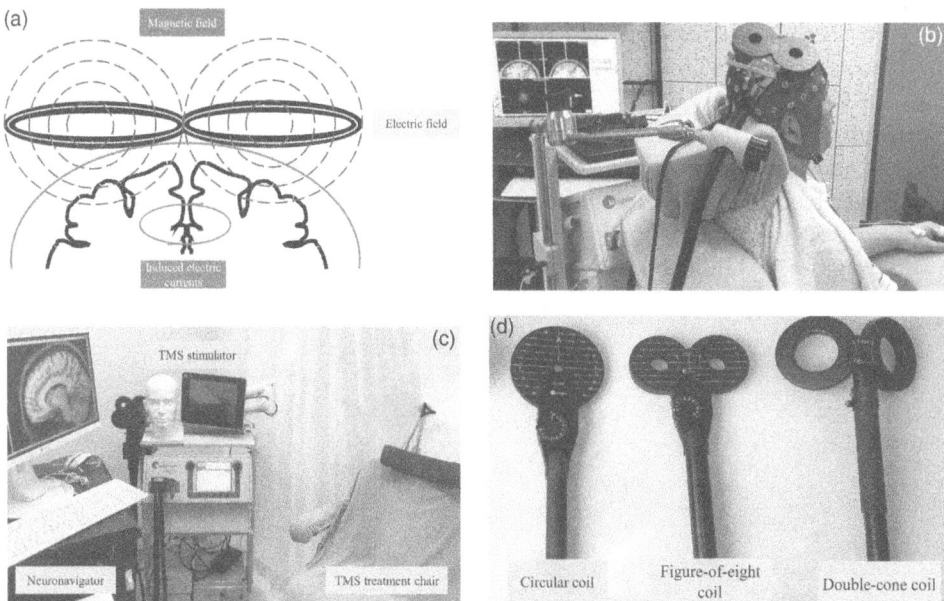

Figure 13.3 (a) The mechanism of TMS: A pulse of electrical current is sent through a wire coil placed over the participant's scalp to generate a rapidly changing magnetic field. The magnetic field further induces a secondary current in the brain cortex underlying the scalp to activate the neurons. (b) A demonstration of a human experiment with TMS. (c) TMS laboratory facilities: a neuronavigator, a TMS stimulator and magnetic coils, and a treatment chair. (d) Various types of customized TMS coil: a circular coil, a figure-of-eight coil, and a double-cone coil

on its delivery pattern, intermittent theta burst stimulation (iTBS) can facilitate cortical excitability, while continuous theta burst stimulation (cTBS) can inhibit cortical excitability (Huang et al., 2005). Figure 13.3b–d demonstrate a human experiment with TMS and typical TMS laboratory facilities.

Brain modulation is now commonly used as a hybrid approach in combination with conventional rehabilitation as a priming stimulation to enhance neuroplasticity in facilitating either cognitive or motor recovery after stroke. A local clinical study demonstrated that low-frequency rTMS applied to P5 of the contralesional hemisphere in stroke clients with left unilateral neglect combined with sensory vibration cueing emitted through a wristwatch device on the hemiplegic arm was better than rTMS alone and conventional rehabilitation in reducing unilateral neglect (Yang et al., 2017). Another local study investigated the effects of a ten-session priming intermittent theta burst stimulation (iTBS, an alternative form of rTMS), relative to non-priming iTBS and sham stimulation, combined with a customary robot-assisted training, on improving upper limb motor functions in clients with stroke using a randomized controlled trial (Zhang et al., 2022). The findings showed that priming and non-priming iTBS were both superior to sham stimulation in enhancing treatment gains from rehabilitative robot-assisted training, and clients with a higher functioning upper limb might experience more benefits from priming iTBS (Zhang et al., 2022). rTMS could be applied as an adjunct and noninvasive therapy that reduces cravings for illicit drugs and potentially helps to reduce consumption. In a recently published meta-analysis (Zhang et al., 2019), numerous studies suggested that an excitatory rTMS either to the left or right dorsolateral prefrontal cortex (DLPFC) could reduce cravings for substances.

Transcranial direct current stimulation

tDCS is another neuromodulation technique. During the administration of tDCS, a pair of electrodes (anode and cathode) are placed on the participant's scalp, and a weak electric current (0.5–2 mA) is delivered via the electrodes to the underlying brain cortex (Figure 13.4a). The after-effects of tDCS are polarity specific, i.e., the cortex

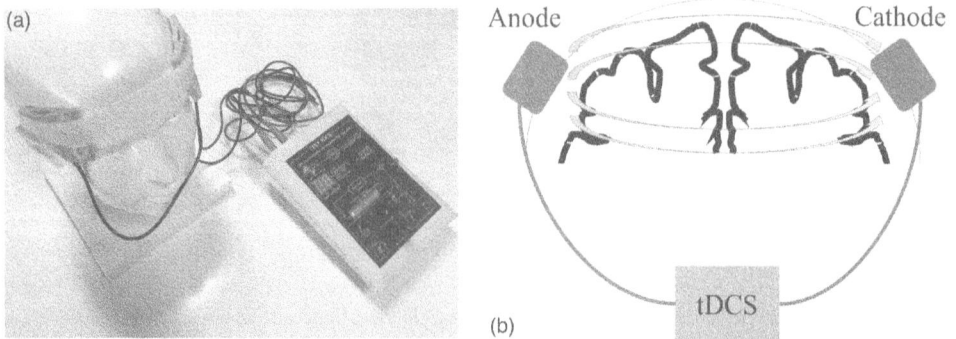

Figure 13.4 (a) The tDCS device: A direct current stimulator with two electrodes. (b) The mechanism of the tDCS: Direct electric currents flow across the cortex, with the cortex underlying the anodal electrode being depolarized and facilitated by the inward current, while the cortex underlying the cathodal electrode is hyperpolarized and suppressed by the outward current

underlying the anode can be facilitated, while the cortex underlying the cathode can be inhibited (Feng et al., 2013) (Figure 13.4b).

The timing-dependent interaction factor of using tDCS to facilitate cognitive or motor recovery should be considered in clinical applications. Current evidence shows that tDCS can be used as a form of stimulation-based priming, and thus can boost recovery induced by conventional rehabilitation training. A local study demonstrated that a concurrent-tDCS priming approach with conventional training seemed to be more advantageous and time-efficient in a clinical trial combined with mirror therapy than prior-tDCS priming, i.e., tDCS applied before training (Jin et al., 2019). On the other hand, a recent systematic review and meta-analysis showed that tDCS improved the memories of people with dementia in the short term; it also seemed to have a mild positive effect on memory and language in people with MCI. However, there was no conclusive advantage in coupling tDCS with cognitive training for the two populations (Cruz Gonzalez et al., 2018). This was also proved by a local randomized controlled trial, which showed that the combination of tDCS and computer cognitive training did not produce a superior effect on cognitive performance compared to sham tDCS plus computer cognitive training or computer cognitive training alone in people with MCI (Cruz Gonzalez et al., 2021).

Neurophysiological examinations and neuroimaging

Neurophysiological and neuroimaging technologies are not only for disease diagnosis but also provide important outcome indicators for predicting disease prognosis. Besides, neurophysiological or neuroimaging assessments make it possible for evaluating neuroplasticity in response to OT and rehabilitation (Milot & Cramer, 2008).

Electroencephalography

EEG is a well-established neurophysiological technique. During the process, several electrodes are placed on the participant's head to record the electrical activity of the brain, and the signals are amplified and converted into digital signals that can be visualized and processed by computers (Figure 13.5a and b). A spontaneous EEG rhythm can be decomposed into four frequency bands, each with distinct functional meanings: (1) delta (1–4 Hz), detected during slow-wave sleep in adults, (2) theta (4–8 Hz), found

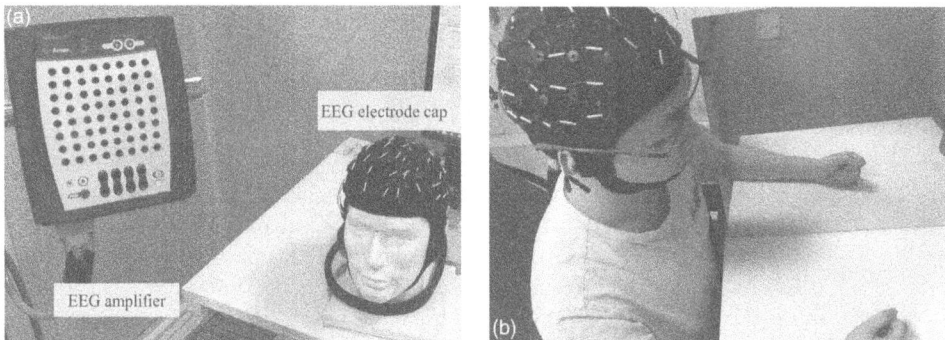

Figure 13.5 (a) An EEG amplifier and a standardized EEG electrode cap. (b) A demonstration of a human EEG experiment

during drowsiness, deep relaxation, or quiet focus, (3) alpha (8–12 Hz), detected during wakeful relaxation with eyes closed, and (4) beta (12–30 Hz), found during active thinking and when mentally alert (Abhang et al., 2016; Kirschstein & Köhling, 2009). Event-related potential (ERP) is a time-locked EEG-evoked response to certain events, such as environmental stimuli and self-initiated behaviors. It indicates how the brain processes afferent signals and makes behavioral responses. It is, therefore, helpful for occupational therapists to understand brain–behavior relationships at millisecond-level temporal resolution (Woodman, 2010).

Functional magnetic resonance imaging and functional near-infrared spectroscopy

The activation of the brain correlates with an increase in cerebral blood flow so that extra glucose and oxygen can be supplied to activate neurons. The increase of local blood flow brings in more oxygenated blood and removes deoxyhemoglobin. The dynamic of brain oxygenation can be reflected in blood oxygenation level-dependent (BOLD) signals using functional magnetic resonance imaging (fMRI) (Buxton, 2013). fMRI allows whole-brain functional imaging at millimeter-level spatial resolution. When administrating an fMRI experiment, participants must perform the given task in upright and supine body positions inside a scanner. Functional near-infrared spectroscopy (fNIRS) has emerged as another neuroimaging tool for measuring cerebral oxygenation. Unlike fMRI, fNIRS estimates the concentration of hemoglobin from changes in the absorption of near-infrared light (Chen et al., 2020) (Figure 13.6a). fNIRS experiments can be carried out in a naturalistic environment (Figure 13.6b).

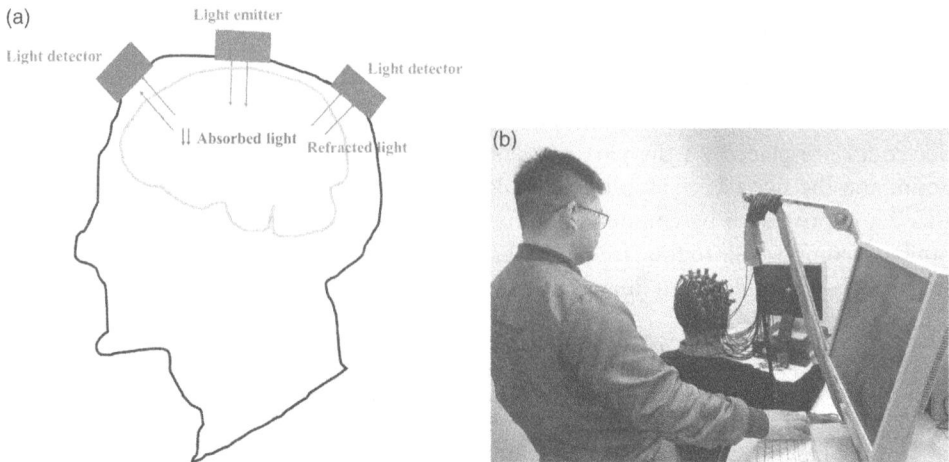

Figure 13.6 (a) The mechanism of the fNIRS: Several light emitter–detector pairs are placed on the participant's scalp. The near-infrared light is emitted into the scalp, which diffuses through the superficial cortex and is absorbed by oxyhemoglobin and deoxyhemoglobin. The refracted light is then collected by the detectors. fNIRS estimates cerebral oxygenation through changes in the absorption of near-infrared light. Near-infrared light in the range of 650–925 nm is absorbed differently by oxyhemoglobin and deoxyhemoglobin: deoxyhemoglobin absorbs the light below 790 nm more strongly, and oxyhemoglobin absorbs the light above 790 nm more strongly (Chen et al., 2020). (b) A demonstration of a human fNIRS experiment

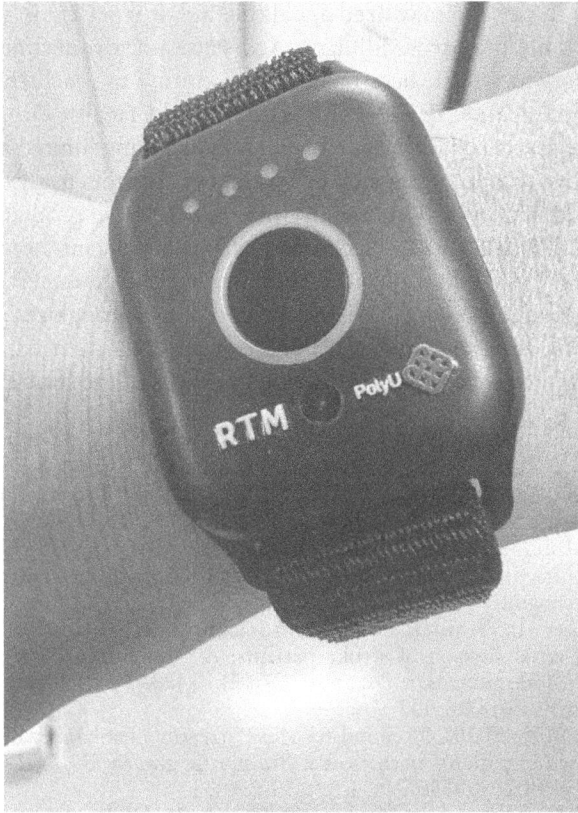

Figure 13.7 Remind-to-Move device

However, fNIRS measurement is limited to the superficial cortex underneath the cortical surface (Ferrari & Quaresima, 2012).

A recent study investigated cortical activation patterns using functional near-infrared spectroscopic topography (fNIRS) in clients with chronic stroke (n = 12) receiving Remind-to-Move (RTM) treatment by comparing them with their healthy counterparts (n = 15) (Bai & Fong, 2020). In this study, all participants, with or without a stroke, wore RTM wristwatch devices (Figure 13.7) under three treatment conditions: (1) RTM, (2) Remind with No-move (RNoM), and (3) Move without reminding (sham). It was found that RTM elicited a higher level of activation than the sham in the contralateral SMA, M1, S1, and DLPFC in clients with stroke, which was also found in healthy adults; however, the effects of RTM were stronger and more widely distributed in healthy adults compared to clients with stroke. In addition, RNoM showed no significantly higher activation than the baseline in those areas in both populations (Bai & Fong, 2020).

Summary

There were roughly 0.53 million individuals with disabilities in 2020, constituting 7.1% of the total population of Hong Kong. This figure does not take into account the aging population who may suffer from aging disabilities such as sarcopenia, low vision, or hearing loss, or those who may need a walking aid or wheelchair. Assistive technology is integral to daily life across all ages. Access to assistive technology is a human right, enabling everyone, regardless of disability status, to reach their full potential (World Health Organization & UNICEF, 2022; World Health Organization, 2024). However, there are several challenges to overcome, including limited access to facilities that provide assistive technology, a lack of awareness about its use, benefits, and availability, and the fact that most users require multiple assistive products (World Health Organization & UNICEF, 2022). Technological advancements necessitate increased collaboration among rehabilitation professionals, healthcare experts, engineers, and designers to develop and implement assistive technology through research and deployment, both in Hong Kong and globally. There is an ongoing need for more trained personnel in OT to provide assistive technology services in the future.

References

Abhang, P. A., Gawali, B. W., & Mehrotra, S. C. (2016). Chapter 2 - Technological basics of EEG recording and operation of apparatus. In P. A. Abhang, B. W. Gawali, & S. C. Mehrotra (Eds.), *Introduction to EEG- and speech-based emotion recognition* (pp. 19–50). Academic Press. https://www.sciencedirect.com/book/9780128044902/introduction-to-eeg-and-speech-based-emotion-recognition

Afsar, S. I., Mirzayev, I., Yemisci, O. U., & Saracgil, S. N. C. (2018). Virtual reality in upper extremity rehabilitation of stroke patients: A randomized controlled trial. *Journal of Stroke and Cerebrovascular Diseases*, 27(12), 3473–3478. https://doi.org/10.1016/j.jstrokecerebrovasdis.2018.08.007

Bai, Z., & Fong, K. N. K. (2020). "Remind-to-Move" treatment enhanced activation of the primary motor cortex in patients with stroke. *Brain Topography*, 33(2), 275–283. https://doi.org/10.1007/s10548-020-00756-7

Bai, Z., Fong, K. N. K., Zhang, J. J., Chan, J., & Ting, K. H. (2020). Immediate and long-term effects of BCI-based rehabilitation of the upper extremity after stroke: A systematic review and meta-analysis. *Journal of NeuroEngineering and Rehabilitation*, 17(1), 57. https://doi.org/10.1186/s12984-020-00686-2

Barker, A. T., Jalinous, R., & Freeston, I. L. (1985). Non-invasive magnetic stimulation of human motor cortex. *The Lancet*, 325(8437), 1106–1107. https://doi.org/10.1016/s0140-6736(85)92413-4

Buxton, R. B. (2013). The physics of functional magnetic resonance imaging (fMRI). *Reports on Progress in Physics*, 76(9), 096601. https://doi.org/10.1088/0034-4885/76/9/096601

Carey, L. (2010). Neuroscience makes sense for occupational therapy. *Australian Occupational Therapy Journal*, 57(3), 197–199. https://doi.org/10.1111/j.1440-1630.2010.00872.x

Cassidy, J. M., & Cramer, S. C. (2017). Spontaneous and therapeutic-induced mechanisms of functional recovery after stroke. *Translational Stroke Research*, 8(1), 33–46. https://doi.org/10.1007/s12975-016-0467-5

Chan, M. K., Tong, R. K., & Chung, K. Y. (2009). Bilateral upper limb training with functional electric stimulation in patients with chronic stroke. *Neurorehabilitation and Neural Repair*, 23(4), 357–365. https://doi.org/10.1177/1545968308326428

Chen, L., Ai, H., Zhuang, Z., & Shang, C. (2018). Real-time multiple people tracking with deeply learned candidate selection and person re-identification. *2018 IEEE International Conference on Multimedia and Expo (ICME)*, 1–6. http://doi.org/10.1109/ICME.2018.8486597

Chen, W.-L., Wagner, J., Heugel, N., Sugar, J., Lee, Y.-W., Conant, L., Malloy, M., Heffernan, J., Quirk, B., Zinos, A., Beardsley, S. A., Prost, R., & Whelan, H. T. (2020). Functional near-infrared spectroscopy and its clinical application in the field of neuroscience: Advances and future directions. *Frontiers in Neuroscience*, 14, 724. https://doi.org/10.3389/fnins.2020.00724

Cook, A. M., & Hussey, S. (2001). *Assistive technologies: Principles and practice* (2nd ed.). Mosby.

Cruz Gonzalez, P., Fong, K. N. K., & Brown, T. (2021). Transcranial direct current stimulation as an adjunct to cognitive training for older adults with mild cognitive impairment: A randomized controlled trial. *Annals of Physical and Rehabilitation Medicine, 64*(5), 101536. https://doi.org/10.1016/j.rehab.2021.101536

Cruz Gonzalez, P., Fong, K. N. K., Chung, R. C. K., Ting, K.-H., Law, L. L. F., & Brown, T. (2018). Can transcranial direct-current stimulation alone or combined with cognitive training be used as a clinical intervention to improve cognitive functioning in persons with mild cognitive impairment and dementia? A systematic review and meta-analysis. *Frontiers in Human Neuroscience, 12*, 416. https://doi.org/10.3389/fnhum.2018.00416

Data.ai. (2022, January 12). *Number of mobile app downloads worldwide from 2016 to 2021 (in billions)* [Graph]. Statista. Retrieved May 2, 2022, from https://www-statista-com.ezproxy. lb.polyu.edu.hk/statistics/271644/worldwide-free-and-paid-mobile-app-store-downloads/

Dionne, T., & Lenker, J. (2019). Developing guidelines for OTs using electrical stimulation (ES) for individuals with spinal-cord injury (SCI). *American Journal of Occupational Therapy, 73*(4, Suppl. 1), 7311520423p1. https://doi.org/10.5014/ajot.2019.73S1-PO3040

Eraifej, J., Clark, W., France, B., Desando, S., & Moore, D. (2017). Effectiveness of upper limb functional electrical stimulation after stroke for the improvement of activities of daily living and motor function: A systematic review and meta-analysis. *Systematic Reviews, 6*(1), 40. https://doi.org/10.1186/s13643-017-0435-5

Feng, W. W., Bowden, M. G., & Kautz, S. (2013). Review of transcranial direct current stimulation in poststroke recovery. *Topics in Stroke Rehabilitation, 20*(1), 68–77. https://doi. org/10.1310/tsr2001-68

Ferrari, M., & Quaresima, V. (2012). A brief review on the history of human functional near-infrared spectroscopy (fNIRS) development and fields of application. *Neuroimage, 63*(2), 921–935. https://doi.org/10.1016/j.neuroimage.2012.03.049

Fong, K. N. K., Chow, K. Y. Y., Chan, B. C. H., Lam, K. C. K., Lee, J. C. K., Li, T. H. Y., Yan, E. W. H., & Wong, A. T. Y. (2010). Usability of a virtual reality environment simulating an automated teller machine for assessing and training persons with acquired brain injury. *Journal of NeuroEngineering and Rehabilitation, 7*, 19. https://doi.org/10.1186/1743-0003-7-19

Fong, K. N. K., & Kwan, R. (2020). Telerehabilitation (remote therapy). In D. Gu, & M. E. Dupre (Eds.), *Encyclopedia of gerontology and population aging* (pp. 1–7). Springer Nature. https://doi.org/10.1007/978-3-319-69892-2_1088-1

Fong, K. N. K., Tang, Y. M., Sie, K., Yu, A. K. H., Lo, C. C. W., & Ma, Y. W. T. (2021). Task-specific virtual reality training on hemiparetic upper extremity in patients with stroke. *Virtual Reality, 26*, 453–464. https://link.springer.com/article/10.1007/s10055-021-00583-6

Ganesan, B., Gowda, T., Al-Jumaily, A., Fong, K. N. K., Meena, S. K., & Tong, R. K. Y. (2019). Ambient assisted living technologies for older adults with cognitive and physical impairments: A review. *European Review for Medical and Pharmacological Sciences, 23*(23), 10470–10481. https://doi.org/10.26355/eurrev_201912_19686

Ganguly, K., & Poo, M.-M. (2013). Activity-dependent neural plasticity from bench to bedside. *Neuron, 80*(3), 729–741. https://doi.org/10.1016/j.neuron.2013.10.028

Haenlein, M., & Kaplan, A. (2019). A brief history of artificial intelligence: On the past, present, and future of artificial intelligence. *California Management Review, 61*(4), 5–14. https://doi. org/10.1177/0008125619864925

Hallett, M. (2000). Transcranial magnetic stimulation and the human brain. *Nature, 406*(6792), 147–150. https://doi.org/10.1038/35018000

Hallett, M. (2007). Transcranial magnetic stimulation: A primer. *Neuron, 55*(2), 187–199. https://doi.org/10.1016/j.neuron.2007.06.026

Hobot, J., Klincewicz, M., Sandberg, K., & Wierzchoń, M. (2021). Causal inferences in repetitive transcranial magnetic stimulation research: Challenges and perspectives. *Frontiers in Human Neuroscience, 14*, 586448. https://doi.org/10.3389/fnhum.2020.586448

Huang, Y.-Z., Edwards, M. J., Rounis, E., Bhatia, K. P., & Rothwell, J. C. (2005). Theta burst stimulation of the human motor cortex. *Neuron, 45*(2), 201–206. https://doi.org/10.1016/j. neuron.2004.12.033

Hung, G. K. N., & Fong, K. N. K. (2019). Effects of telerehabilitation in occupational therapy practice: A systematic review. *Hong Kong Journal of Occupational Therapy, 32*(1), 3–21. https://doi.org/10.1177/1569186119849119

Jin, M., Zhang, Z., Bai, Z., & Fong, K. N. K. (2019). Timing-dependent interaction effects of tDCS with mirror therapy on upper extremity motor recovery in patients with chronic stroke: A randomized controlled pilot study. *Journal of the Neurological Sciences, 405,* 116436. https://doi.org/10.1016/j.jns.2019.116436

Jolliffe, L., Hoffmann, T., & Lannin, N. A. (2019). Increasing the uptake of stroke upper limb guideline recommendations with occupational therapists and physiotherapists. A qualitative study using the Theoretical Domains Framework. *Australian Occupational Therapy Journal, 66*(5), 603–616. https://doi.org/10.1111/1440-1630.12599

Kairy, D., Lehoux, P., Vincent, C., & Visintin, M. (2009). A systematic review of clinical outcomes, clinical process, healthcare utilization and costs associated with telerehabilitation. *Disability and Rehabilitation, 31*(6), 427–447. https://doi.org/10.1080/09638280802062553

Kirschstein, T., & Köhling, R. (2009). What is the source of the EEG? *Clinical EEG and Neuroscience, 40*(3), 146–149. https://doi.org/10.1177/155005940904000305

Knight, K. L., & Draper, D. O. (2013). *Therapeutic modalities: The art and science* (2nd ed.). Lippincott Williams & Wilkins.

Law, M., Cooper, B., Strong, S., Stewart, D., Rigby, P., & Letts, L. (1996). The Person-Environment-Occupation Model: A transactive approach to occupational performance. *Canadian Journal of Occupational Therapy, 63*(1), 9–23. https://doi.org/10.1177%2F000841749606300103

Lefaucheur, J.-P., Aleman, A., Baeken, C., Benninger, D. H., Brunelin, J., Di Lazzaro, V., Filipović, S. R., Grefkes, C., Hasan, A., Hummel, F. C., Jääskeläinen, S. K., Langguth, B., Leocani, L., Londero, A., Nardone, R., Nguyen, J.-P., Nyffeler, T., Oliveira-Maia, A. J., Oliviero, A., & Ziemann, U. (2020). Evidence-based guidelines on the therapeutic use of repetitive transcranial magnetic stimulation (rTMS): An update (2014-2018). *Clinical Neurophysiology, 131*(2), 474–528. https://doi.org/10.1016/j.clinph.2019.11.002

Lefaucheur, J.-P., Antal, A., Ayache, S. S., Benninger, D. H., Brunelin, J., Cogiamanian, F., Cotelli, M., De Ridder, D., Ferrucci, R., Langguth, B., Marangolo, P., Mylius, V., Nitsche, M. A., Padberg, F., Palm, U., Poulet, E., Priori, A., Rossi, S., Schecklmann, M., & Paulus, W. (2017). Evidence-based guidelines on the therapeutic use of transcranial direct current stimulation (tDCS). *Clinical Neurophysiology, 128*(1), 56–92. https://doi.org/10.1016/j.clinph.2016.10.087

Leonard, J., & Kramer, M. A. (1990). Improvement of the backpropagation algorithm for training neural networks. *Computers & Chemical Engineering, 14*(3), 337–341. https://doi.org/10.1016/0098-1354(90)87070-6

Leong, S. C., Tang, Y. M., Toh, F. M., & Fong, K. N. K. (2022). Examining the effectiveness of virtual, augmented, and mixed reality (VAMR) therapy for upper limb recovery and activities of daily living in stroke patients: A systematic review and meta-analysis. *Journal of NeuroEngineering and Rehabilitation, 19*(1), 93. https://doi.org/10.1186/s12984-022-01071-x

Li, C. T. L., Hung, G. K. N., Fong, K. N. K., Cruz Gonzalez, P., Wah, S.-H., & Tsang, H. W. H. (2020). Effects of home-based occupational therapy telerehabilitation via smartphone for outpatients after hip fracture surgery: A feasibility randomised controlled study. *Journal of Telemedicine and Telecare, 28*(4), 239–247. http://dx.doi.org/10.1177/1357633X20932434

Liu, P., Lu, L., Liu, S., Xie, M., Zhang, J., Huo, T., Xie, Y., Wang, H., Duan, Y., Hu, Y., & Ye, Z. (2021). Mixed reality assists the fight against COVID-19. *Intelligent Medicine, 1*(1), 16–18. https://doi.org/10.1016/j.imed.2021.05.002

Madakam, S., Ramaswamy, R., & Tripathi, S. (2015). Internet of Things (IoT): A literature review. *Journal of Computer and Communications, 3*(5), 164–173. https://doi.org/10.4236/jcc.2015.35021

Milot, M.-H., & Cramer, S. C. (2008). Biomarkers of recovery after stroke. *Current Opinion in Neurology, 21*(6), 654–659. https://doi.org/10.1097/WCO.0b013e3283186f96

Moy, A. (1987). Chapter 7 - Which aid? In E. Bumphrey (Ed.), *Occupational therapy in the community* (pp. 74–89). Woodhead-Faulkner Ltd.

O'Keefe, J. A., Orías, A. A. E., Khan, H., Hall, D. A., Berry-Kravis, E., & Wimmer, M. A. (2014). Implementation of a markerless motion analysis method to quantify hyperkinesis in males with fragile X syndrome. *Gait & Posture, 39*(2), 827–830. https://doi.org/10.1016/j.gaitpost.2013.10.017

Ovunc, S. S., Yolcu, M. B., Emre, S., Elicevik, M., & Celayir, S. (2021). Using immersive technologies to develop medical education materials. *Cureus, 13*(1), e12647. http://doi.org/10.7759/cureus.12647

Pantzar-Castilla, E., Cereatti, A., Figari, G., Valeri, N., Paolini, G., Della Croce, U., Magnuson, A., & Riad, J. (2018). Knee joint sagittal plane movement in cerebral palsy: A comparative study of 2-dimensional markerless video and 3-dimensional gait analysis. *Acta Orthopaedica, 89*(6), 656–661. https://doi.org/10.1080/17453674.2018.1525195

Rajawat, A. S., Rawat, R., Barhanpurkar, K., Shaw, R. N., & Ghosh, A. (2021). Depression detection for elderly people using AI robotic systems leveraging the Nelder–Mead Method. In R. N. Shaw, A. Ghosh, V. E. Balas, & M. Bianchini (Eds.), *Artificial intelligence for future generation robotics* (pp. 55–70). Elsevier. https://doi.org/10.1016/B978-0-323-85498-6.00006-X

Ring, H., & Rosenthal, N. (2005). Controlled study of neuroprosthetic functional electrical stimulation in sub-acute post-stroke rehabilitation. *Journal of Rehabilitation Medicine, 37*(1), 32–36. https://doi.org/10.1080/16501970410035387

Rizzo, A. A., Buckwalter, J. G., & Neumann, U. (1997). Virtual reality and cognitive rehabilitation: A brief review of the future. *Journal of Head Trauma Rehabilitation, 12*(6), 1–15. https://doi.org/10.1097/00001199-199712000-00002

Rodgers, M. M., Alon, G., Pai, V. M., & Conroy, R. S. (2019). Wearable technologies for active living and rehabilitation: Current research challenges and future opportunities. *Journal of Rehabilitation and Assistive Technologies Engineering, 6*, 2055668319839607. https://doi.org/10.1177/2055668319839607

Scherer, M. J. (2002). Matching consumers with appropriate assistive technologies. In D. A. Olson, & F. DeRuyter (Eds.), *Clinician's guide to assistive technology* (p. 4). Mosby.

Schroeder, A. S., Hesse, N., Weinberger, R., Tacke, U., Gerstl, L., Hilgendorff, A., Heinen, F., Arens, M., Dijkstra, L. J., Pujades Rocamora, S., Black, M. J., Bodensteiner, C., & Hadders-Algra, M. (2020). General Movement Assessment from videos of computed 3D infant body models is equally effective compared to conventional RGB video rating. *Early Human Development, 144*, 104967. https://doi.org/10.1016/j.earlhumdev.2020.104967

Statista. (2021, May 25). *Forecast of the number of smartphone users in the world from 2010 to 2025 (in millions)* [Graph]. Statista. Retrieved May 2, 2022, from https://www-statista-com.ezproxy.lb.polyu.edu.hk/forecasts/1143723/smartphone-users-in-the-world

Stoykov, M. E., & Madhavan, S. (2015). Motor priming in neurorehabilitation. *Journal of Neurologic Physical Therapy, 39*(1), 33–42. https://doi.org/10.1097/NPT.0000000000000065

Symbolic artificial intelligence. (2022). In *Wikipedia*. https://en.wikipedia.org/wiki/Symbolic_artificial_intelligence

Tanana, M. J., Soma, C. S., Kuo, P. B., Bertagnolli, N. M., Dembe, A., Pace, B. T., Srikumar, V., Atkins, D. C., & Imel, Z. E. (2021). How do you feel? Using natural language processing to automatically rate emotion in psychotherapy. *Behavior Research Methods, 53*(5), 2069–2082. https://doi.org/10.3758/s13428-020-01531-z

Teasell, R., Salbach, N. M., Foley, N., Mountain, A., Cameron, J. I., de Jong, A., Acerra, N. E., Bastasi, D., Carter, S. L., Fung, J., Halabi, M.-L., Iruthayarajah, J., Harris, J., Kim, E., Noland, A., Pooyania, S., Rochette, A., Stack, B. D., Symcox, E., & Lindsay, M. P. (2020). Canadian stroke best practice recommendations: Rehabilitation, recovery, and community participation following stroke. Part one: Rehabilitation and recovery following stroke; 6th edition update 2019. *International Journal of Stroke, 15*(7), 763–788. https://doi.org/10.1177/1747493019897843

Toh, S. F. M., Fong, K. N. K., Cruz Gonzalez, P., & Tang, Y. M. (2023). Application of home-based wearable technologies in physical rehabilitation for stroke: A scoping review. *IEEE Transactions on Neural Systems and Rehabilitation Engineering, 31*, 1614–1623. https://doi.org/10.1109/TNSRE.2023.3252880

Vallbo, Å. B., & Johansson, R. S. (1984). Properties of cutaneous mechanoreceptors in the human hand related to touch sensation. *Human Neurobiology, 3*(l), 3–14.

Wang, Q., Markopoulos, P., Yu, B., Chen, W., & Timmermans, A. (2017). Interactive wearable systems for upper body rehabilitation: A systematic review. *Journal of NeuroEngineering and Rehabilitation, 14*(1), 20. https://doi.org/10.1186/s12984-017-0229-y

Wood, G., & Whittaker, G. (2022). *Assistive technology in humanitarian settings*. UNICEF. https://www.unicef.org/innocenti/reports/assistive-technology-humanitarian-settings

Woodman, G. F. (2010). A brief introduction to the use of event-related potentials in studies of perception and attention. *Attention, Perception & Psychophysics, 72*(8), 2031–2046. https://doi.org/10.3758/APP.72.8.2031

World Federation of Occupational Therapists. (2014). World Federation of Occupational Therapists' position statement on telehealth. *International Journal of Telerehabilitation, 6*(1), 37–39. https://doi.org/10.5195/IJT.2014.6153

World Health Organization. (2024, January 2). *Assistive technology.* Retrieved October 10, 2024, from https://www.who.int/news-room/fact-sheets/detail/assistive-technology

World Health Organization & UNICEF. (2022). *Global report on assistive technology.* https://iris.who.int/bitstream/handle/10665/354357/9789240049451-eng.pdf?sequence=1

Yang, N. Y. H., Fong, K. N. K., Li-Tsang, C. W. P., & Zhou, D. (2017). Effects of repetitive transcranial magnetic stimulation combined with sensory cueing on unilateral neglect in subacute patients with right hemispheric stroke: A randomized controlled study. *Clinical Rehabilitation, 31*(9), 1154–1163. https://doi.org/10.1177/0269215516679712

Zhang, J. J., Bai, Z., & Fong, K. N. K. (2022). Priming intermittent theta burst stimulation for hemiparetic upper limb after stroke: A randomized controlled trial. *Stroke, 53*(7), 2171–2181. https://doi.org/10.1161/STROKEAHA.121.037870

Zhang, J. J. Q., Fong, K. N. K., Ouyang, R.-G., Siu, A. M. H., & Kranz, G. S. (2019). Effects of repetitive transcranial magnetic stimulation (rTMS) on craving and substance consumption in patients with substance dependence: A systematic review and meta-analysis. *Addiction, 114*(12), 2137–2149. https://doi.org/10.1111/add.14753

Index

Note: **Bold** indicates tables, *italics* indicates figures in the text and page numbers followed by "n" refer to end notes

For Product Safety Concerns and Information please contact our EU
representative GPSR@taylorandfrancis.com
Taylor & Francis Verlag GmbH, Kaufingerstraße 24, 80331 München, Germany